COGNITIVE-BEHAVIORAL SOCIAL SKILLS TRAINING FOR SCHIZOPHRENIA

Cognitive-Behavioral Social Skills Training for Schizophrenia

A **Practical Treatment** Guide

Eric L. Granholm
John R. McQuaid
Jason L. Holden

Foreword by
Kim T. Mueser and Alan S. Bellack

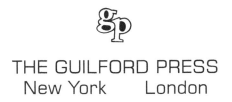

THE GUILFORD PRESS
New York   London

Copyright © 2016 The Guilford Press
A Division of Guilford Publications, Inc.
370 Seventh Avenue, Suite 1200, New York, NY 10001
www.guilford.com

Printed in the United States of America

This book is printed on acid-free paper.

Last digit is print number: 9 8 7 6 5 4 3 2

The authors have checked with sources believed to be reliable in their efforts to provide information that is complete and generally in accord with the standards of practice that are accepted at the time of publication. However, in view of the possibility of human error or changes in behavioral, mental health, or medical sciences, neither the authors nor the publisher, nor any other party who has been involved in the preparation or publication of this work warrants that the information contained herein is in every respect accurate or complete, and they are not responsible for any errors or omissions or the results obtained from the use of such information. Readers are encouraged to confirm the information contained in this book with other sources.

Library of Congress Cataloging-in-Publication Data

Names: Granholm, Eric L., author. | McQuaid, John Robert, 1964–, author. | Holden, Jason L., author.
Title: Cognitive-behavioral social skills training for schizophrenia : a practical treatment guide / Eric L. Granholm, John R. McQuaid, Jason L. Holden.
Description: New York : The Guilford Press, [2016] | Includes bibliographical references and index.
Identifiers: LCCN 2016002390 | ISBN 9781462524716 (paperback : alk. paper)
Subjects: | MESH: Schizophrenia—therapy | Cognitive Therapy—methods | Social Skills | Popular Works
Classification: LCC RC514 | NLM WM 203 | DDC 616.89/8—dc23
LC record available at *https://lccn.loc.gov/2016002390*

About the Authors

Eric L. Granholm, PhD, is Professor of Psychiatry at the University of California, San Diego, and Chief of Psychology and Co-Section Chief of Rehabilitation and Recovery Services at the Veterans Affairs San Diego Healthcare System. Dr. Granholm is an active basic and clinical researcher in the areas of social skills training, cognitive-behavioral therapy for psychosis, mobile assessments and interventions, pupillometry, and cognitive neuropsychology in consumers with schizophrenia. He has conducted eight federally funded clinical trials of cognitive-behavioral social skills training (CBSST) for schizophrenia, has over 100 publications, and has been an investigator on 24 grants to study psychosocial interventions, neurocognition, and functional outcome in schizophrenia.

John R. McQuaid, PhD, is Associate Chief of Staff for Mental Health at the San Francisco Veterans Affairs Medical Center and Professor of Clinical Psychology in the Department of Psychiatry at the University of California, San Francisco. Dr. McQuaid's clinical and research expertise is in the development and use of cognitive-behavioral interventions for psychiatric disorders and health management issues. He has over 60 publications and has served as an investigator or consultant on more than 15 grants in the areas of stress, psychopathology, and psychosocial treatment for psychiatric disorders and behavioral health.

Jason L. Holden, PhD, is a Clinical Research Supervisor in the Department of Psychiatry at the University of California, San Diego. He has been providing clinical services to individuals with psychosis for over 10 years, including cognitive-behavioral therapy, social skills training, and other evidence-based practices. Dr. Holden was a co-investigator on several CBSST clinical trials, a CBSST therapist in these trials, and a supervisor and trainer of other CBSST providers. His research also focuses on ecological momentary assessments and interventions using mobile technology in serious mental illness.

Foreword

Impaired social functioning is a hallmark of schizophrenia, often preceding the onset of frank psychotic symptoms and contributing to impoverished social lives, marginalized and often invisible existence in the community, and difficulties in role functioning in areas such as work, school, and parenting. Medications have little impact on social functioning in schizophrenia, except to control for the most prominent effects of psychotic symptoms on functioning. Only two psychosocial interventions have been demonstrated to improve social functioning in multiple controlled studies: social skills training and cognitive-behavioral therapy. Cognitive-behavioral social skills training (CBSST) is an innovative program that integrates these two approaches into a single, cohesive intervention, in order to improve social functioning in schizophrenia.

Cognitive-behavioral therapy and social skills training are among the oldest and best established psychological interventions for addressing a broad range of problems in functioning, in both clinical and nonclinical populations, with roots dating back to the 1950s and 1960s. Yet despite strong evidence supporting the effectiveness of these approaches for improving social functioning in schizophrenia, and their inclusion in treatment guidelines for the disorder for more than a decade, most clinicians do not know how to do either one, and most clients do not receive either type of intervention. Eric Granholm, John McQuaid, and Jason Holden have created a novel solution to this problem by integrating cognitive-behavioral and social skills training approaches into a unified program: CBSST.

The potential for integrating social skills training and cognitive-behavioral therapy has always been high. Improving social competence through training in social and problem-solving skills is often helpful but not always sufficient to improve social functioning. People's beliefs about their own social potency, and the perspectives of how others view them, can interfere with even the most socially competent individuals deploying their skills in social situations where they need them most. Conversely, believing in one's own ability to be interpersonally effective is crucial to pursuing socially valued roles, but poor social and problem-solving skills can dampen the effectiveness of people's efforts. The role of effective social, problem-solving, and cognitive (appraisal) skills in optimizing social functioning is nicely illustrated in the model described in the first chapter of this book.

CBSST is an innovative psychosocial treatment model that integrates the training of social, problem-solving, and cognitive skills into a single program, with participation driven by the consumer's desire to achieve specific, personally meaningful social goals. The program is flexible, and can be delivered to individual consumers, in groups, or a combination thereof. By developing clear, easy-to-follow guidelines for clinicians, supported by workbooks for consumers containing accessible information and worksheets, Granholm, McQuaid, and Holden have developed an appealing program that can be implemented in any setting in which people receive psychiatric services, including outpatient mental health programs, assertive community treatment teams, supported or supervised residential facilities, or intermediate- or long-stay institutions. Furthermore, CBSST is supported by a growing body of rigorous research showing that the program is effective in helping people achieve their social goals and improving their psychosocial functioning.

CBSST is a new, valuable tool for the social rehabilitation of people with schizophrenia spectrum disorders. The elegance of the integrated CBSST model, combined with the user-friendly program materials including clinical guidelines and consumer workbooks, suit the program to widespread dissemination and implementation. This book provides new hope that after so many years of waiting, people with schizophrenia will finally be able to access effective, evidence-based interventions for improving their social functioning and the quality of their lives.

KIM T. MUESER, PhD
Boston University

ALAN S. BELLACK, PhD
University of Maryland School of Medicine

Preface

Give a man a fish and you feed him for a day.
Teach a man to fish and you feed him for a lifetime.
—*Chinese proverb credited to Lao Tzu,*
the founder of Taoism

This popular Chinese proverb describes the core approach of this book. Cognitive-behavioral social skills training (CBSST) is a psychosocial rehabilitation intervention for consumers with schizophrenia. In CBSST, consumers set specific recovery goals related to living, learning, working, and socializing in their communities of choice, then learn cognitive, communication, and problem-solving skills to achieve these goals. This manual is a practical guide to delivering the CBSST program. CBSST integrates cognitive-behavioral therapy (CBT), social skills training, and problem-solving training, three strong evidence-based practices for schizophrenia. Integrating these interventions strengthens all three. Consumers set specific, motivating goals for their functioning, including the steps they will take to achieve these goals. They then learn skills to work toward their recovery goals. A skills-based cognitive therapy approach is used to teach consumers how to correct inaccurate dysfunctional thoughts that interfere with goal-directed activities, including defeatist expectancies ("It won't be fun"), low self-efficacy beliefs ("I always fail"), and anomalous beliefs ("Spirits will harm me if I go out"). Social skills training is used to teach communication skills to improve assertive engagement in interpersonal interactions, and problem-solving skills training facilitates recovery goal achievement and combats negative symptoms and depression.

This treatment manual is unique among psychosocial treatment manuals for schizophrenia in several ways. First, unlike most other cognitive therapy interventions for schizophrenia, which primarily focus on positive symptoms, the primary focus of CBSST is on recovery goals related to living, learning, working, and socializing. Second, CBSST is unique in bundling together three evidence-based practices—CBT, social skills training, and problem-solving training. Third, CBSST is a simplified, skills-based intervention that is designed to be easy for providers to deliver and consumers to understand. Finally, CBSST can be delivered as group therapy, individual therapy, or in the context of case management (e.g., assertive community treatment).

Evidence-based practices for schizophrenia, such as CBT and social skills training, have been identified and are recommended in best-practice guidelines (Gaebel, Weinmann, Sartorius, Rutz, & McIntyre, 2005; Dixon et al., 2010), but these practices are rarely available to most people with schizophrenia. The field must close the gap between research and service delivery by adapting evidence-based practices for schizophrenia for delivery in community settings. One barrier to their implementation and delivery is the cost associated with existing cognitive therapy models, which typically require a high level of education and extensive training. Consumers with schizophrenia typically do not have the resources to access these interventions, and community mental health systems often cannot afford them. We have challenged the mistaken assumption that CBT for schizophrenia can be delivered only by highly educated, expensive providers. CBSST is designed to be accessible to providers with bachelor's- and master's-level, as well as doctoral-level, education who have experience working with consumers with serious mental illness. CBSST was specifically designed to be a simple, step-by-step, skills-based intervention that can be delivered with high fidelity by novice providers. As such, CBSST has the potential to improve significantly the access of the millions of consumers with schizophrenia to these evidence-based treatments.

This is a practical treatment manual that describes a step-by-step process of learning skills to facilitate recovery goal achievement. The manual includes suggested provider scripts, diagrams that can be used to describe concepts and teach, and exercises and games designed to teach while having fun and maintaining consumer engagement. Also included are CBSST Consumer Workbooks, which contain summaries of all the skills and worksheets for at-home practice (homework). As such, CBSST is relatively easy to implement with high fidelity by clinicians at almost any level of education and experience.

This book is intended to have broad appeal to counselors, care coordinators, case managers, substance abuse counselors, employment/vocational rehabilitation specialists, social workers, psychiatric nurse specialists, psychologists, and psychiatrists working with consumers with schizophrenia, schizoaffective disorder, or other serious mental illnesses. Clinicians with at least a bachelor's degree in a mental health-related field (or less, if experienced with this population) will likely find this treatment manual accessible. This CBSST manual is also appropriate for several types of students, including students in certificate programs and graduate programs in substance abuse, vocational rehabilitation, occupational therapy, social work, psychology, and psychiatric nursing and psychiatry, as well as practicum trainees, interns, postgraduate fellows, and residents from these disciplines.

HOW THIS BOOK IS ORGANIZED

This CBSST treatment manual is divided into three main parts. Part I (Chapters 1–4) describes the theoretical background, research evidence, outcome and fidelity assessments, and guidelines for the implementation of CBSST. Chapter 1 provides the rationale for bundling CBT, social skills training, and problem solving into CBSST to improve functioning and overviews the specific skills modules. Chapter 2 briefly describes research supporting the efficacy of these interventions, including three clinical trials of CBSST that have demonstrated its efficacy for improving functioning in schizophrenia. Practical considerations about how to start a CBSST group and adapt CBSST to the unique needs of different clinical settings are discussed in Chapter 3. Assessments to measure treatment outcomes and evaluate the fidelity of CBSST delivery are described in Chapter 4.

Part II (Chapters 5–9) is a practical guide to delivering the CBSST program. Setting goals is a key component of any effective psychosocial rehabilitation program. In the CBSST program, treatment is guided by recovery goals. Chapter 5 describes the goal-setting process of identifying a long-term recovery goal that is personally meaningful to the consumer, and breaking that goal down into short-term goals and goal steps that can be accomplished each week. Chapters 6–8 then provide practical, session-by-session guidance on delivering the three CBSST modules: Cognitive Skills, Social Skills, and Problem-Solving Skills. Chapter 9 provides tips on adapting CBSST to special populations and overcoming some common challenges clinicians might face in delivering CBSST.

Part III contains consumer workbooks for each of the three skills modules. Each workbook can be copied and given to consumers at the start of its respective module. Alternatively, the workbook pages can be treated as handouts and distributed on a session-by-session basis. Appendices A–C provide additional assessment measures; experiential games that can facilitate learning and engage consumers in treatment by making learning fun; and additional useful handouts.

With the recovery movement, there is growing realization among consumers and providers that people with schizophrenia can achieve meaningful recovery and improved quality of life when offered effective treatments. Effective psychosocial treatments for schizophrenia have been identified but are rarely delivered in the context of busy, underfunded mental health systems. The evidence for the efficacy of CBSST has been evaluated by the Substance Abuse and Mental Health Services Administration and was found to be sufficient to list CBSST on the National Registry of Evidence-Based Programs and Practices website (*http://nrepp.samhsa.gov*). We hope this practical CBSST manual will help increase the availability of cognitive-behavioral, social skills, and problem-solving interventions for consumers with serious mental illnesses to help them learn the skills needed to achieve their recovery goals.

Acknowledgments

The body of work contained in this book would not have been possible without the contributions, inspiration, and support from many individuals. We would like to extend our deepest gratitude to the following:

- Our families, for their support and patience while we worked many late evenings and weekends and spent time away from our homes and loved ones to present our work and train other clinicians.

- The many research lab staff and colleagues who contributed to our clinical trials research and the development of cognitive-behavioral social skills training (CBSST), especially Dr. Fauzia Simjee McClure, Dr. Cathy Loh, and John Borges, who contributed to early drafts of the Consumer Workbooks; the many bright and dedicated therapists, interns, and fellows who have contributed to the development of CBSST and provided services for the consumers in our research projects and clinic; and Dr. Dilip Jeste, who initially encouraged us to begin developing CBSST.

- The many providers we have trained from the San Diego County Mental Health System, including the Community Research Foundation and Telecare Corporation; the University of Calgary and Alberta Health Services in Calgary, Canada, including Dr. Rory Sellmer and Jason Stein; the Maryland Psychiatric Research Center in the University of Maryland School of Medicine and the Spring Grove Hospital Center in the Baltimore Mental Health System; the Veterans Affairs Healthcare Systems in Minneapolis and Ann Arbor; the Centre for Addiction and Mental Health in Toronto, Canada; and Seoul National University Hospital in Seoul, South Korea. The constructive comments and feedback from these providers about the CBSST interventions and the Consumer Workbooks, especially the creative and engaging games they created, have been invaluable.

We would especially like to thank the many consumers who participated in CBSST groups in our clinical trials and treatment programs. Their commitment and dedication to our research projects, desire to help other consumers, and strength and courage to overcome many life challenges have taught us many valuable lessons that have inspired us to try to become better clinicians, refine the CBSST program, and more broadly disseminate CBSST with the hope that it will continue to help consumers make meaningful changes in their lives.

CBSST is, in part, based upon work supported by the Department of Veterans Affairs, Veterans Health Administration, Office of Research and Development, Rehabilitation Research and Development Service (VA Merit Review Grant Nos. 324/426, O3341-R, and E4876-R to Dr. Granholm); the National Institute of Mental Health (Grant Nos. NIMH R01MH071410 and R01MH091057 to Dr. Granholm); and the University of California, San Diego Advanced Center for Innovations in Services and Interventions Research (ACISIR; Grant No. NIMH P30MH66248 to Dr. Dilip Jeste). The content is solely the responsibility of the authors and does not necessarily represent the official views of the Department of Veterans Affairs, the University of California, or the National Institutes of Health.

Contents

PART I

Background, Research Evidence, and Implementation

CHAPTER 1

Improving Functioning in Schizophrenia

Functioning refers to the degree of success that a person has in interpersonal relationships, educational, vocational, or parenting role activities, and self-care and independent living. Poor functioning is present in many mental disorders but is particularly common in schizophrenia (Morrison, Bellack, Wixted, & Mueser, 1990; Harvey et al., 2012; Harvey & Strassnig, 2012). Functional impairments in schizophrenia are present immediately after the first episode (Robinson, Woerner, McMeniman, Mendelowitz, & Bilder, 2004), often even before the first episode (Carrion et al., 2013), continue after successful treatment of psychotic symptoms (Harvey et al., 2012; Robinson et al., 2004), and persist into late life (Harding, 1988; Harrison, Gunnell, Glazebrook, Page, & Kwiecinski, 2001). Consumers with schizophrenia often have difficulty getting their basic needs met, leading to heavy reliance on family members, disability payments (in Western societies), and poor subjective quality of life (Penn, Corrigan, Bentall, Racenstein, & Newman, 1997). Consumers, families, and advocacy groups frequently describe functional impairments as their chief concern. Antipsychotic medications may reduce psychotic symptoms (also called positive symptoms) but have little impact on negative symptoms (e.g., lack of motivation, impoverished speech) and functioning (Bellack, Mueser, Morrison, Tierney, & Podell, 1990; Guo et al., 2010; Kahn et al., 2008; McEvoy, 2008). Thus, schizophrenia treatment has moved beyond pharmacological management of psychotic symptoms to address the more personally meaningful recovery goals of achieving satisfying interpersonal relationships, vocational or educational activities, and independent living.

WHAT IS RECOVERY IN SCHIZOPHRENIA?

The recovery model dates back to the consumer movement that began in the 1960s in the context of deinstitutionalization, which led to a new recovery perspective on how serious mental illnesses are viewed and what the goals of treatment should be. People with mental illnesses objected to the term "patient" and a powerless role in treatment, opting for a role as "consumer" of mental health services (or "service user" in the United Kingdom). Consumers objected to the hopelessness of the mental health system, protesting that disorders such as schizophrenia do not have to be chronic and disabling, citing outcome studies demonstrating functional recovery in a high proportion of consumers (see Table 1.1).

TABLE 1.1. Rates of Recovery in Schizophrenia

Long-term follow-up studies			
Authors	Country	Sample	Recovery rates
Harrow et al. (2005)	USA—Chicago	Chronic	45%
Tsuang et al. (1979)	USA—Iowa	Chronic	46%
Harrison et al. (2001)	WHO—International	Mostly first episode	48%
Ciompi (1980)	Switzerland—Berne	Chronic	53%
Huber et al. (1975)	Germany—Bonn	Mixed	53%
Bleuler (1968)	Switzerland—Zurich	Chronic	57%
Ogawa et al. (1987)	Japan—Urban	Mostly first episode	64%
Harding et al. (1987)	USA—Vermont	Chronic	68%
Loebel et al. (1992) and Lieberman et al. (1993)	USA—New York	First episode	74%
Nuechterlein et al. (2006)	USA—Los Angeles	First episode	79%
Whitehorn et al. (1998)	Nova Scotia—Halifax	First episode	89%
McGorry et al. (1996) and Edwards et al. (1998)	Australia—Melbourne	First episode	91%
Meta-analytic reviews			
Authors	Number of studies	Sample	Recovery rates
Jääskeläinen et al. (2013)	50	Mixed	14%
Warner (2004)	114	Mixed	38%
Hegarty et al. (1994)	320	Mixed	40%
Menezes et al. (2006)	37	First episode	42%

Note. Based in part on Liberman (2008) and Liberman and Kopelowicz (2005).

This new recovery perspective has led to a shift from a treatment focus on symptoms and disease to a rehabilitation and recovery focus on consumer strengths, community functioning, quality of life and recovery. Recovery is a multidimensional construct that includes the different perspectives of professionals and consumers, objective and subjective criteria, clinical and functional outcomes, as well as personal experiences and values (Frese, Knight, & Saks, 2009; Liberman & Kopelowicz, 2005; Leucht & Lasser, 2006). Clinicians and researchers often define recovery with objective criteria for symptom reduction and functioning, such as competitive employment and independent living. Consumer-based groups often conceptualize recovery as a personal journey or the subjective process of coping with illness over time. Consumers emphasize subjective indicators such as quality of life, purpose, self-value, hope, and persistence despite challenges presented by mental illness. The Substance Abuse and Mental Health Services Administration (SAMHSA; *http:// samhsa.gov*) consensus definition of recovery is "a process of change through which individuals improve their health and wellness, live a self-directed life, and strive to reach their full potential." Reaching our full potential is a goal of most everyone, not just individuals with mental disorders.

In research on outcome in schizophrenia, recovery is typically defined as meeting the following objective criteria for a sustained duration of time (e.g., 6 months or 2 years): (1) remission of symptoms and (2) a degree of success in functioning, including (a) engagement in age-appropriate instrumental role activities (e.g., work, education, or family caregiving), (b) independent care of self and home, (c) participation in satisfying interpersonal interactions with a partner, family and/or friends, and (d) recreational activities in the community (Faerden, Nesvåg, & Marder, 2008; Harvey & Bellack, 2009; Liberman & Kopelowicz, 2005; Leucht & Lasser, 2006). Expert workgroups have developed consensus criteria for both remission of symptoms and functional remission in schizophrenia (Andreasen et al., 2005; Harvey & Bellack, 2009; Leucht & Lasser, 2006). Complete recovery implies being *both* relatively free of symptoms and able to function in the community, socially and vocationally, for a sustained duration of time. A scientific definition of recovery, therefore, is a more demanding and longer-term achievement than symptom remission or functional remission alone.

Table 1.1 shows that, in long-term follow-up studies of 10–20 years, recovery rates in individuals with schizophrenia have consistently ranged from approximately 45 to 65%, with much higher recovery rates in some studies (Liberman & Kopelowicz, 2005; Liberman, 2008). A number of meta-analyses of outcome studies in schizophrenia have found similar recovery rates (see Table 1.1). According to a meta-analysis of 114 studies published between 1904 and 2000 (Warner, 2004), approximately 38% of individuals with schizophrenia achieved social recovery (economic and residential independence and low social dysfunction), and 22% achieved "complete" recovery (no symptoms and return to premorbid levels of functioning). A meta-analysis of 320 studies from 1895 to 1992 (Hegarty, Baldessarini, Tohen, Waternaux, & Oepen, 1994), found that approximately 40% of individuals with schizophrenia were considered recovered after follow-ups averaging 5–6 years, and a higher recovery rate (49%) was found in studies completed after 1955, probably due in part to the development of antipsychotic medications in the 1950s. In another meta-analysis of 37 studies of first-episode psychosis, Menezes, Arenovich, and Zipursky (2006) found that 42% of individuals with schizophrenia recovered. In contrast, in a recent meta-analysis of 50 studies, Jääskeläinen et al. (2013) found that only 13.5% individuals with schizophrenia recovered.

Differences in rates of recovery across outcome studies may be due to a number of factors. First and perhaps foremost, the definition of recovery used in the study impacted the recovery rates. Researchers that found higher recovery rates defined recovery as symptom remission and/or functional remission at a specific follow-up assessment, and did not require a specific duration of recovery (e.g., remission at consecutive assessments over time). Researchers who required both symptom and functional remission and a longer duration of stable remission (e.g., 2 years in the meta-analysis by Jääskeläinen et al., 2013) found much lower rates of recovery. Outcome studies, therefore, showed that individuals with schizophrenia can achieve high rates of recovery but may experience fluctuations in recovery over time (Harvey & Bellack, 2009). Defining recovery as functional stability over long periods of time may be an unreasonably high expectation. For example, economic fluctuations such as recessions, layoffs, housing market crashes, and foreclosures may lead to fluctuations in functioning in both mentally ill consumers and healthy individuals. Anyone who has a job at one point, loses it after a year, then gets another job 6 months later would not have stable functioning over a 2-year period. Dynamic changes from remission to disability and back to remission are more consistent with the conceptualization of recovery as a process or journey (Frese et al., 2009).

Another factor that may contribute to variation in recovery rates across outcome studies is availability of comprehensive psychiatric rehabilitation programs, including programs that combine pharmacotherapy with psychotherapy (Menezes et al., 2006; Liberman, 2008). Antipsychotic medications alone have little impact on daily functioning (Bellack et al., 1990; Guo et al., 2010; Kahn et al., 2008; McEvoy, 2008). Stage of illness may also be an important factor. The early intervention movement is based in part on the notion that younger first-episode consumers with shorter duration of illness have better rates of recovery if the person receives comprehensive psychiatric rehabilitation that bundles evidence-based medication protocols with evidence-based psychosocial rehabilitation programs (Birchwood, Todd, & Jackson, 1998; McGorry & Yung, 2003).

In reading this information about recovery in schizophrenia, consider your own attitudes and expectations about recovery in the consumers you serve. The success of participants in cognitive-behavioral social skills training (CBSST) will be impacted by provider attitudes and beliefs about severe mental illnesses such as schizophrenia. Hopeful providers are a key to recovery. If providers do not believe people with schizophrenia can achieve their recovery goals, it will be difficult for them to teach people with schizophrenia to believe in themselves. People who expect to succeed will try new tasks, take on more difficult tasks, and put forth more effort to achieve their goals, because they expect to succeed. This is true for both providers and individuals with mental illness. Providers and consumers who expect success work harder to achieve recovery goals. This chapter section on recovery is about cognitive therapy for the therapist. Use the evidence presented here to challenge mistakes in thinking, such as "people with schizophrenia cannot get a job, partner, home of their own, or serenity."

From a *Time* magazine interview with Elyn Saks, author of *The Center Cannot Hold* and a person with schizophrenia:

> There are lots of misconceptions about schizophrenia, [like that] people can't hold jobs, certainly not high-powered jobs. . . . Can't have close friends and family. Can't live independently. A lot of those have some truth; they're true of a certain portion of people with schizophrenia. But it seems to me that a lot more than is now the case could be leading far more gratifying [lives]. When you tell someone, "you're not going to be able to work," or "scale down your expectations," then they do. And yet work gives most people so much of a sense of well-being, productivity. You're taking away from someone a thing that could be an important tool in their recovery by having these kind of negative expectations. (August 27, 2007)

KEY DETERMINANTS OF FUNCTIONAL OUTCOME

In order to develop treatments to help individuals with schizophrenia achieve recovery goals, it is necessary to understand what determines a successful or poor functional outcome in schizophrenia. Surprisingly, positive symptoms are only a weak determinant of functional outcome, whereas negative symptoms (e.g., anhedonia, amotivation, asociality) are strongly associated with poor functioning and are an unmet treatment need in a large proportion of consumers (Kirkpatrick, Fenton, Carpenter, & Marder, 2006). Another established predictor of poor functional outcome is neurocognitive impairments in attention, memory, and executive functions such as problem-solving and abstract reasoning abilities (Green, 1996; Green, Kern, Braff, & Mintz, 2000; Green, Kern, & Heaton, 2004; Kurtz, Moberg, Ragland, Gur, & Gur, 2005). However, the relationship between neurocognitive deficits and poor functional outcome is at least partially mediated by several factors (see Figure 1.1). One factor is social cognition, which refers to mental processes involved in the perception, interpretation, and processing of social information, including emotion processing, social perception, theory of mind, mental state attribution, and attributional style or bias (Green et al., 2008; Pinkham et al., 2014). A recent meta-analysis of 112 studies found consistent impairment on a variety of social cognition tasks in individuals with schizophrenia (Savla, Vella, Armstrong, Penn, & Twamley, 2013),

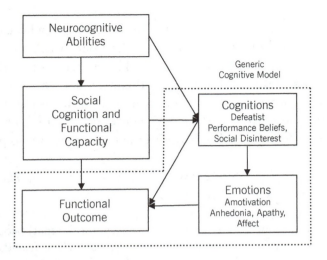

FIGURE 1.1. Key determinants of functional outcome in schizophrenia. Key determinants that are addressed by CBSST are shown. The generic cognitive model that guides CBT is highlighted to show that cognitions can influence functioning behaviors directly or through their impact on emotions and motivation.

and another recent review indicated that social cognition is a mediator between neurocognitive abilities and functional outcome in 14 of 15 studies (Schmidt, Mueller, & Roder, 2011).

Poor neurocognitive abilities are also associated with poor skills competence in several domains, including shopping, managing money, using public transportation, and assertive communication skills—all of which are skills needed to function independently in the community. These functional capacities are typically measured in research projects that ask participants to role-play or perform tasks in laboratory simulations (e.g., read a bus schedule, initiate and maintain a conversation, call a doctor, or shop for items in a simulated grocery store). Better neurocognitive abilities can facilitate better learning of social-cognitive and functional skill capacities, which in turn are associated with better real-world functioning.

Attitudes and motivation can also influence real-world functioning. The key premise of the generic cognitive model that guides cognitive-behavioral therapy (CBT) is that cognitions influence behaviors and emotions. Based on the cognitive model, Beck and colleagues (Beck, Rector, Stolar, & Grant, 2009; Grant & Beck, 2009) have proposed that specific attitudes or cognitions can influence real-world behaviors directly or through their impact on emotions and motivation. Several studies have indicated that cognitions such as defeatist performance beliefs (e.g., "Why try? I always fail") and attitudes of social disinterest (e.g., "I'm better off alone") are endorsed more strongly by consumers with schizophrenia than by healthy controls and are associated with poor functioning and negative symptoms, even after accounting for depression (Couture, Blanchard, & Bennett, 2011; Granholm, Ben-Zeev, & Link, 2009; Grant & Beck, 2009; Green, Hellemann, Horan,

Lee, & Wynn, 2012; Horan et al., 2010; Quinlan, Roesch, & Granholm, 2014). Furthermore, defeatist beliefs have been found to mediate the relationship between neurocognitive abilities and negative symptoms and functioning (Grant & Beck, 2009; Green et al., 2012; Horan et al., 2010; Quinlan et al., 2014). Such findings support the model proposed by Beck and colleagues (Beck et al., 2009, Grant & Beck, 2009) that neurocognitive impairments contribute to discouraging, everyday failure experiences (e.g., poor grades in school, poor work performance) that lead to low expectations for success and defeatist performance beliefs that in turn, lead to negative symptoms such as amotivation, asociality, and poor functioning.

In social learning theory (Bandura, 1986, 1997), self-competency beliefs are central to motivation for achievement and engagement in goal-directed activities. People who expect to succeed are more willing to try new tasks, choose harder tasks, and expend more effort, because they think they will succeed (Avery, Startup, & Calabria, 2009; Bandura, 1997; Wigfield & Eccles, 2000). Rector, Beck, and Stolar (2005) proposed that dysfunctional attitudes about failure and the personal costs of expending energy can lead to passivity and avoidance of activities that require effort, as a defense against anticipated failure and negative evaluations by others. This avoidance and lack of effort manifests as diminished motivation (avolition–apathy), loss of pleasure (anhedonia–asociality), and lack of engagement in goal-directed functioning activities. Consistent with this, social anhedonia and reduced positive affect have been linked to poor functional outcome in several studies of schizophrenia and schizotypy (Bellack et al., 1990; Bellack, Sayers, Mueser, & Bennett, 1994; Granholm, Ben-Zeev, Fulford, & Swendsen, 2013). Taken together, these findings suggest that attitudes of social disinterest, defeatist performance beliefs, and the negative emotional and motivational consequences of these beliefs, can negatively impact real-world functioning in people with schizophrenia. These connections among cognitions, emotions, and functional outcome are consistent with the generic cognitive model of the reciprocal direct effects that thoughts have on feelings and behavior, as highlighted in Figure 1.1. By addressing defeatist beliefs in treatment, therefore, consumers may increase motivation and effort directed at activities of social engagement and goal-directed functioning in the community.

Figure 1.1 shows the key determinants of functional outcome that drove the development of CBSST, but it does not show all the factors that contribute to functioning in schizophrenia. Several other personal factors have been associated with poor functional outcome in schizophrenia, including greater severity of depression, poorer insight, and comorbid substance use disorders (Bowie, Reichenberg, Patterson, Heaton, & Harvey, 2006; Ventura, Hellemann, Thames, Koellner, & Nuechterlein, 2009; Friedman et al., 2001; Robinson et al., 2004; Twamley et al., 2002; Wiersma et al., 2000). In addition, community context and environmental factors clearly can influence functional outcome (e.g., a weak economy, social support, institutional resources and hindrances). In the United States, for example, a strong predictor of unemployment is the receipt of disability compensation (Rosenheck et al., 2006), which can produce a disincentive to seek work. Seeking employment above the minimal level allowed by the rules associated with insurance and disability payments can compromise both compensation and health insurance, which may be too great a financial risk for someone without a strong, stable work history. Stigma among employers can also reduce opportunities for individuals with mental disorders. The family can also support recovery. To address determinants of functional outcome that are not addressed by CBSST, a comprehensive psychiatric rehabilitation program would ideally include choices of other forms of individual and group therapy, pharmacotherapy, family therapy, cognitive remediation, vocational rehabilitation, supported employment, educational resources, supported housing, community linkages, recovery coaching, and case management.

CBSST COMPONENTS AND THEIR RATIONALE

We developed CBSST to address the personal factors shown in Figure 1.1. CBSST is a recovery-oriented psychosocial rehabilitation intervention designed to improve functioning and negative symptoms in consumers with schizophrenia (Granholm, McQuaid, McClure, Pedrelli, & Jeste, 2002; Granholm et al., 2005; McQuaid et al., 2000). CBSST comprises three modules—(1) Cognitive Skills, (2) Social Skills, and (3) Problem-Solving Skills—each consisting of six sessions, though the number of sessions delivered varies depending on the unique needs of different consumers and treatment settings (see Chapter 3). Social skills training is used to improve communication skill capacities; problem-solving training is used to address neurocognitive impairments related to solving problems and developing goal-directed action plans; and cognitive therapy is used to challenge defeatist beliefs that interfere with communication skills performance and goal-directed actions in the real world. Consumers set specific functioning goals in the domains of living, learning, working and socializing, and they identify the steps they will take to reach these goals. CBSST is based on the recovery model, and recovery goal setting is at the core of the intervention. Training in social communication skills and problem-solving skills focuses on using these skills to achieve functional recovery goals. Training in thought-challenging skills helps consumers correct inaccurate defeatist beliefs, including low expectations ("It won't be fun"), low self-efficacy beliefs ("I always fail"), and anomalous beliefs ("Spirits will harm me") that interfere with skills performance. By challenging these beliefs, consumers may increase motivation and effort directed at using their improved skills to engage in community functioning activities. The treatment's components are described in more detail next.

Cognitive Skills

The premise of CBT is that cognition, the process of acquiring information and forming beliefs, can influence feelings and behavior. CBT for schizophrenia originally developed out of work by Aaron T. Beck as early as the 1950s and includes a range of approaches with a variety of treatment elements, including the collaborative understanding of target problems or symptoms; developing specific cognitive and behavioral strategies to cope with these problems or symptoms; and testing the accuracy of defeatist beliefs, key beliefs that maintain delusional thinking, and distressing beliefs about voices. In CBSST, the primary targets of cognitive interventions are defeatist performance beliefs and psychotic symptoms that interfere with the individual's functioning goals (e.g., challenging beliefs about the power of a voice when the voice threatens to harm a consumer if he or she goes to a job interview). Through cognitive therapy, consumers learn to identify and modify thoughts, misinterpretations of experiences, and thinking patterns that contribute to maladaptive behavior or distressing feelings.

CBT for psychosis assumes that (1) hallucinations and delusions are not fixed and can be modified when targeted for intervention; (2) situational factors can exacerbate or ameliorate psychotic symptoms; and (3) the content of psychotic symptoms can be meaningful when placed in the context of the individual's prior experiences and beliefs (Beck & Rector, 2000). A primary goal of CBT for psychosis is to help consumers become more cognitively flexible, to change the way they evaluate their symptoms, and to consider alternative explanations for psychotic experiences (e.g., objective distancing and reappraisal of failure experiences and psychotic symptoms by examining evidence). Exercises and homework assignments (e.g., thought records and experiments) are used to examine the evidence for and against thoughts and interpretations of events and symptoms. For example, to reduce distress or compliance with command hallucinations, one might challenge beliefs about the power or control of voices by conducting experiments involving activities that exacerbate hallucinations (e.g., imagining a stressor) or ameliorate hallucinations (e.g., humming; listening to music) to demonstrate that voices can be controlled. A defeatist belief such as "Nobody would want to talk with me" might be challenged by examining evidence for and against it or by asking about family, roommates, and other group members, who might like to talk with the individual. If just one person, such as a group member or therapist, says that he or she likes to talk with the individual, the belief is proven to be inaccurate. By reevaluating evidence and considering more positive interpretations, positive symptom severity, distress, and dysfunction may be reduced in CBT.

In CBSST, cognitive-behavioral techniques are simplified and taught as skills. The "3C's" (Catch It, Check It, Change It) comprise the primary cognitive skills set. "Catch It" consists of catching automatic thoughts, labeling them as helpful or unhelpful, and using feelings as red flags to identify problematic thoughts. "Check It" consists of checking unhelpful thoughts for "mistakes in thinking," examining evidence, and conducting behavioral experiments to gather evidence. "Change It" involves generating alternative, more helpful thoughts. In addition, providers make use of alternatives therapy, Socratic questioning, guided discovery, thought chaining, and behavioral experiments throughout all the modules when problem beliefs appear to interfere with progress toward goals.

Social Skills Training

Social skills deficits in occupational, interpersonal, and recreational situations are strongly associated with poor social functioning in consumers with schizophrenia (Mueser & Bellack, 1998). Social skills training is an evidence-based psychosocial intervention that teaches social skills to improve social functioning (Bellack, Mueser, Gingerich, & Agresta, 2004). Although skills training programs vary considerably in content, duration, and delivery setting, they share a core set of strategies for training skills, which are based on social learning theory (Bandura, 1969). These core strategies include goal setting, providing a rationale for training skills that links specific skills to consumer goals, role modeling, behavioral rehearsal (repeated role-play practice of skills), lots of positive reinforcement, corrective feedback, shaping, and homework assignments to help promote generalization and use of skills in the community. The social skills module in CBSST uses all of these strategies. The following basic communication skills are the primary focus: active listening, expressing pleasant and unpleasant feelings, making positive requests, and asking for help with goals. Through repeated in-session role plays and "at-home practice" assignments, these skills can be applied to starting and maintaining conversations, assertiveness, conflict management, communal living, friendship and dating, communicating with health providers, and vocational and work interactions.

Role plays in CBSST provide a unique opportunity to test out beliefs that can interfere with successful skills practice in the community. As such, cognitive therapy interventions are combined with social skills training. Role plays can be used as behavioral experiments during sessions to elicit and test out beliefs such as "I won't be able to do it well" or "It won't work." Providers can point out how these low expectations for success can reduce the likelihood that consumers will try to use skills in the community and learn that their low expectations might be mistaken. For example, prior to trying a new skill in group, consumers are asked to rate their expectation of success versus failure on a scale of 1 to 10, and to rerate their performance after practicing the skill. These self-ratings typically increase following skills practice, because consumers typically perform better than they expected. Therapists can point out that initial low expectations for success were mistakes in thinking that can interfere with goals (e.g., "You sold yourself short; you are a lot better at this than you thought you would be. If you think you cannot do this well, will you be less likely to try it out?"). In this way, CBT and social skills training skills can be combined to challenge thoughts that are barriers to successful skills performance.

Problem-Solving Training

Problem-solving deficits in consumers with schizophrenia are associated with poor community functioning and quality of life (Grant, Addington, Addington, & Konnert, 2001; Kelly & Lamparski, 1985; Revheim et al., 2006). Problem-solving training is a therapy developed to improve problem-solving skills for consumers with serious mental illness. It is evidence-based and has been widely used for a variety of clinical problems in psychiatry, social work, and counseling, including schizophrenia, depression, childhood disorders and parenting, and cognitive rehabilitation (D'Zurilla & Nezu, 2010). In the treatment of schizophrenia, it is most commonly included as a component of other interventions, such as family therapy, CBT, and social skills training interventions rather than a stand-alone intervention.

Problem-solving training teaches a systematic strategy both to solve immediate problems and prepare individuals to deal with future problems on their own. Complex problems are broken down into manageable, attainable steps. A similar systematic, stepwise approach is used in most problem-solving interventions: (1) The problem is identified in specific behavioral terms; (2) possible solutions are generated through brainstorming; (3) solutions are evaluated, and the best solution is selected; and (4) the solution is implemented, evaluated, and revised, as necessary. The CBSST Problem-Solving skills module uses a similar five-step strategy called SCALE, an acronym for the following steps: **S**—Specify the problem; **C**—Consider all possible solutions; **A**—Assess the best possible solution; **L**—Lay out a plan; and **E**—Execute and evaluate. Since many individuals with serious mental illness have some degree of cognitive impairment, SCALE was developed as a mnemonic aid to assist them in recalling the steps and to provide structure and guidance to solving problems that can often seem overwhelming. The acronym SCALE also underlines the importance of goal setting and attainment: "Problem solving can help you SCALE a mountain of problems to achieve your goals."

Neurocognitive Compensatory Strategies

Given the link between neurocognitive impairments and poor functional outcome, several neurocognitive compensatory strategies are included in CBSST. The literature on cognitive remediation interventions has generally examined compensatory, environmental, and restorative approaches to treatment, each of which has its strengths and weaknesses (Medalia & Bellucci, 2012; Medalia & Choi, 2009; McGurk, Twamley, Sitzer, McHugo, & Mueser, 2007). Compensatory strategies teach consumers how to use external aids and strategies to "work around" their deficits. Environmental strategies involve manipulations of the environment to decrease cognitive demands. Restorative approaches emphasize improvement of underlying cognitive deficits, often through extensive laboratory-based practice of rudimentary skills. Cognitive remediation studies have found improvements in cognitive functioning in consumers with schizophrenia, especially in attention, memory and abstraction, and flexibility functions (Twamley, Jeste, & Bellack, 2003; Wykes, 2008). The cognitive remediation components of CBSST primarily include strategy-oriented compensatory aids and environmental manipulations. Laboratory-based practice of rudimentary skills is not included.

It is important to emphasize that cognitive therapy is not cognitive remediation. It is possible that cognitive therapy might lead to improvements in neurocognition, but neurocognition is not the primary treatment target of CBT. Cognitive remediation focuses on rehabilitation of specific neurocognitive functions (e.g., memory, attention), and CBT trains consumers to use metacognitive strategies to identify and challenge dysfunctional thoughts. Perris and Skagerlind (1994) pointed out that cognitive remediation and CBT have several factors in common and may lie on a continuum from more "molecular" to more "molar" approaches. At one end, cognitive remediation targets specific problems of neurocognitive processing, and at the other end, CBT targets more global cognitive constructs, such as thinking about experiences and self-concept.

Cognitive therapy and problem-solving training interventions attempt to improve metacognitive belief evaluation processes, cognitive flexibility, inductive reasoning, and abstract thinking. As noted earlier, problem-solving training, which is a significant focus of CBSST, is a verbal mediation strategy that is widely used to compensate for abstraction/flexibility deficits associated with frontal lobe damage. CBSST also incorporates several cognitive compensatory aids. Therapists are encouraged to use multiple presentation modalities to provide information: lecture, extensive writing on dry-erase boards, posters describing skills, laminated wallet cards describing skills, participant workbooks, and group discussion. Acronyms such as SCALE and the 3C's are also taught to help consumers remember skills. Repetition of information is a cornerstone of the intervention: Basic themes are repeated throughout a session; a summary is provided at the end of each session; and the entire content is presented twice. To compensate for motivational and attentional deficits, therapists can use behavioral rewards (token economies, happy face tokens) to reinforce attention to task and participation. In summary, like cognitive remediation, CBSST involves repeated practice of skills, behavioral rewards for attention to task, training compensatory strategies for memory and attention deficits, self-instruction and inductive reasoning strategies applied to thinking and social perception, and hypothesis testing and problem-solving training to promote cognitive flexibility.

SUMMARY

Despite the presence of functional impairments throughout the illness course in schizophrenia, research has shown that functional recovery is not only possible but also a promising target for intervention. CBSST was designed to address key factors that influence functional outcome in schizophrenia, such as dysfunctional attitudes, low motivation, social skills deficits, and problem-solving and neurocognitive impairments. CBSST teaches cognitive skills, social skills, problem-solving skills, and uses cognitive compensatory strategies to help consumers with serious mental illness overcome barriers to achieving their recovery goals. Chapter 2 reviews the evidence base for these CBSST components.

CBSST as an Evidence-Based Practice

Substantial research supports the efficacy of a range of evidence-based practices for schizophrenia. The term "evidence-based practice" refers to interventions found to be effective at improving outcome(s) in a specific illness in multiple randomized clinical trials conducted by independent research teams using highly rigorous and standardized interventions and methodology. Best practice guidelines and nationalized health care systems recommend or mandate several evidence-based apsychosocial interventions as part of a comprehensive treatment program for schizophrenia (Gaebel, Weinmann, Sartorius, Tutz, & McIntyre, 2005; Dixon et al., 2010; Mueser, Deavers, Penn, & Cassisi, 2013). For example, the types of CBT and social skills training interventions in CBSST are among the recommendations made by the Schizophrenia Patient Outcomes Research Team (PORT; Dixon et al., 2010), a project sponsored by the National Institute of Mental Health to develop evidence-based treatment guidelines for schizophrenia in the United States. Additional recommended evidence-based practices include assertive community treatment (ACT), behavioral family therapy, supported employment, and illness self-management. All of these evidence-based psychosocial interventions can play an important role in functional recovery from schizophrenia.

CBSST includes PORT-recommended CBT and social skills training interventions but differs from other evidence-based psychosocial interventions recommended by PORT in several ways. ACT is a case management model that uses a team treatment approach with shared, low caseloads, and community-based service delivery that attempts to reduce hospitalizations, maintain housing, and improve daily living skills. It is more like a system of care delivery than a form of psychotherapy such as

CBSST, but ACT providers can deliver psychotherapy interventions such as CBSST as a part of their team-delivered services (see Chapter 3). Behavioral family therapy and family psychoeducation interventions might involve single-family or multiple-family sessions but typically focus on the whole family (not just the consumer), provide education about schizophrenia and treatments, and teach communication skills and problem-solving strategies to reduce stress and prevent relapse. The communication skills and problem-solving approaches in family interventions are similar to those in CBSST, but CBSST does not specifically involve the family. Supported employment is an intervention to help consumers obtain competitive work. The only requirement for participation is a desire to work (no consumers are excluded), and the provider goes into the community to assist with rapid job search and placement and provides follow-along supports to facilitate work performance. In contrast to supported employment, CBSST is more focused on training skills, does not require provider activities in the community and, although the long-term recovery goal of many consumers in CBSST is competitive employment, CBSST is not exclusively focused on work. Illness self-management programs, like Illness Management and Recovery (Gingerich & Mueser, 2011), include psychoeducation about schizophrenia and treatments for schizophrenia, teach strategies to promote medication adherence, help consumers develop a relapse prevention plan (identifying triggers and action plans), and teach coping strategies for persistent symptoms (including cognitive and behavioral strategies). As in CBSST, an important component is setting long-term, meaningful recovery goals; breaking goals down into manageable steps; and using goals to motivate active involvement in skills learning. Some cognitive-behavioral techniques are also used to teach coping skills in illness self-management, but CBSST is less focused on symptoms, relapse prevention, medication adherence, and illness management.

Integrated psychosocial rehabilitation programs with these recommended psychosocial interventions can reduce the cost of mental health treatment for consumers with schizophrenia. For example, VanMeerten and colleagues (2013) examined the cost savings of adding psychosocial rehabilitation programming, including CBSST, to an outpatient program at a large Midwestern Veterans Affairs Medical Center. Consumers with serious mental illness received family psychoeducation (49%), wellness management and recovery (41%), and supported employment, and the majority (81%) received CBSST. Mental health costs for consumers enrolled in the integrated program were significantly reduced, primarily due to a 9% reduction in hospitalization days, with a $17,739 reduction in costs per hospitalized consumer per year.

OUTCOME RESEARCH ON CBT

Over 50 randomized clinical trials of CBT for schizophrenia have been conducted. Improvements have been found in reduced psychotic symptom severity, delusional conviction, anxiety, and depression relative to standard care and other active psychosocial interventions (Burns, Erickson, & Brenner, 2014; Gould, Mueser, Bolton, Mays, & Goff, 2001; Sarin, Walin, & Widerlöv, 2011; Rector & Beck, 2012; Tarrier, 2010; Turkington, Kingdon, & Weidon, 2006; Wykes, Steel, Everitt, & Tarrier, 2008; Thase, Kingdon, & Turkington, 2014; Turner, van der Gaag, Karyotaki, & Cuijpers, 2014; Zimmerman, Favrod, Trieu, & Pomini, 2005; but see Jauhar et al., 2014). The most recent meta-analysis by Turner and colleagues (2014) included 48 studies of 3,295 consumers and concluded that CBT is more effective at reducing positive symptoms than standard care or supportive contact interventions. One study found large significant improvements in total symptoms for CBT relative to treatment as usual in consumers who had chosen not to take antipsychotic medications (Morrison et al., 2014). An influential meta-analysis of 35 clinical trials of CBT for psychosis (Wykes et al., 2008) showed that although the vast majority of studies focused on symptoms such as hallucinations and delusions as the primary treatment target, CBT also improved functioning. Wykes and colleagues found that the average effect size (range: 0.20 = "small"; 0.50 = "medium"; 0.80 = "large") for improvement in functional outcome (effect size = 0.378) was similar to that for positive symptoms (effect size = 0.372). In addition, they found comparable small-to-medium effect sizes for improvements in negative symptoms (effect size = 0.437), social anxiety (effect size = 0.356), and mood (effect size = 0.363). We (Granholm et al., 2009) also reviewed 18 CBT trials that included at least one functioning measure and found that approximately two-thirds of the studies showed significant gains in functioning, even when functioning was not the primary target. Some negative meta-analyses have found minimal or no benefit for CBT relative to active supportive therapies when only end of treatment assessments were included (Jones, Hacker, Cormac, Meaden, & Irving, 2012; Lynch, Laws, & McKenna, 2010; Newton-Howes & Wood, 2013), but a recent debate at the Institute of Psychiatry in London rejected the assertion that CBT for psychosis has been "oversold" (Maudsley Debates; *www.kcl.ac.uk*). Importantly, greater benefits have been found at 6-month to 5-year follow-ups than at the end of treatment (Gould et al., 2001; Sarin et al., 2011; Turkington et al., 2008; Zimmerman et al., 2005). The consistently replicated finding that CBT improves outcomes relative to standard care (typically only pharmacotherapy and case management in the United States), suggests that existing services for schizophrenia can be improved by adding CBT.

There is also preliminary evidence that CBT is effective as part of an early intervention approach in consumers with recent-onset schizophrenia (Birchwood et al., 1998; Marshall & Rathbone, 2011), as well as a possible approach to preventing psychosis in prodromal/high-risk populations (Addington, Marshall, & French, 2012). A 50% reduction in risk of developing psychosis was found in a meta-analysis of seven trials of clinical high-risk individuals receiving CBT and not taking antipsychotic medication (Hutton & Taylor, 2014).

OUTCOME RESEARCH ON SOCIAL SKILLS TRAINING

Numerous clinical trials have shown that social skills training improves social skills in consumers with schizophrenia. Benton and Schroeder (1990) conducted a meta-analysis of 27 social skills training clinical trials of consumers with schizophrenia and concluded that it improved acquisition and durability of skills such as basic conversation skills, assertiveness, and medication management. In the most recent meta-analysis of 22 randomized clinical trials of social skills training for schizophrenia, Kurtz and Mueser (2008) found a large effect size for proximal content-mastery outcomes (effect size = 1.20); moderate effect sizes for intermediate outcomes, including performance-based measures of social and daily living skills (effect size = 0.52), community functioning (effect size = 0.52), and negative symptoms (effect size = 0.40); and small effect sizes for more distal outcomes such as other symptoms (effect size = 0.15) and relapse (effect size = 0.23). Pfammatter, Junghan, and Brenner (2006) reviewed 19 randomized clinical trials of social skills training for schizophrenia, and found significant benefits for skills acquisition (effect size = 0.77), assertiveness (effect size = 0.43), social functioning (effect size = 0.39), and general psychopathology (effect size = 0.23). The consistently replicated finding that social skills training improves outcomes relative to standard care suggests that existing standard services for schizophrenia can be improved by adding social skills training.

OUTCOME RESEARCH ON PROBLEM-SOLVING TRAINING

CBSST also includes a module on problem-solving training. The evidence for the efficacy of problem-solving training in consumers with schizophrenia is much more limited than the evidence for CBT and social skills training for schizophrenia. This is in part due to the fact that problem-solving training has typically been bundled with other interventions rather than studied as a stand-alone treatment. For example, it has been combined with CBT, social skills training, cognitive remediation, illness management and recovery, and family interventions, all of which have been shown to be effective psychosocial treatments for schizophrenia (Medalia, Revheim, & Casey, 2002; Mueser et al., 2006; Pharoah, Mari, Rathbone, & Wong, 2006; Tarrier et al., 1998; Liberman, 1991). A Cochrane review (Xia & Li, 2007) of the available literature on the effectiveness of problem-solving training as a stand-alone intervention for individuals with schizophrenia found only three small trials that met inclusion criteria (Bradshaw, 1993; Mayang, 1990; Tarrier et al., 1993). All three trials showed some benefits, but the authors concluded that there are currently too few studies to determine whether problem-solving training is an effective intervention when delivered as a stand-alone intervention. Two additional trials compared problem-solving training as a stand-alone intervention with cognitive and social cognitive training interventions and found that both interventions produced similar improvements in functional capacity or social functioning in consumers with schizophrenia (Rodewald et al., 2011; Veltro et al., 2011).

OUTCOME RESEARCH ON CBSST

CBSST was originally developed, manualized, and pilot-tested as a group therapy for middle-aged and older people with schizophrenia (Granholm et al., 2002; McQuaid et al., 2000). In an initial small pilot study (Granholm, McQuaid, McClure, Pedrelli, & Jeste, 2002), we found that group CBSST improved functioning and resulted in medium to large effect sizes for symptom reductions in older consumers with schizophrenia. This pilot study demonstrated the feasibility, acceptability, and preliminary efficacy of CBSST in this population, and justified larger clinical trials. We have since conducted three randomized clinical trials comparing CBSST with standard care, alone (typically only pharmacological treatment and case management), and standard care plus supportive contact control conditions (Granholm et al., 2005, 2007; Granholm, Holden, et al., 2013; Granholm, Holden, Link, & McQuaid, 2014). Given the general effectiveness of CBT and social skills training interventions, which are included in CBSST, it is not surprising that all three of our clinical trials demonstrated that CBSST was more effective at improving functional outcome in consumers with schizophrenia than standard care alone or standard care plus supportive group therapy control conditions. The Substance Abuse and Mental Health Services Administration evaluated the evidence for the efficacy of CBSST and listed CBSST on the National Registry of Evidence-Based Programs and Practices website (*http://nrepp.samhsa.gov*).

CBSST versus Standard Care in Middle-Aged and Older Consumers

In our first clinical trial (Granholm et al., 2005), 76 middle-aged or older consumers with schizophrenia or schizoaffective disorder were randomly assigned to standard care (typically medication management with some case management) or standard care plus CBSST. CBSST was delivered in 24 weekly 2-hour group therapy sessions for 6 months. Transportation was provided to and from group meetings. The mean age of consumers was 54, and most were European American (79%), male (74%), high school–educated (mean = 12.6 years), not married (96%), unemployed (97%), living in assisted housing (62%), and had been ill for approximately three decades. Positive symptoms were well controlled by medications, with 53% of the total sample reporting no current hallucinations or delusions at baseline. Blind assessments of multiple outcomes were completed at baseline and end of treatment (6 months), including CBSST skills mastery, functioning, and positive and negative symptoms.

The results of this first clinical trial were promising. Only four consumers did not engage in CBSST (i.e., dropped out before attending four sessions), and CBSST session attendance was excellent. The mean number of sessions attended was 22

(92%) of the 24 sessions offered (95% confidence interval = 21–23). The mean percentage of homework assignments completed was 75% (95% confidence interval = 66–84%, range = 0–100%). Figure 2.1 shows that at the end of treatment, consumers with schizophrenia in CBSST showed significantly greater skills mastery (Comprehensive Modules Test; Liberman, 1991), functional outcome (Independent Living Skills Survey; Wallace, Liberman, Tauber, & Wallace, 2000), and cognitive insight (i.e., self-reflective and flexible thinking on the Beck Cognitive Insight Scale; Beck, Baruch, Balter, Steer, & Warman, 2004) relative to consumers in standard care (treatment as usual). Consumers in CBSST, therefore, were able to learn cognitive and behavioral skills, showed improved functional outcome, and became more flexible and objective in their thinking (improved cognitive insight). No significant improvements were found for symptoms, but symptoms were not the primary target of treatment (functioning was the target), and symptoms were relatively well controlled in the majority of patients at baseline.

In a follow-up study of consumers 1 year after treatment ended, the improvements in skills mastery and functioning were maintained (Granholm et al., 2007). Given that functional impairments persist in this older outpatient population, despite relatively good pharmacological control of psychotic symptoms, the significant maintenance at 1-year follow-up of improvement in functioning is quite noteworthy. The medium treatment effect size for functioning at 12-month follow-up

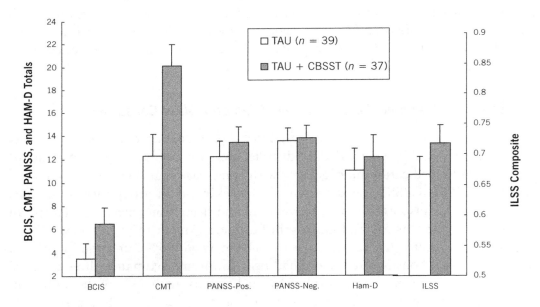

FIGURE 2.1. Outcomes for CBSST versus standard care in middle-aged and older consumers. Outcomes for middle-aged or older consumers with schizophrenia or schizoaffective disorder in treatment as usual (TAU) or TAU + CBSST at the end of 6 months of treatment (adjusted for baseline) on the Beck Cognitive Insight Scale (BCIS), Comprehensive Modules Test (CMT), Positive and Negative Syndrome Scale (PANSS), Hamilton Rating Scale for Depression (HAM-D), and Independent Living Skills Survey (ILSS). Significantly better outcomes were found in CBSST for BCIS, CMT, and ILSS.

(0.50) was slightly stronger than effect sizes found for most outcomes in trials of CBT for schizophrenia (0.36–0.44; Wykes et al., 2008), similar to effect sizes for community functioning in social skills training trials (0.52), and comparable to the general effectiveness of CBT in meta-analytic studies of other disorders (effect size = 0.65; Lipsey & Wilson, 1993).

CBSST versus Supportive Contact in Middle-Aged and Older Consumers

Our first CBSST clinical trial showed that CBSST is more effective than standard care, but the research design did not control for nonspecific therapist contact; that is, it is possible that the additional weekly contact with a caring therapist and other group members, rather than the specific CBT and social skills training skills trained, led to the benefits observed. We therefore conducted a second trial (Granholm, Holden, et al., 2013) comparing CBSST with an active goal-focused supportive contact control condition. CBSST was delivered in 36 weekly two-hour group therapy sessions over 9 months (3 months longer than in our first trial). As in our first trial, a driver picked up consumers in both treatment groups at their homes and drove them to the hospital where group therapy was provided. The goal-focused supportive contact intervention was an enhanced supportive contact control condition that provided the same amount of therapist and group contact as CBSST (weekly 2-hour group therapy sessions for 36 weeks). As in CBSST, the primary focus of goal-focused supportive contact was on setting and achieving functioning goals (e.g., living, learning, working, and socializing), and goals were systematically broken down into short-term goals and goal steps. Sessions were semistructured and consisted of check-in about distress and potential crisis management, followed by a flexible group discussion about setting functional goals and working toward them with minimal therapist guidance.

Middle-aged and older consumers with schizophrenia or schizoaffective disorder (N = 64) were randomly assigned to either CBSST or goal-focused supportive contact. Similar to the participants in our first trial, the mean age of participants in this trial was 55, and most were European American (66%), male (55%), high school educated (mean = 12.5 years), not married (95%), unemployed (95%), living in assisted housing (69%), and had been ill for approximately three decades. Blind assessments of multiple outcomes were completed at baseline, midtreatment, end of treatment (9 months), mid-follow-up, and 9 months after treatment ended, including CBSST skills mastery, functioning, and positive and negative symptoms.

The results of this second clinical trial replicated the first trial. On average, consumers in CBSST attended 30.3 (84%) of the 36 group therapy sessions offered, and consumers in goal-focused supportive contact attended 29.6 (82%) of the 36 sessions. Consumers in CBSST showed significantly greater skills mastery (Comprehensive Modules Test) and functional outcome (Independent Living Skills Survey; see Figure 2.2) relative to consumers in goal-focused supportive contact. These findings replicated the results of our prior trial and showed that the benefits of CBSST

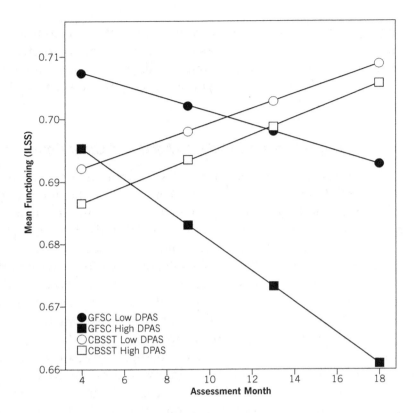

FIGURE 2.2. Outcomes for CBSST versus supportive contact in middle-aged and older consumers. Functioning (Independent Living Skills Survey [ILSS]) trajectories across assessments for middle-aged and older consumers with schizophrenia or schizoaffective disorder in CBSST and goal-focused supportive contact (GFSC) with baseline Defeatist Performance Attitude Scale (DPAS) scores set to high (58) and low (42) values (higher scores indicate greater severity of defeatist performance beliefs). The figure shows a negative effect of more severe defeatist attitudes on functioning in the GFSC group, but this negative impact was mitigated by CBSST treatment. From Granholm, Holden, Link, McQuaid, and Jeste (2013). Reprinted with permission from Elsevier.

cannot be attributed to nonspecific therapist factors alone. Self-reported everyday functioning improved to a greater extent in CBSST than in goal-focused supportive contact, suggesting that specific CBT and social skills training interventions were more potent interventions to improve functioning than goal setting and supportive contact alone.

In addition, for both treatment groups, similar significant improvement was found for experiential negative symptoms (amotivation and asociality), anxiety, depression, life satisfaction, and positive self-esteem, but improvements in CBSST were not significantly greater than improvements in goal-focused supportive contact for these secondary outcomes. This suggests that an active psychosocial intervention such as goal-focused supportive contact that includes at least supportive contact, and systematic recovery-oriented goal setting can be beneficial to consumers with schizophrenia for reducing symptom distress and increasing motivation, self-esteem, and overall subjective life satisfaction. This may point to the power and importance of focusing on recovery goals as a key component of psychosocial interventions. It is important to note that functioning improved to a greater extent in CBSST than in goal-focused supportive contact, suggesting that training in cognitive-behavioral and social skills is more potent than goal setting and supportive contact alone to improve functioning.

This study also provided some evidence that defeatist performance beliefs (discussed in Chapter 1) are associated with change in functioning in CBSST. Figure 2.2 shows the trajectories of functional outcome across the study assessment time points for consumers in each treatment group divided into high and low severity of defeatist attitudes on the Defeatist Performance Attitude Scale (Cane, Olinger, Gotlib, & Kuiper, 2006) at the time they entered the study. Figure 2.2 shows a negative effect of more severe defeatist attitudes on the functional beliefs (e.g., "Why bother trying? I'll just fail") over time in the goal-focused supportive contact group, but this negative impact appeared to be mitigated by CBSST treatment; that is, the severity of defeatist attitudes only impacted outcome in goal-focused supportive contact, where there was no treatment to try to challenge and change these attitudes. The added benefit of CBSST relative to goal-focused supportive contact appeared to be greatest for consumers with more severe defeatist attitudes, especially at 18-month follow-up. A large treatment group difference was found in consumers with more severe defeatist attitudes at the time they started the trial (effect size = 1.11), but only minimal treatment benefit was found in consumers with less severe defeatist attitudes (effect size = 0.18). Furthermore, the extent to which consumers showed a reduction in severity of defeatist attitudes during CBSST treatment was significantly correlated with improvement in functioning at 18-month follow-up. These findings are consistent with the determinants of functional outcome presented in Chapter 1 and suggest that CBT interventions such as CBSST that target defeatist performance beliefs can lead to improvement in functioning in consumers with schizophrenia.

CBSST versus Supportive Contact in Nongeriatric Consumers

Both of our prior CBSST trials focused on middle-aged and older consumers who had been ill for three decades on average. We therefore carried out a third clinical trial to test the efficacy of CBSST in a younger, more representative sample. Consumers (ages 18–65) with schizophrenia or schizoaffective disorder (N = 149) were randomly assigned to either group CBSST or the group goal-focused supportive contact intervention used in our second clinical trial described earlier. Similar to our second trial, CBSST and goal-focused supportive contact were both offered in 36 weekly 2-hour group therapy sessions over 9 months. Consumers were approximately 15 years younger on average than consumers in our prior two trials (mean age = 41 years) but were similar with regard to other demographics. Most consumers were European American (57%), male (66%), high school educated (mean = 12.3 years), not married (91%), unemployed (79%), and living in assisted housing (48%).

Blind assessments of multiple outcomes were made at baseline, midtreatment, end of treatment (9 months), mid-follow-up, and 12 months after treatment ended, including CBSST skills mastery, functioning, and positive and negative symptoms.

The results of this third clinical trial replicated and extended the findings of our prior two trials. Like the older consumers in our prior clinical trials, this more representative sample of consumers in CBSST showed significantly greater skills mastery and better functional outcome relative to consumers in goal-focused supportive contact (see Figure 2.3). In addition, consumers in CBSST showed higher rates of functional milestone achievement (work, education, and independent living), which are very difficult to impact through available treatments, such as those discussed at the start of this chapter. A greater proportion of consumers in CBSST were working in paid or volunteer jobs (CBSST = 38%; goal-focused supportive contact = 23%), engaged in education activities (CBSST = 21%; goal-focused supportive contact = 5%), and living independently (CBSST = 35%; goal-focused supportive contact = 26%) at the end of treatment, although only the difference in education activities was statistically significant ($p < .05$). Experiential negative symptoms (amotivation and asociality) and defeatist performance attitudes also improved to a significantly greater extent in CBSST relative to goal-focused supportive contact (see Figure 2.3). Consistent with the determinants of functional outcome described in Chapter 1, these corresponding improvements in defeatist attitudes, negative symptoms, and functioning suggest interventions such as CBSST that reduce the severity of defeatist performance beliefs can help to improve negative symptoms and functioning in consumers with schizophrenia.

Session attendance in this third trial was much poorer than the excellent attendance found in our prior two trials. On average, participants who initially engaged in treatment (attended at least one session) attended only about half of the 36 sessions offered in this trial (CBSST: mean = 14.8, standard deviation = 9.8, range = 1–34; goal-focused supportive contact: mean = 17.4, standard deviation = 12.4, range = 1–36; the groups did not differ significantly). This level of average attendance did provide exposure to most of the content in the three CBSST modules (three six-session modules would be 18 sessions), but the three modules were designed to be repeated for a total of 36 sessions, so consumers did not receive the intended second exposure to the modules. It is possible that some consumers dropped out because they lost interest in repeating the module content or did not need to repeat the modules because they were doing well and achieving their goals. A second exposure to the modules may not be necessary for all consumers. Monthly booster sessions were also offered for 12 months after treatment ended, but the majority (60%) of participants did not attend any booster sessions. Unlike our prior two trials, transportation to group therapy was not provided in this third trial. We believe this was the primary factor contributing to poor attendance. This trial was conducted in California in San Diego County, where long travel distances and a limited public transportation system (primarily buses with connections and some trolley service) are barriers to participation. Providing transportation increases the cost of providing

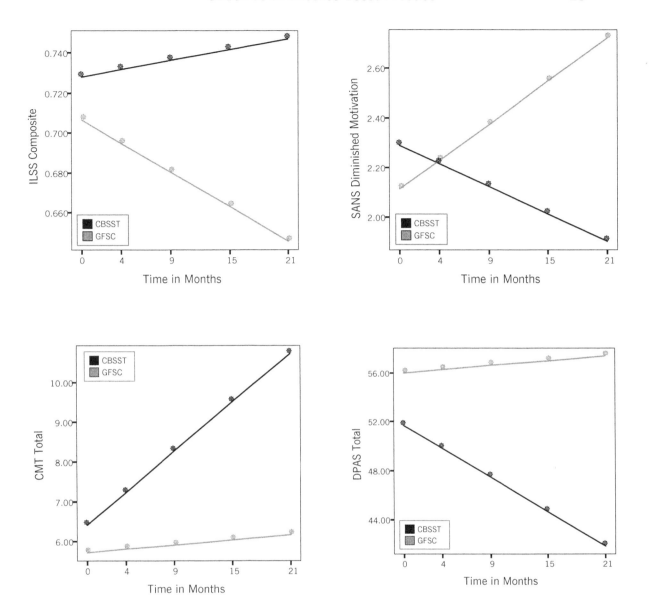

FIGURE 2.3. Outcomes for CBSST versus supportive contact in nongeriatric consumers. Outcome trajectories across assessments were significantly better for CBSST relative to goal-focused supportive contact (GFSC) for functioning (Independent Living Skills Survey [ILSS]), negative symptoms (Scale for Assessment of Negative Symptoms [SANS] Diminished Motivation Factor), dysfunctional attitudes (Defeatist Performance Attitude Scale [DPAS]), and CBSST skills acquisition (Comprehensive Modules Test [CMT]). Improvement is indicated by increasing scores for the ILSS and CMT, and decreasing scores for the DPAS and SANS. From Granholm, Holden, Link, and McQuaid (2014). Reprinted with permission from the American Psychological Association.

psychosocial interventions such as CBSST, but transportation costs may be offset by savings associated with improved functioning (e.g., fewer hospitalizations, productive work, reduced caregiving demands). Providing transportation to increase attendance in treatment programs may also increase billable services in some systems.

It is important to note that despite poor attendance, outcomes were still significantly better in CBSST relative to goal-focused supportive contact. In addition, we found that the number of sessions attended was not significantly correlated with outcome in CBSST ($r = -.14$, $p = .349$), suggesting that a second exposure to the CBSST modules may not result in additional gains for all participants. In contrast, greater attendance was associated with better outcome in goal-focused supportive contact ($r = .34$, $p = .015$). In skills-based interventions, consumers may learn and use skills that can be applied in the absence of a therapist, but when skills are not trained in supportive therapy, longer contact with a therapist may be required for meaningful gains, which can increase the cost of providing supportive contact interventions.

CBSST in Assertive Community Treatment

We have begun to examine the efficacy of CBSST in individual rather than group therapy sessions in the context of standard ACT visits in the community. ACT a well-validated treatment model for people with serious mental illness and is one of the few evidence-based psychosocial treatments for schizophrenia that is widely implemented in community mental health programs throughout the United States (Drake, Bond, & Essock, 2009; Mueser, Bond, Drake, & Resnick, 1998). The ACT model is a team treatment approach with shared, low caseloads, and community-based service delivery focused on reducing hospitalizations, maintaining housing, and improving daily living skills. Although ACT has been found to reduce hospitalizations, homelessness, and legal problems, existing approaches have not been found to make meaningful improvements in everyday functioning in consumers with schizophrenia (Mueser et al., 1998). Enhancing ACT by adding CBSST may improve its impact on functional outcome. Given the prevalence of ACT teams throughout community mental health systems in the United States, implementing CBSST on these teams provides a unique opportunity for broad dissemination of evidence-based psychosocial rehabilitation interventions.

Based on advice from focus groups with ACT team providers in the San Diego County Mental Health System, we adapted CBSST as a team-delivered individual therapy intervention that can be provided by ACT teams in the community. We conducted a pilot study (Granholm, Loh, Link, & Jeste, 2010) to determine whether these teams could deliver the intervention with adequate fidelity after relatively minimal training and supervision. The secondary goals of the study were to determine whether CBSST delivered by case managers could improve client outcomes and to identify factors that facilitated or hindered successful implementation of CBSST by the teams. The intervention was only 12 sessions, in contrast to 24–36 sessions of

CBSST in our prior clinical trials, and focused on cognitive skills. Although this may not have been an adequate dosage of therapy to produce meaningful change in community functioning, we chose this low dosage of CBSST because it provided an adequate sample of sessions (3 months) for training discussions in supervision and assessment of fidelity, which was the primary aim of the study.

Sixteen staff members from two ACT teams in the San Diego County Mental Health System were recruited as therapists. These individuals had bachelor's degrees (most commonly) or master's degrees and 3–5 years of experience working as mental health care providers. Sixteen clients with a chart diagnosis of schizophrenia or schizoaffective disorder who were assessed on the outcome measures on at least two occasions were included in data analyses (mean age = 44.3 years; 81% male; 69% European American; 100% residing in assisted living facilities). Clients were followed for 24 weeks (12 weeks of therapy plus 12 weeks of follow-up). Therapists were asked to provide 12 manualized 30-minute sessions of CBSST to each client at sites convenient to clients and therapists, including board-and-care facilities, residential treatment, clubhouses, and other community settings (e.g., coffee shops), and to record the sessions. Clients continued to receive other standard ACT services throughout therapy and follow-up.

The ACT model is a team treatment model, so clients typically had different therapists deliver different sessions, depending on which team provider visited the client that week. Continuity of treatment (e.g., sharing information between therapists about homework assignments) was managed in the standard morning meetings that are part of the ACT model. The therapists attended an 8-hour training workshop, then received face-to-face group supervision every other week (six meetings) with a psychologist experienced with the intervention. This group supervision was conducted during the standard morning team meeting. Fidelity was assessed using the Cognitive Therapy Rating Scale for Psychosis (Haddock et al., 2001), with "adequate competency" defined as a total score of 30 or greater (Turkington, Kingdon, & Turner, 2002). The average fidelity rating for the therapists (mean = 32, standard deviation = 9.7) was comparable to acceptable standards, and 60% of the therapists achieved adequate fidelity (Cognitive Therapy Rating Scale for Psychosis total > 30; Haddock et al., 2001). All but one of the therapists with Cognitive Therapy Rating Scale for Psychosis fidelity scores below 30 achieved scores greater than 20, so they may have reached adequate fidelity with minimal additional supervision training. Therapists commented that the supervision component contributed to their CBT knowledge and skills level to a greater extent than the didactic workshop, and this was also our impression. Thus, CBSST was generally delivered with adequate fidelity by community therapists with little or no prior experience with CBT. It is important to emphasize that CBSST is a simplified skills-based intervention, not a complex formulation or case conceptualization–driven CBT intervention, which can be delivered by less experienced therapists with minimal training. There is also evidence from effectiveness trials that CBT and social skills training delivered in community mental health settings improves outcomes, and community therapists can deliver these interventions with adequate fidelity (Glynn et al., 2002; Lincoln et al., 2012; Morrison et al., 2004; Pinninti, Fisher, Thompson, & Steer, 2010; Turkington et al., 2014).

FACTORS ASSOCIATED WITH BETTER TREATMENT OUTCOME

Few studies have examined the factors that predict outcome in CBT and social skills training. Several possible factors include consumer characteristics (e.g., motivation, cognitive impairment, insight, delusional conviction, type and severity of symptoms, duration of illness, demographics), therapist characteristics (e.g., skills, experience with CBT and social skills training, assumptions about psychosis and recovery), and components of the therapy itself (e.g., more cognitive vs. behavioral emphasis, duration, individual or group format, setting/adjunctive treatments).

Consumer Characteristics

Although some consumer characteristics have been associated with poorer outcome in CBT and social skills training, currently there is not sufficient evidence to indicate which consumers are more likely to benefit from CBSST. Therefore, there is no screening session in the CBSST program in which assessments are administered to determine who should receive treatment.

Several consumer characteristics have been associated with improvement in CBT for psychosis. Lower levels of delusional conviction (Garety et al., 1997; Brabban, Tai, & Turkington, 2009) and greater insight (Naeem, Kingdon, & Turkington, 2008; Perivoliotis et al., 2010) have been associated with better positive symptom outcomes in CBT, but little is known about whether these factors predict better functional outcome in CBT. Studies are mixed with regard to the impact of symptom severity, with some studies indicating that recent hospitalizations (Garety et al., 1997) and greater symptom severity (Morrison et al., 2004) were associated with *better* outcomes. Greater motivation to reduce symptom distress might make more symptomatic consumers better candidates for CBT. In clinical trials of social skills training, number of hospitalizations, months of prior inpatient care, and positive symptom severity have not been found to moderate outcome (Dilk & Bond, 1996; Heinssen, Liberman, & Kopelowicz, 2000; Kurtz & Mueser, 2008). These findings suggest that more symptomatic consumers can benefit from CBSST. Better outcomes have also been found in females relative to males (Brabban et al., 2009) and white relative to nonwhite consumers (Rathod, Kingdon, Smith, & Turkington, 2005). Longer duration of illness, longer duration of untreated psychosis, and older age have also been associated with poorer outcome in some CBT trials (Drury, Birchwood, Cochrane, & Macmillan, 1996; Morrison et al., 2004, 2012; Tarrier et al., 1998). Older consumers, and consumers with severe and persistent negative symptoms (deficit syndrome) and cognitive impairments have also shown a poorer response to social skills training treatment (Heinssen et al., 2000; Kurtz & Mueser, 2008). However, as described earlier, our clinical trials of older consumers with schizophrenia (age > 50) demonstrated significant benefits for functioning in CBSST, suggesting that older consumers with chronic illness for three decades should still be offered CBSST.

Neurocognitive Impairment

Referring clinicians may not recommend psychotherapy interventions such as CBSST for people with psychotic disorders due to the assumption that neurocognitive impairments in memory, attention, and problem-solving abilities, which are common in these individuals, might be a barrier to success in psychotherapy. This may not be an accurate assumption. While neurocognitive impairment has been associated with reduced skills learning and poorer treatment outcome in social skills training interventions, neurocognitive impairment has not been found to moderate treatment outcome in CBT for schizophrenia (Kurtz, 2011; Garety et al., 1997; Granholm et al., 2008). In social skills training, deficits in verbal memory, executive functioning, and sustained attention have been associated with poor attendance and poor skills acquisition (McKee, Hull, & Smith, 1997; Mueser, Bellack, Douglas, & Wade, 1991; Kern, Green, & Satz, 1992; Smith et al., 1999; Ucok et al., 2006; Silverstein, Schenkel, Valone, & Nuernberger, 1998; Kurtz, 2011), but most researchers did not examine whether neurocognitive impairment differentially impacted outcome relative to a control group, which is required for moderation. In fact, some studies have found that more severe neurocognitive impairment was associated with *better* outcome in CBT (Garety et al., 1997; Kurtz, 2011). We (Granholm et al., 2008) have found that effect sizes for the difference between CBSST and standard care on functional outcome measures were similar for participants with relatively mild (effect size = 0.44–0.64) and severe (effect size = 0.29–0.60) neurocognitive impairment. Participants in CBSST therefore showed comparable benefit relative to those in standard care, regardless of severity of neurocognitive impairment. Adding CBSST to standard care improved outcome even for participants with severe impairment. Thus, consumers with neurocognitive impairment should still be offered CBSST and may even be more likely to benefit than consumers without neurocognitive impairment.

Therapy Characteristics

Even less is known about the relationships between therapist and therapy characteristics and outcome in CBT or social skills training. According to expert consensus (Morrison & Barratt, 2010), therapist assumptions about psychosis, homework, and active behavioral change strategies are important components of CBT for psychosis. Some CBT approaches involve the development of a shared conceptualization of the nature of illness (e.g., Sensky et al., 2000), while others are more skills-training behavioral approaches (e.g., Granholm et al., 2005). In their meta-analysis, Wykes et al. (2008) found modestly better outcomes in therapies with greater behavioral emphasis, suggesting that behavioral components (e.g., skills training, experiments to test beliefs, taking action toward recovery goal steps) are at least as important as cognitive interventions. Wykes et al. also reported that outcomes did not differ significantly between group and individual therapy formats. Social skills training can also be delivered in group or individual formats. Thus, while there are advantages to individual (e.g., more time for personalized formulation) and group (e.g., normalizing and supportive socialization opportunities) formats, there is no evidence that one format is superior to the other.

Engaging support persons, such as family members or case managers, in the treatment process can improve the effectiveness and generalizability of social skills training. For example, when family members are made aware of the skills taught in session, they can reinforce the use of those skills and provide opportunities for consumers to practice skills at home. This can have a direct impact on family communication, problem-solving, and coping strategies (Kopelowicz, Zarate, Gonzalez Smith, Mintz, & Liberman, 2003). An approach called *in vivo* amplified skills training involves case managers creating opportunities and prompting the use of skills learned in social skills training in the community, then offering encouragement and reinforcement for real-world skills performance (Liberman, Glynn, Blair, Ross, & Marder, 2002). Encouragement, creating opportunities for skills performance in the real world, and reinforcement for practicing skills in relevant situations are key components of social skills training. Finally, targeting specific problems (e.g., employment), diagnoses (e.g., substance use), and age cohorts can also improve the efficacy of social skills training (Kopelowicz, Liberman, & Zarate, 2006).

Given the cost and burden of delivering psychosocial interventions such as CBSST, it is important to identify the minimal therapy dosage needed to improve outcomes. A recent meta-analysis found that CBTs that were 20 sessions or longer had better outcomes than shorter approaches (Sarin et al., 2011), but number of sessions was not associated with positive symptom outcome in another meta-analysis of CBT for schizophrenia (Gould et al., 2001). Duration of treatment in trials of CBT for psychosis has ranged from 5 weeks to 9 months and averaged 13.6 weeks (Gould et al., 2001). Shorter treatments have generally been used in acute phases, whereas longer durations have been used for more chronic populations. Some studies have found that brief CBT for psychosis (6 to 10 sessions in 4 months) can be effective, but no study has yet compared brief versus standard duration (12–20 sessions in 4–6 months) therapies (Naeem, Farooq, & Kingdon, 2014).

In a meta-analysis of nine randomized controlled trials of social skills training for schizophrenia by Pilling et al. (2002), the mean duration of treatment was 26.8 weeks (6.7 months; range = 4–104 weeks), and in the meta-analysis by Kurtz and Mueser (2008), treatment duration ranged from 8 to 312 hours (mean = 67.2 hours, standard deviation = 75.4) delivered over 2 to 104 weeks (mean = 19.3 weeks, standard deviation = 22.7). Duration of treatment has either not been significantly associated with outcome or, paradoxically, shorter duration and lower intensity (fewer sessions per week) of training has produced larger effects (Kurtz & Mueser, 2008). In our third CBSST trial discussed earlier, we found improved functional outcome in consumers with schizophrenia with only 15 sessions delivered, on average, and the number of sessions delivered was not significantly correlated with functional outcome.

SUMMARY AND FUTURE DIRECTIONS

Identifying treatments to improve functioning and reduce negative symptoms in consumers with schizophrenia is an important public health goal. The results of our three randomized clinical trials demonstrated that CBSST is an effective psychosocial intervention to improve these outcomes in consumers with schizophrenia. Increasingly, best practice guidelines and nationalized health care systems are recommending or mandating CBT and social skills training for schizophrenia (Gaebel et al., 2005; Dixon et al., 2010). Despite their demonstrated efficacy and recommended use, CBT and social skills training are largely unavailable in the United States, and implementation barriers in other countries also limit access to these evidence-based practices. Even in the United Kingdom, where guidelines strongly recommend its use, up to 90% of eligible consumers with psychosis are not offered CBT (Thase et al., 2014). Improving the dissemination and implementation of evidence-based practices such as CBSST into real-world clinical practice is an important public health goal. We (Granholm et al., 2010) have found promising results in our preliminary trial implementing CBSST in the context of the ACT delivery model. Other research groups have also found that providers with minimal education (e.g., bachelor's-level case managers) in the United States and Canada can deliver similar CBT and social skills training interventions with good fidelity and positive outcomes in their consumers with schizophrenia (Bellack et al., 2004; Lincoln et al., 2012; Pinninti et al., 2010). By adapting evidence-based psychosocial rehabilitation interventions such as CBSST to existing, widely available treatment systems for consumers with schizophrenia (e.g., ACT), implementation barriers may be reduced, and access to these interventions may be increased for consumers with schizophrenia. CBSST is a simplified practical program of step-by-step cognitive, social, and problem-solving skills learning to facilitate recovery goal achievement. As such, it is relatively easy to implement with high fidelity and is broadly appealing to clinicians at almost any level of education and experience.

CHAPTER 3

Getting Started

This chapter describes the CBSST treatment structure and session structure, and offers advice on training providers and implementing the CBSST program in different settings. The chapters that follow in Part II provide detailed practical guidance on setting goals and teaching the skills in each module.

TREATMENT STRUCTURE

The length, frequency, and number of sessions delivered depend on a number of factors, including treatment format (e.g., individual, group, or case management), available staffing, specific service delivery system limitations (e.g., short-stay hospitalizations, insurance or other payer limits), and consumer characteristics (e.g., age, neurocognitive impairment, comorbidity, severity of disorganization, positive and negative symptoms). This treatment manual provides a general structure but the CBSST program can be adapted to the specific needs of consumers and clinical settings. The three CBSST modules offer a flexible menu of skills from which specific interventions can be selected or emphasized.

Duration and Frequency

Each CBSST module consists of a goal-setting session, followed by a sequence of five sessions that build upon each other to teach a skills set. Thus, there are a total of six sessions per module and 18 sessions to complete all three modules. We have recommended that consumers receive all three modules, then repeat the sequence a second time, for a total of 36 sessions. However, as described in Chapter 2, we have found that significant gains in functioning can be achieved with only one exposure to each of the three modules. For some consumers, one exposure to the modules may be sufficient to learn the skills, but others may need a second exposure. For example, older consumers with longer duration of illness and consumers with more severe neurocognitive impairments may need additional practice, while younger consumers with recent onset of illness can typically learn the skills with one exposure. Repeating the modules provides extra practice to compensate for cognitive impairment. It is important to stress that while the same general skills are taught during the second exposure to a module, the skills are applied to different thoughts, problems, and social situations arising in the lives of consumers at different times. This is not simply rote repetition. During their second exposure to the content, consumers already have a working understanding of the skills, so providers can encourage greater application of the skills to working on goal steps in the real world. Younger consumers with more recent onset of illness might be become bored or be put off by a full repetition of the modules, so adding a couple sessions at the end of each module might be a more effective way to maintain engagement, while still providing some additional sessions to practice skills in the real world.

The content in each module session can typically be delivered in 60 minutes in a group format with about six consumers. Less time is typically required in an individual format, and more time is required in groups with more than six consumers. Some consumers (e.g., those with more severe cognitive impairment, disorganization, or negative symptoms) may require longer sessions or multiple sessions to master each skill. If transportation, staffing, group room availability, and consumer engagement are not major concerns, 60- to 90-minute sessions twice per week are ideal and provide more frequent opportunities for skills practice and interactions outside the home. For consumers with transportation challenges (e.g., older consumers, long distances, limited public transportation), longer sessions once per week can improve engagement. For longer 2-hour groups, we recommend taking a 15- to 30-minute refreshment or lunch break between the first and second hour. We recommend that providers share these breaks together with consumers in a public place (e.g., the hospital cafeteria) in order to prompt and observe skills practice in the real world, and we encourage providers to seek out similar opportunities to facilitate skills generalization to real-world settings.

If possible, we recommend supplementing the initial group goal-setting session with an individual goal-setting session. Consumers with severe negative symptoms, cognitive impairment, and hopelessness about change often need more time to plan goals than a group session permits. The merits of individual versus group formats are discussed further in the next section.

Group versus Individual Format

CBSST was originally developed as a group therapy, but the intervention can be delivered in an individual therapy format, combined group and individual therapy, or in the context of intensive case management service delivery models (e.g., assertive community treatment). Most clinical trials of CBT for psychosis used an individual format, but promising results have been reported using group and combined group and individual formats (Wykes et al., 2008). The vast majority of social skills training studies have used group therapy, but training can be delivered effectively in an individual format (Kurtz & Mueser, 2008). Our CBSST trials, discussed in Chapter 2, used group therapy or combined group and individual therapy. In a meta-analysis of clinical trials using CBT for consumers with schizophrenia (Wykes et al., 2008), consumers in group treatment did not differ significantly from consumers in individual treatment on any outcome. Another review of CBT for psychosis studies (Granholm et al., 2009) also found similar improvement in functioning in group and individual therapy for schizophrenia, with four of six group therapy studies (66%) and eight of 12 individual therapy studies (66%) showing significant improvement in functioning on at least one measure.

An individual format provides more time to develop fully a detailed case formulation and set personalized recovery goals. Involving consumers in the process of personalized goal setting is a key component of effective psychosocial rehabilitation treatment planning. In an individual format, all of the discussions and interventions are directly relevant to the consumer, so that he or she receives more direct attention and intervention time. Some consumers also refuse to engage in groups (e.g., due to paranoia or social phobia).

There are also several advantages to a group format. Groups are more efficient than individual therapy, because treatment can be provided for a greater number of patients per hour of provider time in groups. Groups also provide a shared identity with others, and some consumers report that the perception of "not being alone" with their challenges is itself beneficial. Groups can also impact social support systems and allow practice of communication and other social skills with peers. Groups can provide social reinforcement for change, which may be important for interventions that target social functioning. Confronting or observing others in groups can also provide better insight into one's own symptoms, skills deficits, and dysfunctional attitudes.

Given that both therapy formats have advantages, and that both are acceptable in community practice, the best approach may be to combine individual and group formats. If time and resources allow, we have found it helpful to provide individual goal-setting sessions (or "recovery coaching" sessions) at the start of group therapy and about every 6 weeks or 3 months thereafter to review goal progress. Adding individual goal-setting sessions adds the benefit of personalizing treatment without the increased amount of provider workload that weekly individual therapy requires. With eight consumers per group, for example, four participants would be assigned to individual sessions with one of the two group providers, resulting in four additional hours of individual therapy per provider about every 3 months (only 2 additional hours with 30-minute individual sessions). These individual sessions focus on developing personalized treatment goals and the specific steps needed to achieve goals, as well as on tracking completion of goal steps using a goal-tracking form (see Chapter 5). Additional personalized feedback, formulation development, and practice of CBSST skills can also be provided in individual sessions. This combined individual and group therapy procedure is consistent with the types of goal setting, treatment planning, and progress reevaluation occurring in many psychiatric rehabilitation settings.

Group Size

A minimum of four to a maximum of 10 consumers per group is optimal. Groups at the lower end of this range are recommended for consumers with greater severity of disorganization, negative symptoms, neurocognitive deficits, or functional impairments, who may require a slower pace of training. Larger groups with more impaired consumers can present challenges to setting personalized goals effectively, allowing sufficient skills practice (e.g., each group member performing role plays three times a session), and assigning personalized at-home practice assignments during limited session time.

Group Cohesion and Pacing

The pace at which consumers learn skills can vary greatly. Some consumers can progress quickly and find some skills too simplistic, while others require repeated exposure to the content and find the skills challenging to learn and apply in daily life. As a result, some consumers need to repeat the modules, or they require longer or multiple sessions to learn skills, while others may not. When admitting consumers to a group, therefore, providers should strive for homogeneity of members. Clients with more severe cognitive impairments, disorganization, or negative symptoms may require a slower learning pace. It is not always possible, however, to predict an individual's learning pace, nor is it feasible to create multiple homogeneous groups, so providers with diverse learners in the same group must attempt to establish an average pace that may be a bit fast for the slowest learners, but a bit slow for the fastest learners.

To maintain the interest of fast learners and provide extra help for slower learners, providers can elicit the help of consumers who understand the skill to help teach others. For example, more advanced members can explain specific steps, write all the information on the board, help others fill out worksheets, and present their at-home practice as a great example of how to apply skills in the community successfully. This can improve self-efficacy in fast learners and is a useful training approach that engages all group members in the activity when they otherwise might become bored or fall behind. Providers should not feel bound to the manual. If consumers have gained maximum benefit from the skill, providers can move on to a new module at a faster pace. If consumers are struggling to learn skills, providers can spend additional sessions teaching the content.

Group Leaders

Smaller groups may be led by one provider, but there are several advantages to having two providers, even in smaller groups. For example, role plays in the social skills module involve two actors, so each provider can take a different role in modeling effective communication in social interactions. A second provider can also step out of group to intervene with a consumer in crisis, while the other provider continues with the lesson. Finally, with two trainers, one is available to run the group when the other is away, so that the session is not canceled and training continuity is maintained.

Settings

CBSST can be delivered in a variety of settings, including hospital inpatient or outpatient settings and mental health outpatient programs in the community. In our clinical trials, we have also effectively delivered CBSST at board-and-care homes, assisted living facilities, clubhouses, and other settings in communities where consumers live to reduce barriers to engagement (e.g., transportation access) or the stigma associated with coming to a mental health setting. As discussed below, CBSST can also be delivered at the consumer's home, in a coffee shop, or other community locations in the context of ACT or other forms of case management.

The group room should be large enough to seat 10 people comfortably in a circle or in rows, with sufficient personal space between members. A large dry-erase board or flipchart is essential for teaching skills content and reviewing at-home practice (homework) examples and class exercises. Writing on the board, asking consumers to write on the board, and using other forms of media (e.g., poster boards, laminated wallet cards with skills information, workbooks, handouts, homework forms) can compensate for memory problems and other forms of cognitive impairment.

Modular Rolling Admissions

One barrier to engagement in traditional group therapy is that a minimum number of consumers must be recruited to a start group, which can lead to a significant waiting period before initiating treatment. For example, with closed groups and a regimented sequence of 12 weekly sessions, consumers wait up to 3 months before entering treatment at the start of the next group sequence. Alternatively, completely open enrollment can be disruptive to group cohesion and process, and learning skills that build on each other from session to session is difficult. To address these issues, CBSST uses a modular rolling admissions design adapted from the work of Muñoz, Ying, Perez-Stable, and Miranda (1993). This is a hybrid structure that admits new consumers at the start of each new skill module, which is relatively frequent. This maintains group member cohesion as the skill is trained. Each module is designed to be a self-contained skill set. Skills learning in one module is not dependent on learning the skills in any other module, so participants can enter a CBSST group at the beginning of any module. In the first session of every module (described in detail in Chapter 5), the CBSST intervention is explained, recovery goals are set, a treatment contract is established, and the concept that our thoughts can influence our feelings and goal-directed actions is introduced. The next five sessions of each module then build on each other to teach a skills set. These sessions are described in Chapters 6, 7, and 8 and in the Consumer Workbooks in Part III. Since consumers can start treatment at the beginning of any module, the longest wait time to enter treatment is 6 weeks (the number of sessions in one module) assuming weekly sessions, or only 3 weeks assuming sessions twice a week. If two groups are run simultaneously with staggered entry points, the wait to begin treatment is cut in half.

CBSST in ACT

The manualized CBSST intervention is a practical, step-by-step curriculum that can be taught by almost any provider within an ACT team in the context of regular case management visits provided in the community. Conducting individual therapy in the community provides a unique opportunity for *in vivo* skills practice and thought challenging in real-world environments. This may strengthen the intervention by improving generalization of skills to community environments. Using an individual therapy format, each session can be tailored to the unique needs of consumers by selecting about 30 minutes of relevant core session content and teaching skills during regular case management visits at community sites that are convenient to consumers and team providers. This may include residences, board-and-care facilities, parks, coffee shops, or clubhouses, or while driving consumers to appointments. The ACT model is a team treatment model, so consumers may have different providers deliver different sessions, depending on which team provider visits the consumer that week. Continuity of treatment (e.g., sharing information between providers about goals, homework assignments, hot cognitions, and skills acquisition progress) can be managed by exchanging information during the standard team morning meetings or by keeping a "team copy" of each consumer's workbook, with notes from the previous session that are passed between providers.

Neurocognitive Compensatory Strategies

As described in Chapter 1, cognitive therapy and problem-solving training interventions attempt to improve metacognitive belief evaluation processes, cognitive flexibility, inductive reasoning, and abstract thinking. Problem-solving training, which is a significant focus of CBSST, is a verbal mediation strategy that is widely used to compensate for abstraction/flexibility deficits associated with traumatic brain injury and frontal lobe damage. Repetition of information is also a cornerstone of the intervention. Basic themes are repeated throughout a session, a summary is provided at the end of each session, and the three modules are often presented twice. The following list of mnemonic aids and other cognitive compensatory strategies can be used to help consumers learn and remember skills, and complete at-home practice assignments:

- Provide Consumer Workbooks to use outside sessions (see Part III).
- Use the acronyms for skills ("3C's" and "SCALE," described in subsequent chapters).
- Ask consumers or support persons to place Post-it notes or other reminders around the home to prompt at-home skills practice.
- Give consumers laminated pocket-size cue cards displaying key points for skills or other reminders (e.g., a favorite mistake-in-thinking card).
- Encourage note taking on pads, handouts, or workbooks.
- Practice and reinforce skills use (a lot!).
- Use behavioral rewards (token economies, happy face tokens/gold star stickers) to reinforce attention to task and participation.
- Use multiple media, such as writing on a whiteboard or flipchart and displaying skills steps on posters.

SESSION STRUCTURE

All sessions, including the goal-setting sessions at the start of each module, follow the same standard session structure shown in Table 3.1. Each session starts with collaborative agenda setting, followed by review of at-home practice assignments from the previous session. A new skill is then introduced and practiced in session, followed by another at-home practice assignment to be completed by the next session. At the end of the session, providers briefly summarize the content and ask for feedback from consumers.

TABLE 3.1. Standard Session Structure for the Skills Modules

- Set the Agenda Collaboratively (2 minutes).
- Review At-Home Practice (10 minutes).
- Introduce the New Skill (5 minutes).
- In-Session Skills Practice (30 minutes).
- Assign At-Home Practice (10 minutes).
- Summarize the Session (1 minute).
- Ask for Consumer Feedback (2 minutes).

Set the Agenda Collaboratively

Each session begins with collaborative agenda setting. Providers write the agenda for the session on a pad or whiteboard and ask consumers whether they would like to add anything to the agenda. Each session's agenda is also listed in the consumer workbooks in Part III. Some providers use a check-in process at the beginning of the session to ask consumers about their week, offer support, and ask about symptoms, but this type of check-in process can be quite time-consuming and leaves insufficient time to train new skills. During check-in, ask consumers one-by-one to say how they are feeling that day and whether they have a crisis or concern to add to the agenda (e.g., serious symptom exacerbations, suicidal or homicidal ideation, serious life events, other concerns or problems). This provides an opportunity to screen for and manage potentially serious crises. It may be necessary for one provider to step out of group with a consumer to assess and intervene (e.g., hospitalization), allowing the other provider to continue with skills training. Consumer agenda items are opportunities to link the skills to the consumer's problems, concerns, and goals, as described in Part II. Each agenda item reported by consumers is then written down on the agenda.

If the agenda list grows too large to complete during a session, a negotiation must take place in which providers and consumers decide which items must be covered during the limited time available and which items can be put on the top of the agenda in the next session. In this way, the agenda can be used as a time-management tool. If discussions carry on too long or consumers bring up topics during the class that are not on the agenda, providers can point to the agenda and say, "We agreed to try to get through all of this today, and I'm concerned that we are going to run out of time. Do you mind if we move on to the next topic and put this discussion on the agenda for next week?"

The goal of the check-in is not to problem-solve all concerns or provide case management, which would consume too much time to allow for sufficient skills training. The purpose is to screen for crises, and to empower and engage consumers in planning their session. The check-in process can consume too much class time if providers are not careful to contain the discussions. Problems should not be discussed in detail or solved during check-in; rather, they should be placed on the agenda for possible focus during the group. Providers can model a brief check-in for consumers, and role plays can be used to teach consumers to shorten check-ins, if necessary. It can also help to put specific questions on the board to help consumers focus on only the specific content expected for check-ins (e.g., "How do I feel today?"; "Do I need help with something?"; "Am I in a crisis or thinking about harming myself?").

One of the important skills that providers develop with practice is relating agenda items offered by consumers to the skills content for that session. Consumer content can be used as the topic for a role play, for thought challenging, or for a

PROVIDER TIP

Link Skills to Consumer Concerns during Agenda Setting

- Ask consumers what they would like to add to the session agenda.
- Say, "I'm glad you brought that up. We were planning to work on a skill that can help with that today."
- Use the concern raised by the consumer as the topic for the role-play, thought-challenging, or problem-solving exercise planned for that session.

problem-solving exercise. The provider's goal during collaborative agenda setting is to find a way to say, "I'm glad you brought that up. We are going to learn a skill that can help you with that today." Consumers are typically much more engaged and motivated to work on personal problems rather than impersonal examples from the manual. Collaborative agenda setting provides an opportunity to link skills to consumer concerns. Agenda items from consumers should not be viewed as competing with skill training for session time. The skills in CBSST can help consumers solve their problems, manage a crisis, resolve interpersonal conflict, reduce suicidal ideation, cope with symptoms, or otherwise be applied to almost any other concern offered by consumers for the agenda.

Review At-Home Practice (Homework)

Homework is crucial to facilitate skill use outside of session, so that the skill generalizes to everyday life. Consumers must use their newly learned skills outside of group to improve their functioning and quality of life. Consumers who complete more homework assignments have shown greater skills learning and have better outcomes in clinical trials of interventions such as CBSST. Research with a variety of consumer populations has shown that CBT interventions that include homework assignments help clients improve up to 60% more than those in treatment without homework. When talking with consumers, we prefer the term "at-home practice" rather than "homework" to emphasize the importance of skills practice outside of sessions and to reduce the negative connotation that can be associated with "homework" assignments (e.g., being graded in school).

Promoting homework adherence can be challenging, and adherence can vary considerably among consumers, but high adherence rates can be achieved. In our clinical trials, about 80% of consumers completed 80% or more of the homework assignments. There are a number of strategies providers can use to promote adherence. First, and perhaps most important, the provider must make at-home practice an important part of the treatment milieu by *always* assigning at-home practice at the end of *every* session and *always* reviewing at-home practice assigned in the last session at the beginning of *every* session. If at-home practice is an occasional rather than integral part of each session, it will lose its importance and be viewed as optional. Reinforcement of homework completion during homework review through positive attention and praise to those who complete homework can also facilitate homework completion. Providers must be clear that homework completion is expected. Noncompliance with homework assignments should be the topic of thorough problem solving to identify obstacles to help consumers complete the next assignment. If someone forgot the assignment, spend time in group asking that participant to generate a plan to help him or her remember, such as putting the CBSST workbook in an obvious place, using Post-it notes as reminders, setting alarms, or asking someone to remind him or her. No excuse should be accepted without generating a plan to overcome it by the next class. The group leader's stance in this discussion should not be to criticize, scold, or punish. Rather the leader should be genuinely interested in understanding what got in the way, so that solutions might be found.

Introduce and Practice the New Skill

Most of each session is devoted to introducing a new skill and having consumers practice it, ideally by applying it to their personal goals. As described in Chapters 6, 7, and 8, it is best to minimize time spent lecturing and instead engage consumers through games, exercises, provider modeling, and behavioral practice strategies. The general philosophy of CBSST is that people learn by practicing skills more than by listening to providers talk. The consumer workbooks in Part III summarize the basic didactic information for the skills in each session.

Assign At-Home Practice

New at-home practice of the skill is assigned before the end of every session. To improve motivation for completing homework assignments, it is important to link at-home practice with the consumer's goals, as described in Chapters 6, 7, and 8. Providers must explain that completing at-home practice activities facilitates goal achievement (e.g., "The more you practice initiating conversations, the better you will become at talking with women, and ultimately have a girlfriend"). To explain the importance of practice in the real world, metaphors can also be helpful. For example, riding a bike or playing a musical instrument is at first difficult and requires work and concentration, but with practice, these skills eventually become automatic and can be performed with little effort. This is the principle underlying CBSST. Eventually skills become overlearned through practice in session and at home, such that people can use the skills with little effort to achieve their goals.

Cognitive impairments and poor understanding of the homework assignment may also interfere with homework completion. To determine whether homework assignments are clearly understood, providers can ask consumers to complete an example of the homework in session with guidance. The consumer workbooks in

PROVIDER TIP

Musical Instrument Analogy to Encourage At-Home Practice

"It's like learning how to play the piano or guitar. If you practice playing the guitar only while you are at your lesson with your guitar teacher, you might eventually learn how to play the guitar, but you will learn a lot faster and play a lot better if you also practice at home between lessons. If you really want to achieve your goal of learning how to play guitar, you have to practice at home.

"It works the same way in this class. If you practice the CBSST skills only here with us, you might eventually learn how to use the skills to achieve your goals, but you will learn a lot faster and do them a lot better if you also practice at home. If you really want to achieve your goals, you have to practice the skills at home."

Part III contain worksheets for each session's assignment, and each worksheet contains space for in-session practice of the assignment. Offer suggestions throughout the process and set the at-home practice goals collaboratively. To establish a clear plan, agree on a specific day, time, and place for homework completion (e.g., on Tuesday at 2:00 P.M. with Joe at my board-and-care home). Discuss in detail whether consumers have access to necessary resources (e.g., people, places, and even seemingly trivial things, like pen and paper). Encourage consumers to review the session content again at home in their workbooks or handouts and session notes. Stress that at-home practice does not take very long to complete. Most homework assignments are estimated to take about 5–15 minutes.

Summarize the Session and Ask for Consumer Feedback

Periodic summaries at key points during the session, as well as at the end of the session, are helpful in several ways. Summarizing and asking consumers whether they understand the material ensures that both provider and consumers have a mutual understanding. It also communicates empathy, slows down the pacing of the session, allows time for reflection, and prompts the consumer to collaborate. Summarizing

PROVIDER TIP

Assessing Motivation for At-Home Practice

Ask consumers to rate on a scale of 0–100% how likely they are to complete each at-home practice assignment. Draw a line on the board with anchors of 0%, "definitely will not complete it," to 100%, "positively will complete it," and ask each consumer to put a mark on the line.

- 90–100%: The person is motivated to complete it.
- < 90%: The person is not sold on it, so reevaluate obstacles.

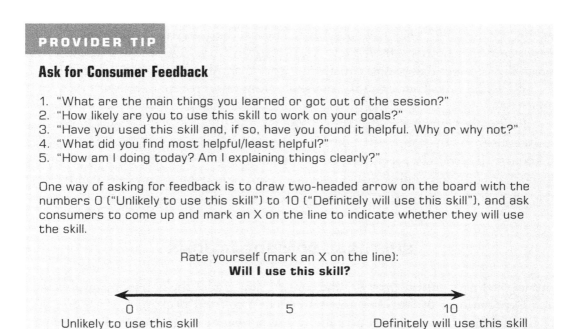

PROVIDER TIP

Ask for Consumer Feedback

1. "What are the main things you learned or got out of the session?"
2. "How likely are you to use this skill to work on your goals?"
3. "Have you used this skill and, if so, have you found it helpful. Why or why not?"
4. "What did you find most helpful/least helpful?"
5. "How am I doing today? Am I explaining things clearly?"

One way of asking for feedback is to draw two-headed arrow on the board with the numbers 0 ("Unlikely to use this skill") to 10 ("Definitely will use this skill"), and ask consumers to come up and mark an X on the line to indicate whether they will use the skill.

Rate yourself (mark an X on the line):
Will I use this skill?

0   5   10
Unlikely to use this skill   Definitely will use this skill

also provides opportunities to modify the agenda (flexibility) and can help the provider make adjustments. When you are stuck, summarize. Asking for feedback allows for assessment of progress and whether any modifications in treatment are necessary. Check in with consumers to determine whether they comprehend the skills and find them useful, so that adjustments can be made to facilitate learning.

Graduation

The last session of a module might be a graduation session, if any consumers have completed the intervention. If so, begin to prepare consumers for graduation prior to the last session. The introductory session of the consumer's final module (six sessions before graduation) is a good time to begin discussions and focus on what goal steps can be accomplished in the final six sessions. When preparing for graduation, emphasize mastery of skills, as well as persistent problems and potential problems that may need to be managed. Identify the skills that can be used to address those problems. Emphasize continuation of practice skills to achieve goals.

The agenda for the final session should include some time for graduation celebrations. We give consumers who completed treatment a graduation certificate, like a diploma, and often provide refreshments for a celebration during this last session. About 15 minutes can be set aside at the end of the session to award the certificate and celebrate achievements. Ask consumers who are graduating to describe what goal steps they have achieved. The 7–7–7 Goal Jackpot! Worksheet, discussed in Chapter 5, can be helpful here. Involve other group members in this discussion by asking what changes they have observed. This can be a very rewarding and positive experience that boosts self-efficacy. Also focus on work that needs to be done and normalize the fact that people can always work toward goals, not just when they are in a class like this. They can take the skills from the three modules with them and continue to apply them in their lives.

Follow-up "booster" sessions may also be helpful, although we have found that most consumers in groups often do not take advantage of available booster sessions. Of course, if resources permit and additional ongoing support is needed (e.g., a crisis has occurred, or a member just started a job or relationship), providers can be flexible and allow consumers to repeat an additional module.

CULTURAL CONSIDERATIONS

Broadly defined, culture provides the context that guides the development of beliefs and expectations. By learning about someone's cultural background, we can better understand factors that contribute to the person's current beliefs. For example, culturally informed and sanctioned religious beliefs and practices can influence the content and perceived origin of auditory hallucinations (e.g., voices are angels or the devil), the type and structure of delusions (e.g., "I'm being punished for my past sins"), or coping strategies for these symptoms. Culture can influence a consumer's willingness to accept and engage in prescribed treatment approaches, such as psychotropic medication, the relationship the consumer has with a provider (e.g., some cultures see health care providers as experts who dispense advice and the consumer as a passive participant in therapy), or the use of specific skills (e.g., using Making Positive Requests to request a change in a parent's behavior toward the consumer when cultural beliefs about the family structure and the role of individual family members may be inconsistent with the treatment approach).

Cultural awareness is also particularly important when teaching social skills. For example, in most Western European cultures, eye contact is considered a sign of attentiveness, directness, sincerity, or understanding. However, in many cultures, such as Hispanic, Asian, Middle Eastern, and Native American cultures, making direct eye contact may be disrespectful, shameful, aggressive, or rude. Additionally, a lack of eye contact in those cultures does not mean that a person is not paying attention to the listener and, in some cultures, women may particularly avoid eye contact with men, because it can be perceived as a sign of sexual interest. There are some gestures used in the United States that may have a different meaning or even be offensive to people in other cultures. Using certain finger or hand movements means "come here, please" to some, but the same gesture is used to summon dogs in some cultures and may be very offensive. In some Middle Eastern cultures, for example, the thumbs-up gesture, which indicates approval or that all is well in some Western cultures, is vulgar, and nodding one's head down indicates agreement, while nodding up signals disagreement. Interestingly, facial expressions may be more universal. In the 1870s, Charles Darwin first proposed that all cultures express emotions universally with their faces. This assertion has since been supported by several studies, including the work of Paul Ekman, who suggested that there are six universal facial expressions: anger, disgust, fear, happiness, sadness, and surprise. He then later expanded the list to include amusement, contempt, contentment, embarrassment, excitement, guilt, pride in achievement, relief, satisfaction, sensory pleasure, and shame (Ekman, 1999).

Perhaps the best way to determine the meaning of nonverbal behaviors and beliefs about appropriate and inappropriate verbal communication in the context of an individual consumer's cultural background is to ask. We have found it very informative to ask, "In your family or the community where you grew up, how would this be perceived (or would it be OK to do/say this)?" A good time to initiate a conversation about how the various forms of nonverbal communication might be perceived differently in different cultures is in Session 2 of the Social Skills Module, when these skills are introduced.

COGNITIVE-BEHAVIORAL TECHNIQUES

Providers need to know how to use a number of key cognitive-behavioral techniques throughout the skills modules. These include Socratic questioning, alternatives therapy, thought chaining, and behavioral experiments, described below and used in all the modules. In addition, role playing (also called behavioral rehearsal) is the main technique used in the Social Skills Module. It is described in detail in Chapter 7. Behavioral activation, which includes activity scheduling, is used in problem-solving training and is described in Chapter 8.

Socratic Questioning and Guided Discovery

In CBSST, Socratic questioning is a form of guided discovery used to create doubt about the accuracy of dysfunctional beliefs that can interfere with goal achievement. Socratic questioning can be used to help consumers become more aware of their thoughts and the logic behind their actions and feelings. It helps people figure things out on their own rather than being told the answer. People are more likely to remember and understand the connections among thoughts, feelings, and behaviors if they are guided to discover them on their own rather than being told by a provider who is doing all the talking.

Providers should not give advice or argue points. This can be experienced as being told, "Your thoughts are distorted!" In Socratic questioning, the tone of the discussion remains neutral, collaborative, and curious rather than judgmental. Ask open-ended questions phrased so that people cannot respond with "yes" or "no."

Socratic questioning may be used at almost any stage of therapy, and it may be particularly useful when resistance is detected. Some types of Socratic questioning and examples are defined below.

Conceptual Clarifying Questions

Encourage people to think about what they are thinking. Ask for more detail or clarifying questions to identify mistakes in thinking:

> "What exactly does this mean?"
> "How does this relate to what we have been talking about?"
> "What do we already know about this?"
> "Can you give me an example?"
> "Are you saying _____ or _____?"

Probing Assumptions

Probe the assumptions or evidence upon which the person is basing his or her beliefs. The following questions will be helpful in later discussions about checking a thought for accuracy:

> "You seem to be assuming _____; is that right?"
> "What else could we assume?"
> "How did you decide this was true?"
> "How can we verify or disprove that assumption?"
> "What would happen if . . . ?"
> "If _____ is true, what does that mean about _____?"
> "If _____ is not true, what does that mean?"

Probing Rationale, Reasons, and Evidence

People often base their beliefs on very little or even erroneous evidence. The following questions are helpful in examining the reasons why people may hold a particular belief:

> "Why is that happening?"
> "How do you know this?"
> "What do you think causes . . . ?"
> "How might it be refuted?"
> "Why?" (Keep asking why.)
> "What evidence is there to support what you are saying?"

Exploring Alternative Viewpoints and Perspectives

Most arguments are given from a particular position. Show that there are other, equally valid viewpoints by asking the following questions:

"Another way of looking at this is. . . . Does this seem reasonable?"
"Are there other ways of looking at this?"
"What if you compared . . . and . . . ?"
"What is the difference between . . . and . . . ? How are they similar?"
"What are the strengths and weaknesses of . . . and . . . ?"
"Why is it better than . . . ?"

Probing Implications and Consequences

Even if a thought is accurate, it may not be helpful with regard to goal achievement. Ask the person about the utility of the thought. Ask the following questions to help him or her examine the possible consequences of a belief with regard to impact on feelings and goal-directed actions:

"Does that make you more or less likely to [action]?"
"How does that make you feel?"
"What are the implications of . . . ?"
"How does . . . affect . . . ?"
"How does . . . fit with what we learned before?"
"Why is . . . important?"

Developing Links between Beliefs

Use "thought chaining" to uncover links between beliefs:

"And if that is/is not true, then _____ is/is not true. . . . And if that is/is not true, then _____ is/is not true. . . . And if that is/is not true. . . ."

Once you understand these links, challenge the "weakest" link. Weaker links are usually more peripheral beliefs, not beliefs near an emotionally charged core belief about the self or at the core of a delusion.

Example

The following dialogue illustrates Socratic questioning, thought chaining, and alternatives therapy. The latter is a technique used to help consumers brainstorm alternative thoughts or alternative explanations for events and situations. The consumer in the following dialogue got off the bus on the way to class because he thought a man on the bus was following him and going to harm him.

PROVIDER: How did you know he was following you?

CONSUMER: He was in the FBI?

PROVIDER: Why did you think he was in the FBI? [The provider avoids asking challenging questions about why the FBI would be following the consumer, because this is an emotionally charged discussion too close to the core delusional belief.]

CONSUMER: He had a gun under his coat.

PROVIDER: So, you assumed that, if he had a gun, he must be in the FBI?

CONSUMER: Yes, FBI agents carry guns. [At this point, the provider could have discussed alternative types of people who might carry guns, but this is still a limited group of people mostly comprised of police and other officials like FBI agents, so the provider asks on.]

PROVIDER: Did you see his gun? Why did you think he had a gun?

CONSUMER: He had a bulge under his coat that looked like a gun.

PROVIDER: What else could have caused a bulge in his jacket besides a gun? [The provider begins alternatives therapy at this point with this assumption, because it is easier to challenge.]

CONSUMER: I don't know, maybe a wallet or a phone?

PROVIDER: So, if you are not sure it was a gun, then maybe he was not in the FBI, and if he was not in the FBI, maybe you were not being followed that day on the bus. Maybe some days you can ride the bus without being followed. [Thought chaining: Break one link and the logic breaks down.]

In this example, the provider used phrases such as "How did you know . . . ?" and "Why did you think . . . ?" to help the consumer examine his thinking and become aware of the lack of solid evidence for his beliefs. The following chain of thoughts emerged: If "bulge = gun," then "gun = FBI," then "FBI = I'm followed" and, ultimately, the core delusional belief that federal agencies have him under surveillance and want to keep him quiet about government secrets he knows. The provider had several choices of thoughts to challenge (in this case by using alternatives therapy) in this thought chain. The provider did not select the highly emotionally charged core delusional belief (e.g., did not ask, "Why would the government want to follow you?"). Rather, the provider worked at the perimeter of this core belief, choosing the weakest link in the chain that interfered with goal-directed behavior (riding the bus to a class in this case). Alternatives therapy was used to reduce conviction in the assumption that "bulge = gun," which broke down the rest of the chain: If no gun, maybe not FBI; if not FBI, maybe sometimes it is safe to ride the bus. The goal is to increase the likelihood of riding the bus, not to eliminate all conviction in delusional beliefs. If the FBI is not around *all* of the time, it is *sometimes* safe to go out and engage in productive activities. The more people engage in new, productive activities, the more they will be presented with information and evidence that contradicts anomalous beliefs and move closer to goal attainment.

Behavioral Experiments

Behavioral experiments are planned activities performed by consumers to test out beliefs either in session or for homework. They are a powerful way to challenge maladaptive cognitions and increase productive behaviors in the community. When someone is hesitant to try a new activity due to an interfering cognition (e.g., "It will never work"), say, "Are you willing to do something to test out that thought?"

Behavioral experiments need to be carefully planned; do not just say, "Why not try it out?" Follow systematic steps (see Table 3.2) and be specific about where, when, and what resources will be needed to carry out the activity. The first step is to specify clearly the belief being tested. Write it down in quotes. The belief should be stated in terms that can lead to directly observable consequences. There must be an outcome to observe (e.g., a letter arriving, hearing a voice, someone saying "yes" to an invitation, a roommate doing the dishes). The belief being tested should also be related to personal recovery goals. Test beliefs that interfere with goal-directed activity or cause distress. In the example in Table 3.2, the consumer's belief that his mail was being stolen was part of a larger persecutory system. He believed that several possessions were being stolen. This led to aggressive behavior toward roommates, which interfered with an independent housing goal. These beliefs about theft by roommates were related to a delusion about theft of a large fortune, but the providers avoided this core delusional belief. He and his provider worked instead

---

TABLE 3.2. Steps of a Behavioral Experiment

1. Specify the belief to be tested:
   "Someone is taking my mail."

2. Design an experiment to test the belief:
   Send myself a letter.

3. Get agreement on the conclusion a priori:
   If the letter comes, nobody is taking my mail.

4. Record the results of the experiment:
   The letter arrived.

5. Work with implications for belief accuracy:
   Mail was not stolen, so the belief is inaccurate.

with related, but less emotionally charged, beliefs about roommates stealing things, which were more directly linked to the housing goal.

Step 2 is to design an experiment. This should be done collaboratively with the consumer. Start by asking, "How do you think we could test this out?" Revise the design until the experiment is simple enough that the consumer can carry it out during the session or before the next session.

In Step 3, provider and consumer agree in advance on the experiment's outcome and its meaning. The experiment should result in a clear outcome that either supports or disputes the belief being tested. In the example, a letter was addressed to the consumer's home during a session and mailed by the consumer from the clinic. Provider and consumer agreed that if the letter was delivered, this would be evidence that mail was not being stolen.

Record the results of the experiment (Step 4) and then work with the implications of the new evidence for belief accuracy (Step 5). Ask, "Does this new evidence support or dispute the belief?" Often consumers accept the implications of the evidence, but providers should expect "Yes, but . . ." responses that suggest the disconfirming evidence did not really disprove the belief being tested. That is fine. Firmly held beliefs can be difficult to change. Regroup and redesign another experiment to check for more evidence. In the earlier example, the letter arrived at the consumer's home (evidence that mail was not being stolen), but the consumer said, "Yes, but only letters with a check or money in them are being stolen." Another experiment was then conducted, in which an envelope from the Social Security Administration, which looked like it might contain a check, was sent, and it also arrived, providing more evidence to contradict the persecutory belief.

Ratings of belief conviction (0–100% certain it is true) can be helpful to both consumer and provider, because both will likely observe some reduction in the level of conviction in beliefs following disconfirming evidence, even if there is not full agreement that the belief is inaccurate. Try to remain open and curious about the consumer's beliefs, which can help the consumer become more curious about the possibility that beliefs might be mistaken. Instilling curiosity and an experimental perspective on testing out beliefs is the goal of the behavioral experiment skill, not the complete elimination of all mistaken beliefs.

Experiments also provide an opportunity for experiential learning or learning by doing. Behavioral experiments can be used to increase participation in new activities related to goals. For example, if a consumer wants to make more friends but is afraid of meeting new people because he or she feels inadequate or fears rejection, ask, "Are you willing to do something to test it out?" Then, give the consumer an impromptu homework assignment to talk to one new person that week. Follow up on progress the following week, with careful attention to dysfunctional thoughts that came up during the activity, and whether the outcome (degree of success vs. failure) supported or contradicted thoughts. Activities are typically more successful than expected, which provides ammunition to dispute unhelpful or inaccurate thoughts. For example, if someone thinks no one likes him or her, you could respond that he or she met a new person last week who seemed to like him or her. Get consumers behaving differently and trying new actions toward goals, then deal with the cognitions as they come up.

ADDRESSING PSYCHOTIC SYMPTOMS

While the primary focus of CBSST is not on reducing the severity of psychotic symptoms, CBSST does address delusional beliefs and beliefs about voices that interfere with recovery goal achievement or cause high levels of distress. Research has shown that poor functioning in consumers with schizophrenia is only weakly associated with severity of positive symptoms (delusions and hallucinations). Neurocognitive impairment, negative symptoms, and defeatist performance beliefs are better predictors of poor community functioning. In addition, we often find that hallucination severity and delusional conviction can be diminished by changing the consumer's focus of attention to performing goal-directed behaviors. If you help people increase functioning behaviors and become less isolated, then their daily activities can distract from and often diminish psychotic symptoms. People who isolate and focus all of their attention on voice content and delusional beliefs tend to be more distressed and symptomatic.

When psychotic symptoms appear to interfere with goal achievement, interventions in the Cognitive Skills Module can be used to address them (e.g., the 3C's, mistakes in thinking, behavioral experiments). It is typically helpful to start by reviewing the individual's history and symptoms at the onset of psychotic illness in the context of the initial stressors that may have triggered it. In this discussion, reflections can be used to clarify how the individual gathered evidence to form beliefs (e.g., "So, with all these stressors going on, including your father's death, you suddenly began hearing this voice, and tried to make sense of it. Given that it seemed that nothing else could explain where this voice was coming from, I can see why you decided it was your father talking"). Comments like this emphasize both that data were gathered that lead to a conclusion about an experience (an empirical approach) and that life events contributed to the experience. This can set the stage for gathering evidence that might dispute these long-held conclusions, as well as identify potential relapse triggers for relapse prevention plans.

Behavioral Experiments for Voices

Behavioral experiments for voices can address common general beliefs about control (e.g., "There's nothing I can do to stop my voices"), belief in the voices' omnipotence and power (e.g., "My voices will harm me if I don't do what they say"), and their source as an external agent or not from the self (e.g., "My voices are from demons talking to me"). For example, the consumer can test whether the voices diminish when he or she listens to music or watches TV, or when using other distraction techniques. This provides evidence undermining beliefs about power and control. Consumers can also experiment by not complying with command hallucinations to do a specific action. If there are no negative consequences, then this provides evidence that the voices do not have the power to punish if commands are not followed.

To gather evidence to evaluate anomalous beliefs, behavioral experiments are conducted inside and outside of sessions (at-home practice). For example, one common belief is that a voice is from an external agent who is omnipotent (e.g., the voice of God or a demon). If consumers can control the voices to *any* extent using distraction techniques such as humming, this is discussed as evidence against the external agency and omnipotence of the voices (e.g., "How can simply humming or turning on the TV control God or Satan?"). If medications control or quiet voices to any extent, this also provides evidence that voices can be controlled and are probably not from an external agent with any power (e.g., "How can something you put in your body that changes your brain chemistry control something outside your body?"). If a consumer has voices during the session, you can ask him or her to check with another group member or a provider to verify whether other people can also hear them or try to record them with a digital recorder. If nobody else hears them or they are not captured on the recording, this test provides evidence against external agency beliefs.

The Pie-Chart Technique for Delusional Preoccupation

Delusional preoccupation can also interfere with goal-directed tasks. The pie-chart technique described in Chapter 5 as a goal-setting tool can also be a helpful intervention for delusional preoccupation, reducing the time spent ruminating or engaging in other behaviors related to delusional beliefs (e.g., worry about conspirators, preparing to rescue or protect others). The intent is not to challenge directly or dispute delusional beliefs but to increase time spent on goal-directed rather than delusion-directed behaviors.

Start by drawing a circle on a pad or whiteboard and ask the consumer how much time in an average day he or she spends thinking or acting on the delusion, hallucination, and so forth. Draw a proportional piece of pie (usually nearly all of the pie circle) to represent the amount of time spent this way. Then ask how much time is spent pursuing activities related to life goals and daily tasks, and draw proportional pieces of pie for each activity. Then ask a series of questions related to the chart: "Do you think this amount of time is sufficient to achieve your goals? What might happen if less time was spent thinking or acting on these beliefs? What else would you have time for? What's the worst thing that could happen if you spend 1 hour less each day doing these things? Has that ever happened? What is the best thing that could happen if you spend more time on your goals?"

This exercise can demonstrate to consumers how much time they spend thinking about their delusions, hallucinations, or unhelpful beliefs to the exclusion of other things they want in life. In this way, delusional worry time can be scheduled and minimized, and goal-directed behavior can be increased despite the perceived obstacles related to delusional beliefs.

POSITIVE REINFORCEMENT AND SHAPING

"Positive reinforcement" is defined as a consequence of a behavior that increases the frequency of the behavior it follows. Praising or otherwise rewarding a consumer's skill practice will help increase that skill's use. Shaping is used when teaching a more complicated skill. The skill is broken into smaller steps. Practice of each step is reinforced until it is learned. The next step is then taught and reinforced. Reinforcement is most effective when it immediately follows the desired behavior, is enthusiastic, and is offered frequently. Examples include applause following a role play (always applaud to end a role play), saying, "Good job; you are really learning to do this skill well," or placing stickers, stamps, or gold stars on completed homework assignments. Raffle tickets can also be given out to reward success and desired behavior, with a drawing held at the end of each group session or the end of a module and prizes awarded for one or more winning tickets. Reinforce often the consumer's active participation in group, homework completion, volunteering to "go first" during in-session skill practice, good attendance in sessions, good answers to questions, and other positive behaviors. Reinforcement promotes learning, bolsters self-efficacy, and facilitates engagement in treatment by making group a fun and rewarding place to go.

GENERALIZATION OF SKILLS TO THE COMMUNITY

Despite their mastery of the skills taught in CBSST classes, individuals often do not spontaneously use skills to solve problems in daily life. To promote generalization of skill use in the community, ask consumers to carry a laminated card reminding them of the skill, put Post-it notes up as reminders to try the skill more often during the

PROVIDER TIP

Materials to Promote Skills Performance in the Community

In addition to the Consumer Workbooks, provide other materials to remind consumers to use skills in the community. Provide index cards for participants to write down the names and phone numbers of their primary support persons in order to facilitate interactions with social support systems. If possible, offer to laminate this index card or other wallet-size card with support person contact information. Similar wallet cards can be easily created, displaying the steps of the four communication skills, the 3C's, mistakes in thinking, SCALE, and recovery goals.

week, or use other creative ways to promote skill use in daily life. Enlisting a support person (e.g., family, residential staff, case managers) to prompt skill practice or do at-home practice assignments can also improve generalization. The optimal way to accomplish this is to meet with the support person to describe CBSST and review the skill that you would like them to prompt. If this is not possible, asking a support person to just remind consumers to "do your homework" can help.

PROVIDER TRAINING

Providers with a bachelor's degree in a mental health-related field and experience with severe mental illness, as well as more expert master's- or doctoral-level providers, can learn to deliver CBSST interventions with high fidelity. Most mental health service delivery systems in the United States have many more providers with bachelor's-level or master's-level education than providers with doctoral-level (PhD or MD) education. Learning CBSST is like taking a course in psychosocial treatment, whereby with good training and some supervision, providers learn the skills though practice, regardless of their background, with less experienced providers typically needing more training and practice. No specific credentials are required to deliver CBSST interventions, but scope of practice issues and legal, billing, or clinical service contract requirements may have implications for which providers are selected to deliver CBSST (e.g., billing for CBSST as psychotherapy vs. CBT- and SST-informed illness management or psychoeducation in the context of case management or rehabilitation counseling). These decisions about scope of practice and billing compliance are made by leadership based on the unique circumstances at individual agencies, and we provide no legal or other advice regarding these choices.

The CBT techniques in CBSST focus on practicing simple skills for belief modification (e.g., the 3C's—Catch It, Check It, Change It—thought challenging skill), using a CBT-informed skills training or psychoeducation approach, rather than the complex, formulation-driven approach of traditional CBT. As such, CBSST may require less training and experience in CBT than traditional approaches. For example, we demonstrated that bachelor's-level case managers on ACT teams can deliver the CBSST cognitive therapy interventions with adequate fidelity following only minimal training (Granholm et al., 2010). Other researchers have also demonstrated that community therapists and case managers can deliver CBT interventions to consumers with schizophrenia with adequate fidelity (Turkington et al., 2014; Lincoln et al., 2012; Morrison et al., 2004; Pinninti et al., 2010). Previous research has also shown that staff members from multiple disciplines with minimal education can administer manualized social skills training interventions (Liberman, 1994), like the communication skills training interventions described in detail in Chapter 7.

The amount of experience and education required to deliver evidence-based practices such as CBSST for schizophrenia has not been established, but published recommendations for the dissemination of CBT in the United Kingdom are consistent with our training model (Williams, 2008; Fowler et al., 2009; Rollison et al., 2007). The provider training model we recommend includes (1) an initial 1- or preferably 2-day workshop (7–8 hours per day), including didactics, demonstrations, and role-play practice of skills; (2) a copy of this book, which details the CBSST treatment; (3) weekly-to-monthly skills-focused consultation meetings (30–60 minutes; in-person or via audio or video teleconferencing) using coaching and role-play modeling for 3–12 months after providers start delivering CBSST; (4) review of session audiotapes in consultation meetings; and (5) feedback of fidelity ratings of recorded sessions to monitor fidelity (if needed). This is the training model that has been successful in our prior CBSST clinical research trials. A workshop alone is likely not sufficient to achieve adequate fidelity of CBT and social skills training interventions. Supervision has been reported to be an essential component of CBT training to improve fidelity (Williams, 2008; Fowler et al., 2009; Rollinson et al., 2007), but the minimal number of weeks of supervision required to reach adequate fidelity is not clear and varies with provider prior training and experience. A useful initial approach is to provide supervision with feedback of fidelity ratings to individual providers until they reach a fidelity standard. Additional training information and resources are available at *http://cbsst.org.*

CHAPTER 4

Assessment
Measuring Effects of CBSST

In this chapter, we describe assessments that help administrators and providers measure the effectiveness of the CBSST program. Outcome measures can be selected and administered at baseline when consumers start CBSST treatment and again at regular intervals over the course of treatment (e.g., every 3 to 6 months) to provide a clear sense of consumer progress in treatment on key outcomes. In addition, intervention fidelity measures can be selected to provide information about the effectiveness of provider training and implementation strategies.

While assessment may inform treatment planning to some extent, this is not the primary purpose of assessment in the CBSST program. Treatment is guided by the consumer's personal recovery goals. Part II of this book provides detailed guidance on how meaningful long-term recovery goals are broken down into short-term goals and goal steps, and how skills training is personalized to help consumers achieve their unique recovery goal steps. Although not the primary purpose of assessment in the CBSST program, some assessment measures may inform treatment planning. For example, a consumer with severe dysfunctional attitudes about socializing on a consumer attitude scale, but intact communication skills on a social competence measure, might benefit more from cognitive skills training to challenge dysfunctional asocial beliefs than from social skills training.

Assessment is not used to select consumers for CBSST treatment. As discussed in Chapter 2, research has not clearly identified specific consumer characteristics that reliably predict which consumers are more likely to benefit from CBSST. For example, severity of psychiatric symptoms and neurocognitive impairments do not appear to moderate treatment outcome reliably. Similarly, there is some evidence that consumers with poor insight are less likely to benefit, but there is not suffi-cient evidence to exclude these consumers from treatment. Given the lack of clear evidence about which consumers are more likely to benefit from CBSST, there is no screening session in the CBSST program in which assessments are administered to determine who should receive treatment.

In this chapter we describe assessments to measure functioning, recovery, symp-toms, CBSST skills knowledge, consumer attitudes, provider attitudes, and inter-vention fidelity. Several validated assessment measures will be described for each assessment domain, and validated inexpensive measures that can be used efficiently in the context of a busy clinic will be noted.

FUNCTIONING

The primary treatment target of the CBSST program is functioning. There is some debate in the field about the best way to measure functioning in schizophrenia. Several methods are available, including performance-based skills assessments, interviewer-rated self-report instruments, and objective indicators or milestones. Each assessment method has its own strengths and weaknesses, but for busy clinics with limited staff time and resources, self-report measures and objective indicators may be the best choice.

Self-report questionnaires are convenient to administer and typically do not require a significant amount of staff time; relatively brief instruments with minimal consumer burden are available. These assessments are questionnaires that can be read by most consumers and require "yes" or "no" or Likert-type scale responses (e.g., ratings of how well or how often a behavior is performed on a scale of 1 to 5), although staff may need to read questions to consumers who cannot read or under-stand them on their own. Self-report measures are efficient, inexpensive or free, and do not require special equipment or training. However, there are several drawbacks to using them. The reliability and validity of self-report outcomes can be influenced by several factors, including cognitive impairments that interfere with reading and understanding items or accurately remembering behaviors (typically over the past month), response bias (e.g., social desirability), symptom severity (e.g., disorganiza-tion or auditory hallucinations), and limited insight/introspection ability. Due to these factors, the validity of self-reported functioning has been questioned in con-sumers with schizophrenia. The major concerns with self-report instruments are with scales that ask consumers to rate the quality of their performance of functioning behaviors. Scales that simply ask whether or not a specific functioning behavior was performed, not how well it was performed, do not rely as heavily on neurocog-nitive ability, insight, and response bias. The accuracy of self-reports can also be enhanced by using an interview format and incorporating information from multi-ple available sources. Therefore, the best approach may be to administer assessments in an interview format and formulate aggregate best-estimate ratings (e.g., based on observations, the reports of the consumer, and any available informant or medical record information).

The primary measure of functional outcome we selected for our CBSST clinical trials (see Chapter 2) was a self-report measure called the Independent Living Skills Survey (ILSS; Wallace et al., 2000). The ILSS, a 71-item instrument to measure functioning in multiple domains (appearance and clothing, personal hygiene, care of possessions and living space, food preparation, health maintenance, transportation, money management, leisure and recreational activities, job seeking, job maintenance), requires about 15–20 minutes to administer. Items are scored 0 ("not performed"), 1 ("performed"), or "not able to demonstrate" (e.g., for food preparation items when meals were provided by assisted living staff members), and the average score for items that were not scored "not able to demonstrate" is computed for each domain (domain scores are not computed if more than half the items are missing or scored "not able to demonstrate"). The total score is the average of all available domains. There is also an informant version of the ILSS, if a provider or family member who has frequent contact with the consumer is available. The ILSS is available for free as an appendix in the original publication (Wallace et al., 2000), which is available online (*http://schizophreniabulletin.oxfordjournals.org/content/26/3/631.full.pdf*).

Performance-based skills capacity measures of functioning require consumers to demonstrate skills (e.g., write a check to pay a bill, shop for groceries, start a conversation) in an artificial recreation or simulation of the real world (e.g., role play with props or virtual reality computer simulation) in the clinic. Because consumers actually have to demonstrate the skills rather than report on whether they can perform them, performance-based measures are less likely to be influenced by participant or observer bias, lack of insight, or inability to recall activities. Determining whether or not a consumer can demonstrate skills can also inform treatment (e.g., how much social skills training is needed). However, confirming that a consumer *can* perform skills in the clinic does not guarantee that the consumer *does* perform the skills in the real world. Other measures of functioning may be needed to determine the actual level of skills performance or functioning in the real world.

Commonly used performance-based measures include the Maryland Assessment of Social Competence (MASC; Bellack & Meuser, 1993; Bellack et al., 1994) and the UCSD [University of California, San Diego] Performance-Based Skills Assessment (UPSA; Patterson, Moscona, McKibbin, Davidson, & Jeste, 2001). The MASC is a structured behavioral role-play assessment of the ability to initiate and maintain conversations and resolve interpersonal problems through verbal communication. The MASC can be administered in about 15–20 minutes but requires at least an additional 20 minutes to code and score. The MASC consists of three 3-minute role-play communication scenarios (one conversation initiation and two assertion), during which the consumer interacts with a live confederate who plays a role (e.g., boss, coworker) in a problem-oriented situation (e.g., asking for a work shift change; initiating a conversation). Video recordings of the role plays are coded on dimensions of verbal content, nonverbal communication behavior, and an overall effectiveness score. The measure has three parallel sets of scenarios for multiple administrations. A simplified audio recorded version of the MASC that is easier to score is the Social Skills Performance Assessment (SSPA; Patterson et al., 2001), which requires approximately 12 minutes (administration and scoring). Performance on the MASC or SSPA is a useful outcome measures and may also inform treatment planning, because both measure communication skills similar to the ones trained in the Social Skills Training Module. If consumers perform well on these measures, social skills training can progress more rapidly or be shortened (e.g., with fewer practice role plays of each skill). However, we do not recommend eliminating the Social Skills Training Module for these consumers, because role-play practice can serve as a useful behavioral experiment to help consumers identify and challenge defeatist attitudes that can come up during role plays and interfere with skills performance in the community, as described in Chapter 7.

The UPSA measures performance in a number of domains of everyday functioning (Household Chores, Communication, Finance, Transportation, and Planning Recreational Activities) through the use of props and standardized skills performance situations. For example, on the Finance task, consumers count out given amounts from real currency, make change, and fill out a check to pay a utility bill. On the Communication task, consumers use a phone to make an emergency call, call directory assistance to request a telephone number and call the number, and reschedule a medical appointment. An abbreviated version of the UPSA, referred to as the UPSA–Brief (Mausbach, Harvey, Goldman, Jeste, & Patterson; 2007), is available. This version includes only two of the original UPSA domains, Finance and Communication, and the total score for the UPSA–Brief is highly correlated with the total score of the full UPSA ($r = .91$). The UPSA–Brief requires about 12 minutes to administer (the full UPSA requires 30 minutes). A mobile application has also been developed for an iPad platform (UPSA–M, for mobile) and is as sensitive to functional capacity deficits as the standard version (Moore et al., 2015).

Objective indicators of functioning include milestone achievements such as getting a job, getting married, educational enrollment, and independent living. Objective indicator measures avoid some of the problems noted for self-report measures, because reports can be verified through informants and records (e.g., transcripts, paychecks), although the time needed to verify information can be a significant burden on the staff. Milestones can also require a long period of time to achieve, so objective indicator measures may not change during a typical course of CBSST. The Psychosocial Rehabilitation Toolkit (PSR Toolkit; Arns, Rogers, Cook, & Mowbray, 2001) is an objective indicator measure of work, education, finances, residential independence, and health care service utilization (e.g., hospitalizations) milestones. Consumer progress in each domain is rated on a scale, ranging from the absence of meaningful functioning in the domain to fully independent functioning (e.g., employment: 1 = "no employment," 2 = "nonpaid work," 3 = "sheltered work-shops," . . . , 11 = "independent competitive employment").

Interviewer rating scales involve semistructured interviews with standardized questions and anchors to rate aspects of functioning and typically allow the interviewer to use all available information (consumer responses, direct observation, clinical records, informants, etc.) to make judgements about ratings. Interviewer assessments may be more reliable than self-report measures, but interviews can be lengthy, and significant interviewer training is typically required to ensure reliable, accurate data collection. The Specific Levels of Functioning Scale (SLOF; Schneider & Streuening, 1983) is a 43-item interviewer rating scale (with Consumer and Informant versions) of functioning in the following domains: Physical Functioning (e.g., vision, hearing), Personal Care (e.g., toileting, eating, grooming), Interpersonal Relationships (e.g., initiating, accepting, and maintaining social contacts; communicating effectively), Social Acceptability (e.g., verbal and physical abuse, repetitive behaviors), Community Activities (e.g., shopping, using telephone, paying bills, use of leisure time, use of public transportation), and Work Skills (e.g., employable skills, level of supervision, punctuality). The SLOF can be completed in 15–20 minutes. The National Institute of Mental Health–funded Validation of Everyday Real-World Outcomes study found that the SLOF was the best-functioning measure for people with schizophrenia (Harvey et al., 2011).

The Abbreviated Quality of Life Scale (A-QLS; Bilker et al., 2003), another semistructured interview measure, is a seven-item assessment of subjective and objective aspects of functioning over the past month (e.g., Motivation, Anhedonia, Capacity for Empathy, Active Acquaintances, Social Initiative, Occupational Role Functioning). This scale focuses on assessment of negative symptoms and social functioning in schizophrenia. The full 21-item QLS (Heinrichs, Hanlon, & Carpenter, 1984) is one of the most commonly used measures of social and occupational role functioning in schizophrenia treatment outcome research, but the full scale requires 30–45 minutes to administer. The abbreviated version is well-validated and strongly correlated with the longer version ($r = .98$), and requires only about 15 minutes to administer.

The Birchwood Social Functioning Scale (SFS; Birchwood, Smith, Cochrane, Wetton, & Copestake, 1990) is designed to assess social functioning in people with schizophrenia. The SFS provides broader coverage of social behaviors and less focus on everyday living skills (e.g., hygiene and home care) than the other functioning measures discussed here. A panel of experts on the assessment of functioning rated the SFS the best measure of social aspects of functioning based on multiple factors, including practicality, reliability, sensitivity, and comprehensiveness (Harvey et al., 2011). The SFS assesses six domains of social functioning: (1) Social Engagement/ Withdrawal; (2) Interpersonal Communication; (3) Independence: Performance; (4) Independence: Competence; (5) Recreation; and (6) Prosocial Activities, as well as some information on occupation/employment. Items are scored from 0 to 3; total score may range from 0 to 213. The SFS can be completed in about 20–30 minutes.

RECOVERY

With the recovery movement, outcome assessments have expanded to incorporate recovery-oriented aspects of goal attainment in living, learning, working, and socializing domains, as well as subjective quality of life. The principles of recovery-oriented psychiatric rehabilitation include responsibility, self-determination, empowerment, and the inclusion of individualized and person-centered approaches. These principles reflect the essential philosophy that consumers with serious mental illness can and should be active participants in the goal-setting and rehabilitation-planning process, including measurement of progress toward these rehabilitation goals. This recovery movement approach to rehabilitation has led to the development of several more recovery-oriented outcome measures. For example, the Client's Assessment of Strengths, Interests, and Goals (CASIG; Wallace, Lecomte, Wilde, & Liberman, 2001) was developed as a tool for embedding the measurement of functional outcomes into the process of individualized treatment planning and evaluation. The CASIG allows clinicians to obtain valuable information on domains relevant to treatment planning and rehabilitation goal setting, including Community Functioning, Living Skills, Medication Compliance, Quality of Life, Quality of Treatment, Symptoms, and Frequency of Unacceptable Community Behaviors. One drawback mentioned by the authors is that the measure can be time-consuming to administer, which may make it a less desirable choice in some clinical settings.

The Choice of Outcome in CBT for Psychoses (CHOICE; Greenwood et al., 2010) measure stands as the first psychometrically sound outcome measure specifically for CBT for psychoses that utilizes consumer definitions of recovery and CBT aims. This measure captures important internal elements of recovery, including self-direction, hope, empowerment and coping, and also provides the opportunity to evaluate specific CBT domains, such as normalizing and psychological and behavioral flexibility. This measure is an excellent recovery-oriented measure for programs with a strong focus on CBT.

A measure that provides perhaps the most flexibility and consumer choice in deciding valued outcomes and systematically measuring progress toward achieving these outcomes is Goal Attainment Scaling (GAS), developed as an individualized method of evaluating personalized recovery goal achievement, which involves translating issues and problems into specific goals with specific levels of achievement marked by directly observable indicators. We (Tabak, Holden, & Granholm, 2015) developed and standardized GAS measures for several common recovery goals, with specific indicators of level of achievement (all rated on a 0- to 10-point scale), including Employment, Housing, Relationship, School, Self-Care, Leisure Activities, Recovery from Addictions Goal, Money Management, and Independent Transportation goals. The GAS measure for a Relationship Goal is shown in Figure 4.1 (see Tabak et al., 2015, and *htpp://CBSST.org* for other GAS templates).

To obtain GAS ratings, consumers meet with CBSST providers individually at the beginning of treatment to develop personalized recovery goals that will be the

0	Contemplates meeting new people/re-establishing past relationships
1	**Talks to doctor, case manager, CBSST therapist, or other support person about:** 1. Meeting new people—asks for help in finding venues to meet new people. OR 2. Re-establishing past relationships (family, friendships, etc.).
2	**Independently:** 1. Researches venues for meeting new people—community organizations, and so forth. OR 2. Researches ways to establish contact with family or friends from the past. 3. Finds means of getting to new places (bus; phone numbers).
3	**EITHER:** **1. Goes to a community venue (coffee shop, clubhouse, etc.) to meet new people.** **OR** **2. Meets with family or friend from the past.** BUT → Does not speak to other people when spoken to. AND → Does not initiate conversation.
4	**EITHER:** **1. Goes to a community venue (coffee shop, clubhouse, etc.) to meet new people.** **OR** **2. Meets with/calls family or friend from the past.** AND → Speaks to others when spoken to. BUT → Does not initiate conversation.
5	**EITHER:** **1. Goes to a community venue (coffee shop, clubhouse, etc.) to meet new people.** **OR** **2. Meets with/calls family or friend from the past.** AND → Speaks to others when spoken to. AND → Initiates conversation.
6	**EITHER:** **1. Goes to a community venue (coffee shop, clubhouse, etc.) to meet new people.** **OR** **2. Meets with/calls family or friend from the past.** AND → Initiates plans with someone (asks someone to go do something). BUT → The other person declines to go or no shows.
7	**EITHER:** **1. Goes to a community venue (coffee shop, clubhouse, etc.) to meet new people.** **OR** **2. Meets with/calls family or friend from the past.** AND → Initiates plans with someone (asks someone to go do something). AND → The other person accepts the invitation and shows.
8	**EITHER:** **1. Meets a new friend.** **OR** **2. Re-establishes relationship with family or friends from the past.** AND → Make plans at least once a month.

(continued)

FIGURE 4.1. Goal attainment scaling: relationship goal.

9	EITHER: 1. **Meets a new friend.** OR 2. **Re-establishes relationship with family or friends from the past.** AND → Makes plans at least twice a month.
10	EITHER: 1. **Meets an additional new friend.** OR 2. **Re-establishes another relationship with family or friends from the past.**

FIGURE 4.1. *(continued)*

focus of treatment in the CBSST program (see Chapter 5). Providers then meet with consumers individually at midtreatment (if feasible) and at the end of treatment to use GAS ratings to monitor goal progress. For example, if a consumer only talks with providers about meeting people but has taken no action toward his or her goal at the beginning of treatment, the rating would be 1 (see Figure 4.1). If, at the end of treatment, the consumer is meeting with family or friends at community venues and initiating conversations and plans, the GAS rating would increase to 6. In this way, GAS can be used to quantify and standardize the measurement of progress toward different personalized recovery goals listed on the 7–7–7 Goal Jackpot! Worksheet described in Chapter 5. Using these standardized GAS ratings, we (Tabak et al., 2015) found a statistically significant increase in mean goal attainment during CBSST treatment, with scores increasing from 2.38 (standard deviation = 1.69)—corresponding to "independently researches venues/ways to meet people and establish contact"—at the beginning of treatment to 5.64 (standard deviation = 2.31)—corresponding to "goes to venue or meets/calls family or friends and initiates conversations"—at end of treatment.

Other recovery-oriented instruments are focused on assessing service delivery programs rather than the consumers they serve. For example, the Recovery Assessment Scale (RAS; O'Connell, Tondora, Croog, Evans, & Davidson, 2005) measures the degree to which a program implements recovery-oriented services and identifies strengths and areas of needed improvement. The 36-items of the RAS can be grouped into five domains: Life Goals, Consumer Involvement, Diversity of Treatment Options, Client Choice, and Individually Tailored Services.

SYMPTOMS

Symptom severity and distress can be measured with several commonly used assessments. The well-known Beck Depression Inventory–II (BDI-II; Beck, Steer, & Brown, 1996) and Beck Anxiety Inventory (BAI; Beck & Steer, 1990) are self-report instruments that are easy and fast to administer in a busy clinic, but they do not measure positive and negative symptoms of schizophrenia. The Positive and Negative Syndrome

Scale (PANSS; Kay, Fiszbein, & Opler, 1987) is a widely used 30-item interview that assesses balanced representation of positive and negative symptoms and global psychopathology. The Brief Psychiatric Rating Scale (BPRS; Lukoff, Nuechterlein, & Ventura 1986), another widely used interview measure of global psychopathology, is a 24-item scale that measures positive symptoms, negative symptoms, anxiety, depression, mania, grandiosity and other aspects of psychopathology. Each item is rated by the interviewer on a 7-point scale that ranges from "not present" to "extremely severe" over the past 7 days. In contrast to the PANSS and BPRS, which measure only the severity of psychiatric symptoms, the Psychotic Symptom Rating Scales (PSYRATS; Haddock, McGarron, Tarrier, & Faragher, 1999) is an interviewer-administered measure that assesses severity, as well as other dimensions of hallucinations and delusions, including delusional conviction and beliefs about voices (e.g., external agency, control). All of these interviewer rating scales can be lengthy and require significant rater training to ensure reliable, accurate data collection.

Negative symptom severity can be measured with the Scale for the Assessment of Negative Symptoms (SANS; Andreasen, 1982) or Clinical Assessment Interview for Negative Symptoms (CAINS; Forbes et al., 2010), both also interviewer-administered measures. The CAINS is a relatively new scale that assesses five negative symptoms: Asociality, Avolition, Anhedonia (Consummatory and Anticipatory), Affective Flattening, and Alogia. Items are rated on a 7-point scale, with higher scores reflecting greater pathology. The CAINS may be more effective at capturing experiential deficits (e.g., motivation, interest, desire for social affiliation, and anhedonia) and experiential negative symptoms appear to be most linked to defeatist attitudes targeted in CBSST.

Greater insight and belief flexibility have been associated with better positive symptom response to CBT for psychosis (Naeem et al., 2008; Perivoliotis et al., 2010). Simple self-report measures of clinical and cognitive insight are available. "Clinical insight" is awareness of a mental illness requiring treatment, whereas "cognitive insight" refers to metacognitive processes of reevaluation and correction of distorted beliefs and misinterpretations (i.e., belief flexibility and objective reappraisal of symptoms). The Birchwood Insight Scale (BIS; Birchwood et al., 1994) for psychosis is a very brief self-report clinical insight measure of awareness of illness, need for treatment, and whether consumers attribute symptoms to illness. The Beck Cognitive Insight Scale (BCIS; Beck at al., 2004) is a brief, self-report questionnaire that assesses metacognitive processes (e.g., Self-Reflectiveness and Self-Certainty, or Overconfidence in Beliefs). Improved cognitive insight or belief flexibility may mediate change, especially change in positive symptoms, in CBT for psychosis.

CBSST SKILLS KNOWLEDGE

For ongoing treatment planning, it is helpful to determine whether consumers are learning the CBSST skills. If consumers are not learning the skills, modules can be repeated or the pace of training can be slowed, with more experiential learning games included. We developed a measure to assess the acquisition of specific skills knowledge in CBSST called the Comprehensive Modules Test (CMT). The CMT was originally developed to assess acquisition of specific skills during social skills training modules (Liberman, 1991). We adapted the CMT to assess acquisition of the skills trained in the three CBSST modules. The CMT is an interviewer-administered measure of content trained in CBSST (e.g., "What are the 3C's?"), as well as the application of skills in vignettes. Questions with vignettes were developed to assess mastery of thought-challenging, communication, and problem-solving skills. Partial- and full-credit scoring criteria are included for each item (11 points per module; 33 total). The CMT has been used in previous studies to demonstrate that participants with schizophrenia are able to learn the cognitive and behavioral skills taught in CBSST (Granholm et al., 2005, 2007, 2013, 2014). The full measure can be administered in 10–15 minutes and is provided in Appendix A.

CONSUMER ATTITUDES

As discussed in Chapters 1 and 2, defeatist performance attitudes and social disinterest attitudes appear to be important mechanisms of change that may mediate improvements in negative symptoms and functioning in CBSST. The Defeatist Performance Attitude Scale (DPAS; Grant & Beck, 2010; see Appendix A) is a 15-item subscale of the 40-item Dysfunctional Attitude Scale (DAS; Weissman, 1978). It can be administered in 5 minutes to assess defeatist attitudes about one's ability to perform goal-directed tasks (e.g., "If you cannot do something well, there is little point in doing it at all"; "If I fail at my work, then I am a failure as a person"; "People will probably think less of me if I make mistakes and fail"). We found significantly greater reduction in severity of defeatist performance beliefs on the DPAS in CBSST relative to a supportive contact control group in one clinical trial (Granholm et al., 2014), and reduction in DPAS scores during CBSST treatment was significantly correlated with functional outcome on the ILSS 9 months after treatment in another clinical trial (Granholm et al., 2013). Consumers with greater severity of defeatist performance beliefs on the DPAS (scores > 55) were also more likely to benefit from CBSST (Granholm et al., 2013). We have not yet replicated this finding, but it suggests that the DPAS may prove to be a useful screening tool to select consumers most likely to benefit from CBSST.

Social disinterest attitudes or asocial beliefs about interacting with others can be measured using the Asocial Beliefs Scale (ABS; Grant & Beck, 2009; see Appendix A), a 15-item true–false subscale of the Revised Social Anhedonia Scale (RSAS; Eckblad, Chapman, Chapman, & Mishlove, 1982; Mishlove & Chapman, 1985). In order to tap attitudes of social disinterest more specifically, rather than emotional experiences, Grant and Beck (2009) selected 15 RSAS items with face validity for assessing social disinterest in interacting with others, including "I attach very little importance to having close friends" and "I could be happy living all alone in a cabin in the woods or mountains." Items that reflected emotional aspects of social satisfaction and pleasure or general emotional dysregulation were not included. Items that might reflect the frequency of actual social interactions were also avoided. We found that reduction in social disinterest beliefs on the ABS during CBSST was associated with better functional outcome at end of treatment (Granholm et al., 2009).

PROVIDER ATTITUDES

It may be of interest to mental health treatment agencies or clinical supervisors to measure providers' attitudes toward evidence-based practices and confidence in delivering those interventions. The Evidence-Based Practice Attitudes Scale (EBPAS; Aarons, 2004; Aarons Fettes, Flores, & Sommerfeld, 2009) is a 15-item measure of provider attitudes about the adoption of innovation and, in particular, evidence-based practices. It consists of four subscales: Appeal, Openness, Requirements, and Divergence. The Self-Efficacy Questionnaire, based on the work of Ozer et al. (2004) and Weingardt, Cucciare, Bellotti, and Lai (2009), was developed to assess providers' level of confidence in their ability to deliver evidence-based practices such as CBSST. This questionnaire can provide information about implementation readiness at an agency, which can be used to begin a discussion with staff about potential barriers and facilitators to rolling out an evidence-based practice. Repeated assessments on measures like this can provide information about changes in attitudes and confidence after steps are taken to train and overcome barriers.

INTERVENTION FIDELITY

"Fidelity measures" are checklists and rating scales that assess whether key intervention components (e.g., setting an agenda, challenging dysfunctional thoughts, assigning homework) are delivered. Fidelity ratings are best completed by someone experienced with the intervention, who is already a high-fidelity provider. Ratings are completed by directly observing service delivery or reviewing audio or video recordings of several (e.g., 10) sessions and completing a checklist of observed aspects of the session structure, therapist behavior, and proper effective use of the intervention. Greater intervention fidelity is associated with better consumer outcomes. As discussed in Chapter 3, fidelity measures can be used as a training tool, by feeding back strengths and areas for improvement based on fidelity ratings of specific intervention components. Fidelity ratings can also be used to document an agency's high-fidelity delivery of evidence-based practices.

We have used the Cognitive Therapy Rating Scale for Psychosis (CTS-Psy; Haddock et al., 2001) to rate fidelity of cognitive therapy components of CBSST for consumers with schizophrenia. Fidelity of nonspecific therapist skills (understanding, interpersonal effectiveness) and specific CBT intervention skills (sum of Agenda, Feedback, Collaboration, Guided Discovery, Focus on Key Cognitions, Choices of CBT Interventions, Quality of Interventions, and Homework Items) are rated on the CTS-Psy, which is available in Haddock et al. A total CTS-Psy score of 30 or greater has been used as a cutoff for competent CBT for psychosis (>30) in clinical trials research (Granholm et al., 2005, 2014; Turkington et al., 2002).

We recommend the Social Skills Group Observation Checklist (available in Bellack et al., 2004) to rate social skills training sessions. This checklist is a 17-item scale that assesses session structure, provider characteristics, and correct instruction of role plays. Bellack et al. also include a Social Skills Group Leader Self-Rating Checklist that uses the same items as the observer-rated checklist. Using both the CTS-Psy and Social Skills Group Observation Checklist provides comprehensive fidelity ratings of nonspecific therapist factors, cognitive therapy components, and social skills training components of CBSST sessions.

SUMMARY

There is increasing pressure on treatment delivery programs to implement recommended evidence-based practices and to assess consumer outcomes to document the benefits of these services. Accrediting bodies (e.g., Commission on Accreditation of Rehabilitation Facilities) and many mental health systems require programs to measure outcomes and use data from outcome assessments to inform treatment planning and program development. A great many questionnaires, interviews, and performance-based measures are available to assess functioning, recovery, and symptom outcomes, as well as intervention fidelity and attitudes in consumers and providers, which can impact treatment success. Some of these measures involve significant program resources and consumer burden, but relatively brief, low-cost measures with relatively good reliability and validity are available for use in busy clinical settings. Although all assessment places some burden on staff members and consumers, investing in careful assessment can inform service delivery and improve quality of care and consumer outcomes.

PART II

Practical Guide

CHAPTER 5

Introduction and Goal-Setting Session

ABOUT THIS SESSION

Each of the three skills-oriented modules in CBSST starts with this Introduction and Goal-Setting session. It is Session 1 for each module. Setting recovery goals helps people focus on success, prioritize actions, and follow through with specific goal-directed tasks. In contrast to diagnostically based treatment plans, which tend to focus on symptom reduction and eliminating problems, recovery plans focus on setting living, learning, working, and socializing goals to improve quality of life. Diagnostically based treatment plans tend to be a less flexible approach to treatment, whereas personalized recovery plans tailor skills training to an individual's personal needs and chosen functioning goals. For example, someone with the goal of finding or keeping work should role-play scenarios during social skills training that focus on work-related interactions (e.g., interviewing, asking for a different shift, meeting coworkers). The same person's thought-challenging skills should focus on defeatist attitudes about work (e.g., "I'll never find a job, "I'm going to be fired," "I'm being sabotaged by coworkers"). For someone with a socialization goal, role plays should focus on relevant social interactions (e.g., asking someone to go on a date, meeting someone new, setting limits with roommates or partners). That person's cognitive skills should focus on unhelpful beliefs such as "I'm not likable," "Social interactions are not fun," or "They will laugh at me." The specific skills emphasized during CBSST should also be tailored to the specific strengths and weaknesses of each individual. For example, someone with the goal of finding work who has good communication skills but is hopeless about finding a job may need to focus more on cognitive restructuring skills to reduce defeatist expectations rather than on social skills training. Someone with poor communication skills who is optimistic about finding a job may need to focus more on social skills training. In this way, the CBSST modules can be tailored to personalized recovery goals by focusing rehabilitation on practicing the needed skills most relevant to an individual's goals. Personalized recovery goals guide treatment.

The Introduction and Goal-Setting session repeats at the start of each new skills module. In this session, the CBSST program is briefly described, and the rehabilitation process begins by helping consumers identify recovery goals. If a modular rolling admissions group format is used, new consumers may or may not enter the group during this session. If new members enter, time must be set aside during this session for introductions and orientation to the CBSST program. Experienced members can be called upon to help describe CBSST and share their progress and recovery goal achievements. In addition to the session plan described below, Appendix B offers several goal-setting activities. Any one of these can be used to facilitate the goal-setting process.

We believe the primary goal of this first session is to get newcomers to come to the second session, that is, to engage them in treatment. A good way to do this is to identify recovery goals that would improve someone's life and to be excited and hopeful about the possibility that learning the CBSST skills can help people achieve these goals. A key message of this session, as described below, is that changing our thoughts can change our lives.

PROVIDER PLAN FOR SESSION 1: INTRODUCTION AND GOAL SETTING

- Set the Agenda Collaboratively
- Introduce Newcomers
- Orientation
  - Class Rules
  - Class Contract
- Introduce CBSST and Changing Unhelpful Thinking
- Review At-Home Practice (previous members only)
- Set Goals
  - Identify Long-Term Goals
  - Identify Short-Term Goals and Goal Steps
- Assign At-Home Practice: Setting Goals
- Summarize the Session
- Ask for Consumer Feedback

CONDUCTING THE SESSION

Set the Agenda Collaboratively

In this session, as in every CBSST session, the provider begins by writing a simplified session agenda on the board (or on a notepad if a board is not available in individual sessions). This simplified agenda also appears in the Consumer Workbooks at the start of each session. The agenda for this session is as follows:

- Introductions and Orientation
- CBSST and Changing Unhelpful Thinking
- Review At-Home Practice (previous members only)
- Set Goals
- Assign At-Home Practice: Setting Goals
- Additional (Consumer) Agenda Items?

If this is the first CBSST session for any consumers, the idea of collaborative agenda setting can be introduced in the following way:

> "Each class will begin with setting an agenda, which is our list of things we want to accomplish during class. You can add anything to the agenda that you would like to discuss. For example, if you have any questions about the skills you are learning, problems you are experiencing, or something in your life you would like to get help with, you are welcome to add it to the agenda. Your participation in setting the agenda is very important because each class is intended to help you improve your life."

Introduce Newcomers

The first item on the agenda is introductions. If there are newcomers to class, we recommend that introductions be guided by two statements written on the board:

1. "Tell us your name and something positive about yourself—something you are good at or enjoy doing."
2. "Tell us something you want to get out of the group—one of your goals."

This can get the ball rolling on goal setting. We have found that asking consumers to introduce themselves by sharing something positive can facilitate engagement. People usually prefer to talk about something they enjoy doing rather than describe their history of symptoms and problems. There are exceptions to this, however. Some consumers prefer to talk about symptoms, and others discover for the first time that other people also hear voices or worry about being harmed. This "me, too" experience can help normalize and destigmatize symptoms, and promote connections and engagement in treatment. Although symptoms are not the primary focus of CBSST, symptom discussions should not be discouraged.

We note one caveat when working in a group format. It is important to guide discussions by commenting on the amount of shared time allotted to ensure that all consumers have a chance to introduce themselves. Some consumers may want to share a great deal and may not be interested in moving on to new topics and agenda items. The experience at the beginning of the group will set expectations for the rest of the sessions, particularly new members. Therefore, guide consumers to be aware and respectful of each other's time while still sharing their own perspective; this is an important skill in and of itself. Note that while sharing can feel good and be helpful, it is only one component of the treatment, and the majority of time needs to be dedicated to skills training.

Orientation: Class Rules and Class Contract

We encourage providers to establish class rules during introductions in the first session. The rules might spell out length of treatment, expectations about missed sessions and coming late, confidentiality, what to do in a crisis, rules about aggression, and so forth. We recommend formalizing these rules with a class contract. Doing so will make expectations clear and may make consumers feel more comfortable engaging in activities and discussions. In particular, clearly discuss confidentiality in groups ("what is said here stays here") and limits to confidentiality (e.g., harm to self or others, depending on local setting and state laws). This can facilitate sharing among members. Explicit rules establish a foundation for appropriate and expected behavior in class, including active participation and completion of at-home practice. One way to introduce the idea of a class contract is to ask, "What are some rules we should have to make sure everyone feels safe and comfortable, and gets the most out of this class?" The discussion will likely produce items relevant to a treatment contract. A sample class contract is presented in Figure 5.1.

Introduce CBSST

We typically introduce CBSST by calling it a class (or individual tutoring) in which people learn new skills to achieve their recovery goals. This label avoids the perception that CBSST is "just another therapy group," which can deter engagement in consumers who have been ill for a number of years and in many therapy groups. However, in younger consumers (e.g., recent onset, prodromal, high risk), who already spend much of their time in high school or college, the "class" label can be a barrier to engagement, especially in consumers who are having negative experiences at school. Alternative labels may be preferred, such as groups or social clubs, or ask consumers to label the meetings. The choice of label can either facilitate or deter engagement in CBSST.

I would like to participate in this class. I agree to the following class rules:

1. I will attend this class and follow its rules for the next ____ months. However, I know that my participation in this class is entirely voluntary, and I may choose to stop at any time.

2. I will try to attend every class session and will try to participate actively. I will call the provider(s) before class if I cannot make it to a class session.

3. I will not be late.

4. I will be respectful of others. I will not talk with someone while someone else is talking. I will not shout. I will not hurt anyone, nor will I threaten or yell at anyone.

5. So that I and others in the class can be open and honest, I will not reveal the names of other members or talk about what they say outside of class. The provider(s) will also not release any information about me outside the group without my written consent unless releasing the information is required by law (e.g., is about hurting myself or others).

6. I can achieve my goals by learning CBSST skills through practice. This includes at-home activities that I will do. I agree to work hard to practice in class and complete practice activities at home.

7. The class providers decide what to do if the rules are broken. I agree to follow their decision.

I have read these rules, understand them, and will follow them.

_____   _____   _____
(Print Name)   (Signature)   (Date)

_____   _____   _____
(Provider Name)   (Signature)   (Date)

FIGURE 5.1. Sample class contract.

The provider presents the general philosophy of CBSST as a skills training class that emphasizes how thoughts can influence feelings and actions. He or she briefly describes the three modules, emphasizing that cognitive, communication, and problem-solving skills are taught to help people achieve recovery goals, and that people have to practice the skills at home to do well. The provider can use the following phrasing, which also appears in the CBSST session on goal setting in the Consumer Workbook:

"In CBSST, you will learn how to achieve your personal goals by thinking about your thoughts and learning new skills. You will learn how to change unhelpful thinking, communicate better with others, and solve problems. Plan to participate actively. The more you participate, the more you will get from CBSST. Feel free to ask questions and make comments during discussions, and talk about the program with others. Discussing the material with others will help you improve the skills you learn. It will be very important to practice the skills you learn at home, so that you can reach your goals."

Changing Unhelpful Thinking

People are more likely to learn and remember if you teach by asking questions in a discussion through guided discovery rather than by lecturing. To stimulate discussion about how thoughts can influence feelings and behaviors, describe the following scenario, then ask the following questions, which can also be found in the Consumer Workbook in the session on goal setting:

Scenario: A guy bumps into you on the street and you immediately think he did it on purpose to hurt you.

1. How would this situation make you feel?
2. Would you shout at him or shove him?
3. Would this make you want to be around people more or less?
4. Can you see how the thought influenced your feelings and actions?

During the discussion, try to elicit and label an unhelpful thought, such as "He did it on purpose," and point out that such thoughts are unhelpful because they:

- Can prevent us from working on our goals (e.g., if we isolate to avoid perceived threats) and make us feel bad.
- Make it difficult to tell the difference between real and unreal experiences.
- Make it difficult to have relationships, work, or go to school.

Emphasize that:

- This class will teach how to change inaccurate, unhelpful thoughts that prevent us from achieving our goals.

It is not necessary for consumers to understand this cognitive model fully in this first session; there will be significant focus on learning this in the Cognitive Skills Module. At this point, it is important to be enthusiastic and hopeful about the idea that we have control over our own thoughts and beliefs, so we can change them if we want to, and if we change them, we can change our lives. Instill hope and optimism about this new way of thinking that you will teach and how it can help people achieve their recovery goals.

Review At-Home Practice

The at-home practice assigned in the final session of the previous module is reviewed for consumers who have just completed that module. Reviewing this homework provides both an opportunity to continue teaching the skills from the previous module for previous members and examples for newcomers of the types of skills that are trained in CBSST and the benefits of practicing at home. If this is the first CBSST session for all consumers in a class, then there is no at-home practice to review, so this item can be left off the agenda. Additional guidance on reviewing at-home practice in Session 1 of each module is provided in Chapters 6–8.

Set Goals

Collaborative goal setting is an effective method for encouraging and achieving change in consumers with serious mental illness. This process begins with clarifying which recovery outcomes are most valued by each consumer and deliberately choosing the outcome that would improve his or her quality of life the most. The goal-setting process can be challenging. The ability to formulate and pursue goals is a fundamental ability that may be impaired by mental illness, but people in recovery must overcome this impairment to engage in rehabilitation. Setting personally relevant recovery goals and tracking progress toward achievement of these goals can be a powerful treatment in and of itself.

In the CBSST program, setting a recovery goal that is personally meaningful to the consumer is an essential first step. Recovery goals involve the ability to function in living, learning, working or socializing domains. Specific long-term goals include making a friend, having a boyfriend or girlfriend, moving from a board-and-care facility to independent living, taking a class, or finding paid or volunteer work. The first session of each CBSST module includes goal-setting exercises, and these goals then become the focus of the thought-challenging, communication skills training, and problem-solving interventions in the CBSST program. Linking skills practice to personal recovery goals is motivating—for example: "If you practice the 3C's skill at home, you will get better at changing the unhelpful thoughts that get in the way of you having a girlfriend." This is called "bridging the skill–goal gap." Skills are learned because they help people achieve their recovery goals. If this skill–goal link is clearly explained for each skill, motivation to practice the skills will be increased.

Depending on available resources and time, goal setting can be done in group sessions or in individual sessions that supplement group. We recommend supplementing group sessions with individual goal-setting sessions when possible, but if this is not possible, goals can be effectively set in the group setting. Individual sessions allow more time to develop personalized goals and plan the detailed steps needed to achieve the goal. Consumers with severe negative symptoms, such as apathy, amotivation, or hopelessness about change, may also require more time and individual attention to develop goals. Consumers may also be more open and willing to share hopes and dreams in individual sessions rather than in a group. Periodic individual goal progress sessions (e.g., every 6–12 weeks) can also help to modify goals and set additional short-term goals and goal steps to achieve larger, long-term goals.

Introducing Goal Setting

Providers can use the following sentences to introduce goal setting. This text also appears in the Consumer Workbook for this session, so consumers can read along or providers can ask for a volunteer to read from the workbook:

> "One of the best ways to improve the quality of our lives is to set goals. In today's class, we are going to set at least one personal goal. The purpose of this program is to help you learn skills that will help you reach your goals. The best goals are things that you really, really want, that will improve the quality of your life, like finding a girlfriend or boyfriend, making a new friend, having more fun with friends, reconnecting with family, living independently, taking a class, getting a job, or volunteering. We can break it down into small steps you can do each week to accomplish a long-term goal in the next 6 months to a year. The longest journey starts with the first step. Small steps lead to bigger goals. For example, if you wash the dishes today and pay your own bills tomorrow, then soon you will be someone who takes care of your own apartment."

Identifying Long-Term Goals

Providers can begin a goal-setting discussion by asking consumers to describe individual strengths, how they spend their time, the things they enjoy doing now or used to enjoy doing, and any problems they would like to address. Providers can guide this discussion to explore changes that consumers would like to make in specific areas to enjoy life more. These desired changes can be developed into long-term goals, for example, "Sounds like you are bored staying at home all the time and would like to go out, maybe with a friend, and have fun." Strengths and activities people enjoy can also be transformed into long-term goals, for example, "You are good with computers and like going online. Maybe there is something you could do with computers that you would enjoy, like classes, volunteering, or working on computers somewhere." Allocate a set amount of time for each newcomer to identify a long-term meaningful goal during the first session of each module. To facilitate long-term goal setting, Appendix B includes several goal-setting games and activities.

Identifying Short-Term Goals and Goal Steps

Long-term goals are then broken down into smaller, short-term goals and goal steps. It is often challenging to break down long-term goals into attainable steps, but this is a crucial process to prevent consumers from being overwhelmed by big goals. Breaking down big goals into tasks that can easily be accomplished that day or that week emphasizes that small tasks accomplished immediately lead to larger goal achievements down the road. "A journey of a thousand miles begins with a single step" (Laozi, 1963). Breaking down big recovery goals into specific, attainable steps instills hope and empowers consumers to believe they can achieve big goals one step at a time. The "7–7–7 Goal Jackpot!" timeline process can be used to help consumers learn to do this. Long-term goals likely require 7 or more months to be achieved, short-term goals can be achieved in about 7 weeks, and goal steps can be achieved in 7 days or less— that is, the 7–7–7, Goal Jackpot! Sharing this rule with consumers is a positive way to help them break down big, long-term goals into smaller tasks that can accomplished each week.

Goals and goal steps are written on the 7–7–7 Goal Jackpot! Worksheet, which is included as the at-home practice assignment in the Consumer Workbook in Session 1 of each module. The worksheet is similar to the goal-tracking sheets used in the Illness Management and Recovery Program (Gingerich & Mueser, 2011; Meyer et al., 2010). Figure 5.2 is an example of a partially completed goal worksheet in the Consumer Workbook that can be used as a teaching tool in session. In the example worksheet, Jane describes being lonely and would like to "have a boyfriend" (long-term goal). To achieve this long-term goal, she may need to learn how "improve conversations" (short-term goal), which might involve goal steps to generate possible conversation topics, practice in starting and stopping conversations, and practice in asking someone for a date. Another short-term goal might be to "improve hygiene" to be more attractive to potential partners, with goal steps to shower, brush teeth,

---

PROVIDER TIP

Hit the 7–7–7 Goal Jackpot!

When setting goals, use this timeline to teach consumers how to break down big long-term goals into manageable goal steps that can be accomplished each week:

- Long-term goals can take longer than 7 months to achieve.
- Short-term goals can be achieved in 7 weeks.
- Goal steps are homework assignments that can be achieved in 7 days.

Name: _Jane_   **Date Long-Term Goal Set:** _Oct. 1_

Long-Term (Meaningful) Goal (7 months): _Have a boyfriend_

Short-Term Goals Related to the Long-Term Goal (7 weeks):
(check off steps when you complete them)

1. _Improve hygiene_   **2.** _Improve conversations_

Steps (7 days):

1. Separate clean/dirty laundry ✓
2. Do laundry 2X per week ✓
3. Brush teeth A.M./P.M. ✓
4. Shower daily ✓

Steps (7 days):

1. Draft list of possible topics ✓
2. Practice starting conversations ✓
3. Practice ending conversations
4. Practice asking someone for a date

FIGURE 5.2. Example of a partially completed 7–7–7 Goal Jackpot! Worksheet.

and wear clean clothes. We recommend that providers keep a copy of all goal worksheets. If goal steps are developed as tasks that can be accomplished with 7 days, the worksheet becomes a useful resource to refer to when identifying at-home practice assignments that can be completed before the next class (typically within a week).

The group process can facilitate goal setting if providers encourage new consumers to draw on the experiences of other group members to brainstorm possible goals and goal steps, as well as to problem-solve ways of overcoming obstacles. Group members who have already set goals and worked on goal steps in prior CBSST modules can update their Goal-Setting Worksheets by checking off goal steps achieved and adding additional steps. Celebrate, applaud, and reinforce every step achieved when checking off steps and remind consumers that each step brings them closer to their long-term goal. This provides a model for goal setting and illustrates goal achievement successes to promote hope in newcomers.

Goal-Setting Case Example: Juan

Juan expressed frustration with his current roommate at his board-and-care home: "My roommate always treats me bad. I can't take it anymore." He added that he is very "annoyed" with his board-and-care manager, because the manager intrusively inquires about his activities and interactions with others. When the provider asked Juan if he had discussed these concerns with his roommate or the manager, Juan replied, "No, they'll never listen to me." The provider noted Juan's defeatist expectations about not being able to change the behavior of his roommates and manager, and planned to mention them later when providing a rationale for setting goal steps and describing the skills he will learn in CBSST. It was clear that Juan was dissatisfied with his current living situation, so the provider asked Juan if his primary long-term goal might be to "move into his own apartment." Juan confirmed that it was. Since Juan has had previous experience living independently, the provider and Juan discussed what went well, the skills he already possesses, what went wrong, and skills in need of improvement in order to live independently in an apartment. Part of this conversation is presented below to illustrate how Juan and the provider completed a 7–7–7 Goal Jackpot! Worksheet (see Figure 5.3) and broke down Juan's long-term goal into two short-term goals with related goal steps. Notice how the provider asks questions to develop goals (i.e., uses guided discovery), rather than providing all the answers.

PROVIDER: You mentioned that you lived in an apartment before. Why did you move to the board-and-care?

JUAN: I can't manage my own money. I had a hard time remembering to save enough money to pay my bills or for groceries. Sometimes my landlord would get mad because I paid the rent late, and he eventually kicked me out.

PROVIDER: It sounds like learning to better manage your money would help you achieve your long-term goal of living in an apartment again. Do you agree?

JUAN: Yes, that makes sense.

PROVIDER: OK. Let's write down "Learn to manage money" as one short-term goal. That sounds like something you could learn to do in about 7 weeks. Do you see how we are breaking down a big goal, like moving into your own apartment, which could take 7 or more months to achieve, into more manageable things we can accomplish in about 7 weeks, like learning to manage money? The next step is to break that down even more into things we can do each week, in 7 days or less, to better manage money. We call this the 7–7–7 Goal Jackpot!; you get the big jackpot of achieving the big goal by taking small steps toward the goal each week. What could you do in a week to work toward managing money better? What would you be doing if you were a good money manager?

JUAN: I would pay my rent on time and have money for groceries.

PROVIDER: What do you need to do to be sure you have enough money to pay for these things?

JUAN: I guess I would need to save money and plan a budget.

PROVIDER: OK, so let's put "open a savings account" and "complete a budget worksheet" on the goal worksheet as goal steps. Do you think you could do each of these steps in a week?

JUAN: Well, I don't know how to get a savings account, what bank to go to, or where to get a budget worksheet.

PROVIDER: One of the skills you will learn in the CBSST program is how to solve problems like these. I have seen lots of people learn to use these skills to solve these types of problems in a week, and I'm sure you can do it, too.

Name: _Juan_   **Date Long-Term Goal Set:** _November 19_

Long-Term (Meaningful) Goal (7 months): _Move into my own apartment_

Short-Term Goals Related to the Long-Term Goal (7 weeks):
(check off steps when you complete them)

1. _Learn to manage money_   2. _Improve communication with roommates_

                                          and building manager

Steps (7 days):   **Steps (7 days):**

1. _Open a savings account_ ✓   1. _Negotiate quiet hours with roommates_ ✓

2. _Complete a budget worksheet_ ✓   2. _Learn to express frustration w/roommate_

3. _Check thoughts about managing money_ 3. _Check thoughts about roommates_ ✓

4. _Learn how to get a money order_   4. _Identify ways to practice ADLs at B&C_

Start Date: _November 19_   **Start Date:** _November 19_

Date Reviewed: _January 2_   **Date Reviewed:** _January 2_

Modified/Next Steps: **Modified/Next Steps:**

1. _Withdraw $12 for transit pass_   1. _____

2. _Find out how to get off payee status_ 2. _____

3. _____   3. _____

4. _____   4. _____

FIGURE 5.3. Example of a completed 7–7–7 Goal Jackpot! Worksheet for Juan.

The provider also made note of Juan's statement (thought) that he cannot manage his own money and encouraged Juan to include a goal step to check out thoughts that can interfere with his confidence in managing his own money (see Figure 5.3). The provider will later teach thought-challenging skills in the Cognitive Skills Module, so it is useful to try to add goal steps related to challenging thoughts that will be checked off as homework assignments accomplished in that module. Adding goal steps to "check thoughts about . . ." provides an opportunity to introduce briefly how thoughts are related to actions and feelings (cognitive model) and how this will be a focus of the CBSST program. For example:

PROVIDER: Do you think you are more or less likely to try to manage your own money if you think, "I will mess it up" or "I'm bad with handling my money?"

JUAN: Probably less likely.

PROVIDER: Right! Why try if you think you are just going to mess it up?

JUAN: But it's true; I have messed up with money a lot in the past.

PROVIDER: Maybe, but who knows what the future holds; we can't predict the future. If you learn new money management skills, you might do it well in the future. A common mistake in thinking that we all do is predicting the future, like predicting we will mess it up, when we don't really know what will happen. In the CBSST program we will learn to identify and correct thoughts like this that could be mistakes, so we have a better chance of success. If you change the thought to "I might be able to learn how to manage money," do you think you are more or less likely to succeed at managing money so you can get your own apartment?

JUAN: More likely to succeed, I suppose.

The second short-term goal Juan and the provider identified was to improve communication with his roommate and the board-and-care manager. The provider pointed out that Juan has an opportunity to learn more effective communication skills to improve his living situation as much as possible while still living in the board-and-care and added that these skills will then increase the likelihood of success when he moves into an apartment with a new roommate and apartment manager. Provider and consumer then collaborated to develop goal steps related to expressing unpleasant feelings to a roommate, negotiating rules (e.g., quiet hours), and discussing with the board-and-care manager ways that Juan can practice and take responsibility for more activities of daily living prior to moving to an apartment. These goal steps can later be checked off as homework assignments completed in the Social Skills Module (e.g., expressing unpleasant feelings, making positive requests). These goal steps might be developed as follows:

PROVIDER: We added "Improve communication with roommates and manager" as the second short-term goal. The next task is to think of steps we can take to work on this short-term goal each week. You mentioned that your roommate treats you badly. What is one way that you are treated badly?

JUAN: He won't let me sleep. He is always doing things in our room late at night that wake me up.

PROVIDER: You sound very frustrated with your roommate's behavior. I wonder if we could think of some ways to talk to your roommate about setting some quiet hours in your room. What do you think about that?

JUAN: No way. He's just going to get mad.

PROVIDER: One of the skills we will work on during this class is how to effectively ask people to do things you want them to do and how to express unpleasant feelings, like telling people that what they are doing makes you mad and suggesting what else they can do instead. It might be worth trying these skills to see if they work with your roommate. Would you be willing to just give it a shot, even if we don't know how your roommate will respond?

JUAN: It won't work, but we can try.

PROVIDER: I appreciate your willingness to try and test it out. Let's add "Negotiate quiet hours with roommate" as one of the goal steps under this short-term goal.

At the end of the session, the provider summarized how the skills Juan will learn in CBSST will help him accomplish his long-term goal. Note that Juan's goal worksheet includes goal steps related to the skills trained in the three CBSST modules, which is helpful because the goal worksheet will be used to generate ideas for homework assignments. The provider referred to goal steps related to checking out defeatist expectations about money management and changing the behavior of roommates and managers, and described how CBSST thought-challenging skills will help Juan test the accuracy of those thoughts, how problem-solving skills will help him solve problems related to money management, as well as how learning effective communication skills will help him address concerns with current and future roommates and managers. The provider emphasized that learning skills to achieve these goal steps each week in the CBSST program will lead to achieving the short-term goals they set today, as well as other short-term goals they will set later in the program (e.g., "find an affordable apartment") and eventually the long-term goal of living in his own apartment. The provider assigned homework to generate at least one other step Juan could do in a week to become a better money manager and write it on the worksheet. By the next session, Juan added, "Learn how to get a money order," and when the worksheet was reviewed at the start of the next module 6 weeks later, Juan added two other steps for this short-term goal.

Goal-Setting Case Example: Carol

During the initial goal-setting session, Carol complained of feeling "bored" and "not having any fun" due to limited activities outside her board-and-care home. When asked how she would prefer to spend her day, Carol had some difficulty identifying alternative activities and later admitted it was because of concern about experiencing symptoms (i.e., voices) in the community (e.g., "People will laugh at me because I talk back to the voices"), not being able to use the transit system (e.g., "I will get lost"), and a belief that the "cartels" would harm her if she left her home. The provider asked Carol what she would do if she were better able to manage the voices and more confident that she could leave her board-and-care home without being harmed. However, Carol further explained why she could not do anything to "get rid of the voices" and the multitude of ways the cartels could follow and harm her. The provider used "the magic wand question" and asked what Carol would do if she could wave a magic wand and get rid of the voices and the threat of the cartel.

> PROVIDER: Are you willing to do an exercise together that can be helpful when we think we are stuck or facing impossible barriers preventing us from doing the things we enjoy?
>
> CAROL: Sure. I'll try it.
>
> PROVIDER: Let's pretend that I hand you a magic wand. This wand is very powerful and, when waved, can make all of these concerns go away—the voices would disappear and there would no longer be any threat of harm from the cartels.
>
> CAROL: That would never happen. The cartels are too powerful.
>
> PROVIDER: Maybe not but just pretending that it can, if I waved the wand, what would your future look like? Who would you be talking to? What would you do during the day?
>
> CAROL: Well, I would probably go out more. It's really boring at my board-and-care place.
>
> PROVIDER: What types of activities would you do? Where would you go?
>
> CAROL: Maybe I'd go to the coffee shop by my house or go to a clubhouse.

Carol and the provider continued to brainstorm some possible activities without focusing on the possible barriers. Eventually, Carol acknowledged that she enjoys caring for animals and has had a long-held desire to work with animals at a shelter. Prior to the onset of Carol's symptoms, she briefly held competitive employment positions, but she did not have the desire nor did she feel prepared to start working again. Carol stated that she would feel comfortable with the flexibility of volunteering at a shelter. Based on their conversation, the provider was confident that this was a meaningful long-term goal to Carol and then proceeded to collaboratively identify two short-term goals with goal steps and began working on the 7–7–7 Goal Jackpot! Worksheet (see Figure 5.4).

> PROVIDER: Carol, it sounds like obtaining a volunteer position at an animal shelter is something you would really like to work on. This is a big goal that is easier to achieve if we break it down into short-term goals you can accomplish in about 7 weeks and further break those goals into steps you can take each week, in 7 days to work toward your big goal of working at an animal shelter. We call that the 7–7–7 Goal Jackpot! It's a way to learn how to break big goals into manageable steps to take every 7 days. Thinking back to your previous experiences while working, what might be some of the tasks you will need to do first. What do you need to do to get ready to volunteer?

CAROL: I guess I need to figure out where I can volunteer and how to apply, but it will be hard to find a place that will hire me. I wasn't sick when I worked before. A shelter won't hire someone with schizophrenia.

PROVIDER: Your thoughts about a shelter not hiring you are important and they are certainly something we can talk about further. You mentioned needing to locate some shelters. Maybe a helpful short-term goal is to prepare yourself for employment. This might include identifying some shelters, asking if they have any volunteer positions, and requesting an application. How does that sound?

CAROL: We can try that, but I'm not sure how I can get there.

PROVIDER: You brought up an important point about getting there. If you aren't familiar with the transit system here, we could include a short-term goal about learning how to use the transit system.

CAROL: I've tried it before, but I got lost. I don't want to do that again. It took me a long time to find my way home.

PROVIDER: It sounds like you are thinking you will get lost again. In the CBSST program, we check out thoughts like that to make sure they are correct, because if you expect to get lost again, you probably won't try taking the bus, which can prevent you from working at a shelter. Learning to check unhelpful thoughts like that is a skill we can work on together. As part of this class, we will also discuss a problem-solving strategy that will be very helpful to you while you learn how to use the transit system. Would you like to add this as a short-term goal?

CAROL: Yes. It is something I need to do. I need to do something to get to an animal shelter.

Notice how the provider described some of the skills that will be trained in CBSST as part of the goal-setting process. Anticipating that learning to catch, check and change unhelpful thoughts will be an important focus of treatment, the provider included goal steps to check out thoughts (defeatist expectations) about getting lost on the bus and not getting hired at a shelter. The remaining goal steps for the "Use public transit system" short-term goal were added during a brief discussion about what Carol might need to do to ride the bus (e.g., find bus routes, practice riding the bus, purchase a transit pass). Despite some initial resistance from Carol, the provider also encouraged her to add a goal step for checking her thoughts about how the "cartels" night harm her if she rides the bus, and how "voices cannot be controlled." Carol agreed to do so, but only after the goal worksheet was reviewed at the start of the next module. The provider expected that the thoughts would arise as soon as Carol began working on getting on the bus.

Name: _Carol_   **Date Long-Term Goal Set:** _March 3_

Long-Term (Meaningful) Goal (7 months): _Volunteer at an animal shelter_

Short-Term Goals Related to the Long-Term Goal (7 weeks):
(check off steps when you complete them)

1. _Use public transit system_   **2.** _Prepare for employment_

Steps (7 days):   *Steps (7 days):*

1. _Find bus route to provider office_ ✓   1. _Identify possible shelters_ ✓

2. _Practice bus route to office_ ✓   2. _Role play asking about positions_ ✓

3. _Purchase transit pass_ ✓   3. _Complete an application_ ✓

4. _Check out thoughts on getting lost_ ✓   4. _Check thought "They won't hire me"_ ✓

Start Date: _March 3_   **Start Date:** _March 3_

Date Reviewed: _April 27_   **Date Reviewed:** _April 27_

Modified/Next Steps: **Modified/Next Steps:**

1. _Check thought "The cartels will hurt me"_   1. _Wash clothes_

2. _Check thoughts about voices_   2. _Practice interview_

3. _Practice the bus route to the beach_   3. _Shower for interview_

4. _____   4. _____

Date Reviewed: _____   **Date Reviewed:** _____

FIGURE 5.4. Example of a completed 7–7–7 Goal Jackpot! Worksheet for Carol.

With regard to the "prepare for employment" short-term goal, the provider and Carol collaborated to come up with a few practical aspects of locating and obtaining a volunteer job (e.g., identifying possible shelters and obtaining and completing applications). Carol and the provider also discussed the likelihood of needing to interview for the position, and the provider took the opportunity to introduce briefly the Social Skills Module by providing examples of how communication skills could help (e.g., role playing how to respond to interview questions and making a positive request for an application). The provider also pointed out that Carol had expressed doubts about being hired ("They won't hire me") and suggested that she also include checking out those thoughts as an important goal step that might later be addressed during the Cognitive Skills Module.

SMART Goals

One strategy providers can use to guide goal setting is to set SMART goals. SMART is an acronym that stands for the desirable qualities of goals: <u>S</u>pecific, <u>M</u>eaningful (or <u>M</u>otivating), <u>A</u>greed upon, <u>R</u>ealistic, and <u>T</u>imely.

SPECIFIC GOALS

Goal steps are best stated in specific behavioral terms that can be observed and measured. It should be very clear when the goal or goal step has been accomplished. For example, the goal, "I will keep my room cleaner," is vague. It is not clear what a cleaner room would look like or what would need to happen to achieve the goal. In contrast, the goal, "I will keep my dirty clothes in a hamper, instead of on the floor," is specific and it will be easy to determine whether it is accomplished. Long-term goals (e.g., "move to independent housing") and, to some extent, short-term goals (e.g., "improve home care") are often stated in less specific terms than goal steps, because checking off specific observable achievements in goal steps is evidence that larger goals are being achieved.

PROVIDER TIP

Set SMART Goal Steps

S—Specific   Only goal steps should be clearly articulated in behavioral and measurable terms that can be observed. How will you know the goal has been achieved? What exactly will the consumer *do* if the goal is achieved?

M—Meaningful   Only the long-term goal should be a personally meaningful recovery goal chosen by the consumer. Consumers are more likely to engage in skills practice in session and at home if practice is linked to achieving meaningful, valued goals. The long-term goal is the **M**otivator.

A—Agreed upon   Goal setting is a collaborative process between provider and consumer. Both parties must agree upon the goals if they are to work together to achieve them.

R—Realistic   To increase success experiences, goal steps must be realistic, attainable tasks that are easy to accomplish as homework assignments. It is more difficult to judge whether long-term goals are realistic. We all have limitations, and illness places limits on achievement, but until we try, we cannot know what we can achieve over the long term.

T—Timely   Select target dates for long-term goals, short-term goals and goal steps using the "7–7–7 Goal Jackpot!" timeline.

MEANINGFUL GOALS

A meaningful (or motivating) goal is one that is valued and desired by a consumer who believes it will lead to a real improvement in quality of life. A meaningful goal can motivate engagement in CBSST classes and completion of at-home practice assignments, if the consumer believes that engagement in CBSST will lead to achievement of the goal. We have found that the most meaningful goals are about functioning (e.g., increasing socialization, relationships, leisure activities, independent housing, education, work or volunteering). To assess whether the goal is highly desired and meaningful, we have found it helpful to ask, "Why do you want [the goal]? How would your life be better?" Consumers of all ages, but especially older consumers who have had more experience with the mental health system, may at first offer a goal that they think providers want to hear (e.g., "I want to take my medications more regularly"). They may offer other socially desirable goals that someone *should* want. For example, a consumer might say, "I want to get a job," but upon further questioning, the person may acknowledge no real desire to work, although he or she would like to have more money for recreational activities with friends or to move to better housing. Although our personal value systems as providers may lead us to assume that consumers will highly value work or education goals, we cannot assume that these are goals valued by everyone. We need to keep asking questions until we are convinced the goal is truly valued and meaningful to the individual consumer. Even if goals are highly desired, a defeatist belief (e.g., "I'm too sick to get a job") might interfere with verbalizing the goal. Such defeatist beliefs can be addressed using the cognitive restructuring techniques in the Cognitive Skills Module. Long-term goals might be revised as consumers have the courage to endorse more meaningful goals when defeatist beliefs are changed during treatment.

Only long-term goals need to be personally meaningful; this is less important for short-term goals and goal steps. In fact, many short-term goals and goal steps are often not inherently rewarding. For example, it is a burden to remember to take medications, and taking them can lead to distressing side effects or self-stigma associated with a person being reminded that he or she has a mental illness each time he or she takes them. These barriers to medication adherence can be overcome by focusing on long-term goals that are facilitated by medication adherence (e.g., being able to go to work or function in family roles with medications). In this way, short-term goals or goal steps (e.g., "take medications as prescribed") can be motivated by linking them to achievement of a meaningful long-term goal (e.g., "be a good mother" or "get a volunteer job").

Some consumers may name a long-term goal that is actually a means for achieving a much more valued goal. For example, a consumer says, "I want to lose 20 pounds." This may be a useful short-term goal, but it is not a motivating long-term goal, so ask questions until you arrive at a more meaningful goal. You might ask, "Why do you want to lose 20 pounds?"; "What would be different if you lost weight?"; "How would your life be better?" These questions may reveal that losing

PROVIDER TIP

Meaningful Long-Term Goals Are Motivators

To be sure a goal is personally meaningful, keep asking questions until you are convinced you have arrived at a truly meaningful long-term goal:

- "Why do you want to _____?"
- "What would be different if you achieved _____?"
- "How would your life be better?"

weight will lead to being more attractive in order to *have a girlfriend or boyfriend*, or to being healthier and less fatigued in order to *do fun things with friends* or *be a better parent*. These long-term goals would help motivate someone to lose 20 pounds. The rationale for participating in CBSST classes and practicing at home is that quality of life will be better if a meaningful goal is achieved. A long-term goal that the consumer truly desires and believes will improve his or her life will help motivate active participation. Remind consumers, "If you complete this task at home, you will be one step closer to your goal."

AGREED-UPON GOALS

CBSST is a collaborative learning program, so providers and consumers must mutually agree that the goals are achievable and worth pursuing. Goals that are not agreed upon are usually not achieved. If the provider decides on the goals without consumer buy-in, or consumers choose goals that are not relevant to provider-valued outcomes, then motivation and engagement in the learning process can be reduced in both parties. For example, a goal to stay at home and read a book per week is specific, realistic, time-bound, and could enrich quality of life in some ways, but it may not have obvious relevance to improving community functioning, and it could even have negative consequence by contributing, for example, to social isolation. The provider who asks, "How will your life be better (or how much better) if you read this many books?" can begin a conversation about how meaningful the goal is. Further questioning could lead to a broader educational or recreational goal. Similarly, working on goals related to delusions, such as exorcising demons or fighting against a conspiracy, can distract from working on productive community function activities. Although providers might not agree with such goals, we have found it helpful to avoid direct disagreements, because they can interfere with rapport and treatment engagement. It is possible to agree with goals that are not recovery-oriented by listing them on the 7–7–7 Goal Jackpot! Worksheet as short-term goals, or goal steps, rather than long-term goals. For example, by asking, "What would you do during the day if the demons were exorcised (or the conspiracy was exposed)?" it may be possible to uncover a meaningful long-term recovery goal (e.g., "Well, then

I could go back to school"). A short-term goal that could facilitate attainment of the long-term goal could then be "manage the demons" or "cope with the conspiracy." Related goal steps might include "Figure out if demons can be controlled" or "Find out if they are always watching," based on the rationale that if demons can be controlled or if enemies are not always watching, then work on the long-term goal is sometimes possible. These goal steps can be the target of behavioral experiments and other thought-challenging interventions in the Cognitive Skills Module. Other short-term goals (e.g., "register for a class") that also may be included are more directly related to the long-term goal. In this way, providers can collaborate with consumers to develop an agreed-upon recovery plan that is both consumer- and provider-driven.

REALISTIC GOALS

Goal steps should be simple, realistic, attainable tasks that lead to successful experiences that boost self-efficacy. Goal steps are deliberately developed to be clearly attainable within a week, so that they can be assigned for at-home practice. It is more difficult to estimate the timeline for successful achievement of long-term goals. Keep an open mind. The only way to determine whether a long-term goal is achievable is to try to achieve it. We recommend not discouraging consumers from setting challenging goals, if the goals are meaningful to them. It is more important to focus on whether goal steps and short-term goals are realistic and attainable. Accomplishing goal steps toward short-term goals will likely lead to important improvements in functioning, regardless of whether the larger goal is achieved in the long term.

Consider the consumer who set the long-term goal "to be a rock star." This was a real childhood dream of his, and he enjoyed playing guitar and writing songs in the past. He frequently shared this dream with people, who often responded that it was not a realistic goal. Given that he was highly motivated to work on any tasks related to becoming a rock star, it was agreed that this would be the long-term goal. His short-term goals were to "improve guitar playing," and "join a band." Goal steps included tasks such as "find a used guitar," "save money to buy a guitar," "take lessons," "practice playing," "identify places to meet musicians," "identify places to play for people," "play in front of an audience," "learn to listen to bandmates," "learn to be assertive with bandmates," and "learn to be confident in front of an audience." In CBSST, problem-solving skills were used to accomplish most goal steps related to getting and playing a guitar and finding places to play. Social skills training was used to improve communication and negotiations with bandmates, and cognitive skills were used to challenge unhelpful thoughts about what others (e.g., bandmates, guitar teachers, audiences) thought about him and his playing. Over the course of CBSST, he purchased a guitar and enjoyed playing, went to coffee shops and music stores, and became less isolated. He played guitar and sang for the CBSST group, at a clubhouse, and at coffee shops. He joined a band, began to form friendships, and developed a social network around his music goals. As he focused more attention on his music and was not ruminating alone at home, he became less concerned and distressed about the malicious intentions he attributed to his voices. The steps he took toward his long-term rock star goal led to important changes in his socialization and leisure activities, as well as symptom reductions, which significantly improved his quality of life.

TIMELY GOALS

To help identify a timeline to accomplish long-term and short-term goals and goal steps, we have found the previously discussed "7–7–7 Goal Jackpot!" rule helpful (see the Provider Tip on page 79).

Using Pie Charts to Turn Roles into Goals

One common belief shared by individuals with serious mental illness is that they are defined by illness and disability (e.g., "I'm a schizophrenic, so I can't do normal things"). This thought obviously interferes with recovery goal achievement. If people are consumed by thinking of themselves in only one role, as "a sick person," it is difficult to expect growth and change. A pie chart technique can be used to help consumers become aware of all the roles they currently play in life, as well as potential new roles. New roles can become new goals. The steps for the technique are as follows:

1. Draw a circle on a piece of paper or whiteboard.
2. Write "I'm a schizophrenic" or "I'm a patient" in the middle of the circle.
3. Then, draw another circle and a sequence of pie slices that represent various roles (e.g., brother/sister, mother/father, son/daughter, neighbor, friend, student, employee, artist, musician) to show that people are defined by much more than their illness. Turn new roles into goals. Examples of finished pie charts are shown in Figure 5.5.

Symptom Goals

Often people with serious mental illness initially set goals to stop feeling a certain way (e.g., "I just don't want to be depressed anymore"), stop harmful behaviors (e.g., "I need to stop drinking and using drugs" or "I need to quit smoking"), eliminate psychotic symptoms (e.g., "I want to get rid of my voices" or "I need to stop the government from spying on me"), or stop unhealthy lifestyle behaviors (e.g., "I need to lose weight"). These common "symptom goals" are often addressed in treatment plans, but they are not recovery goals. The CBSST program is more effective when consumers set long-term recovery goals, because consumers are typically

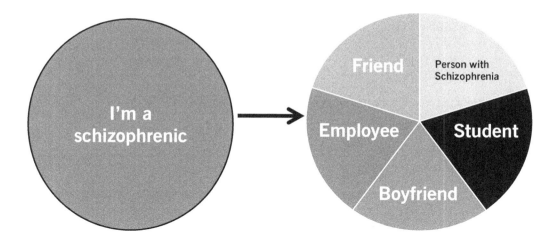

FIGURE 5.5. Example of completed pie charts turning roles into goals.

more motivated to engage in treatment if they believe it will result in a meaningful improvement in quality of life. Although symptom reduction remains an important treatment goal, consumers, families, and advocacy groups frequently describe recovery goals as being of chief concern to them. In the CBSST program, symptoms are addressed as short-term goals when they interfere with long-term recovery goals, but the primary focus is on personally meaningful recovery goals.

A symptom goal can become an obstacle to achieving a recovery goal when consumers believe they cannot work on recovery goals until their symptoms are eliminated. Consumers can get stuck in the mind-set that they cannot move on with their lives until the depression, voices, or delusional concerns are eliminated. They may assume that schizophrenia must be cured before moving on with life goals, so they spend the majority of their time focused on symptoms rather than on community life. Symptom relief is certainly an important part of treatment plans, and actions that can improve symptoms should be discussed (e.g., medication adherence and behavioral coping strategies). However, in CBSST, consumers are encouraged to pursue recovery goals despite their illness. We have found that meaningful, rewarding, social and community function activities can distract from symptoms, reducing their associated distress and severity. Isolation and avoidance of community activities can lead to more attention to voices and delusional beliefs, resulting in increased distress, worsening symptoms, and greater dysfunction. Symptom goals can be reframed as functional recovery goals by asking:

"How would you know you weren't sad anymore?"
"How would your life be different if that happened? What would you do?"
"If you didn't hear any voices, what would you be doing differently with your life?"

For the symptom goal "I want to stop being sad," the conversation might go as follows:

CONSUMER: I want to stop being sad.

PROVIDER: If you woke up happy one day, what would you do that day?

CONSUMER: I would do more things.

PROVIDER: What kinds of things?

CONSUMER: I don't know, going out, like to the movies or with friends.

PROVIDER: OK, so your goal is to go out with friends and do fun activities.

This is similar to the "magic wand" question:

"If I could wave a magic wand and make all your problems disappear, what would you do tomorrow? If you woke up one day and your problems were gone, what would you do differently that day? What would you start to do more of? Would you act differently with other people? When you wake up that day, where are you sleeping? Are you alone in your bed? What would you do first that day and do next, and do next?"

This can stimulate discussion about desired, meaningful relationships and activities.

The "life documentary" question can also help transform symptom goals into recovery goals:

"Suppose I followed you around with a video camera and filmed everything you do in your life for a week, and then, after we work hard in this class and your problems are much improved or even eliminated, we film your life again for a week. What would we see you do in the movie or hear you saying to other people? What would be different about the two movies before and after your problems are solved?"

One strategy for providers to assess whether a goal is a quality-of-life recovery goal is to ask yourself whether it passes the Dead Person Goal Test (Harris, 2009). Goals to stop symptoms or to stop feeling or behaving a certain way are "dead person" goals. Dead people are not targeted by conspiracies, they do not hear voices, get depressed, drink, use drugs or smoke cigarettes, and they lose a lot of weight. Long-term recovery goals are living goals; they are things a living person could do better than a dead person, such as work, go to school, volunteer, live independently, make friends, and have a family. The Dead Person Goal Test can help providers remember to guide goal-setting discussions toward recovery goals.

We do not discuss the Dead Person Goal Test with consumers, because it can be offensive to be told your goal failed any test, but especially a test for goals even a dead person could achieve. It is not helpful to disagree directly with consumers, because this can interfere with rapport and treatment engagement, and even make people angry. A provider once told a consumer that his personally meaningful goal (related to a delusion) was not a good goal, because even a dead person could achieve it. The consumer became angry and dropped out of treatment. As discussed earlier, it is possible to identify a living recovery goal by asking people what they would do differently and how quality of life would be improved if their goal to eliminate symptoms, feelings, or behaviors was achieved. In this way, providers can agree with dead person goals and list them on the Goal-Setting Sheet as short-term goals that can facilitate the achievement of the long-term recovery goal.

Goal-Setting Challenges

Cognitive impairments, negative symptoms, and dysfunctional attitudes can hinder goal setting. Cognitive impairments, like deficits in abstraction and problem solving, can lead to challenges with brainstorming, imagining a different life, and setting specific goal steps to achieve goals. In addition, consumers with severe negative symptoms such as apathy, amotivation, and asociality may have become complacent about the status of their lives. They may be reluctant to set goals due to dysfunctional attitudes such as low expectations for success or a better life. As discussed in Chapter 1, self-competency beliefs are central to motivation to engage in difficult goal-directed activities. People who expect to succeed are more willing to try new tasks, choose harder tasks, and work harder, because they think they will succeed. By acknowledging a goal, consumers must accept the risk of yet another failure. Unfortunately, these problems can be compounded by providers with low expectations for recovery. Many consumers have been advised not to work, not to take classes or take on challenges due to concerns that stress will lead to relapse and hospitalization. The advice may also be due to the misconception that people with schizophrenia are not capable of working or functioning well in society. For these reasons, hopelessness in consumers and providers can be a barrier to goal setting. We have found the following strategies helpful in overcoming these types of goal-setting challenges:

- Use cognitive therapy interventions such as the 3C's, mistakes in thinking, and behavioral experiments in the Cognitive Skills Module to address dysfunctional attitudes that lead to hopelessness and reluctance to set a meaningful goal.
- Use the goal-setting games and activities in Appendix B to activate low-energy consumers and provide a structure and concrete focus to compensate for cognitive impairments.

- Ask people to recall a time in the past when their quality of life was better (e.g., "Was there something you enjoyed doing back then that you are not doing as much now? What did you enjoy about it? Would you like to try to do that again?").
- Ask people to rate their level of satisfaction with different aspects of their life (e.g., "On a scale of 1 to 10, with 10 being the best, rate how satisfied you are with (1) your living situation, (2) school and other enrichment activities, (3) work or volunteer activities, (4) relationships with friends and family, (5) love life, and (6) leisure and recreation activities?" Discussion of areas of dissatisfaction can lead to recovery goals.
- Supplement group sessions with individual goal-setting sessions, which allows a slower pace and more personalized exploration.
- Use the previously discussed pie chart technique to transform roles into goals (see Figure 5.5). Pie charts can be helpful visual aids to compensate for cognitive impairments and help consumers brainstorm and imagine a fuller life with more rewarding roles than just "a schizophrenic" or "a patient."

If consumers seem stuck and find that it is very difficult to set a goal, take a step back, but keep trying and gently say, "It sounds like you believe things are the best they can be? Have you given up on making things better? How do you feel about that?" Try to remind consumers that they can get pleasure from activities (e.g., that they have laughed in session and can enjoy being with others), so they might be able to do things to make their life more enjoyable.

Challenge your own unhelpful beliefs about "unmotivated consumers." Provider appraisals of consumer motivation (e.g., "He is not motivated to come to class or do homework") can interfere with progress. For us as providers, shifting from labels ("unmotivated consumer") to situational descriptions ("an option that a consumer does not find motivating") can reduce our own frustration and hopelessness, and increase empathy, engagement, and effectiveness in our role. Beliefs about unmotivated consumers prevent providers from being good skills trainers. It is normal for interest in working on goals to fluctuate, and nobody is interested in everything all the time. By identifying a meaningful long-term goal that is truly of interest to the consumer, remaining positive about skills learning and goal progress, and addressing thoughts associated with ambivalence, providers can help consumers move from slips in motivation back to goal-directed action. By teaching people that they can succeed, providers can transform "unmotivated consumers" into "motivated consumers." People who expect to succeed are more motivated, willing to try new tasks, choose harder tasks, and try harder, because they think they will succeed. Providers can use cognitive skills to challenge their own inaccurate beliefs about consumer motivation and recovery. Use the data in Chapter 1 to challenge hopeless beliefs about recovery (e.g., "This consumer could never get a job, a home of his or her own, or a friend or partner").

Assign At-Home Practice: Setting Goals

The at-home practice assignment is to continue developing goals and goal steps, and writing them on the 7–7–7 Goal Jackpot! Worksheet at home. During the review of at-home practice at the beginning of the next session, additional session time is allocated to goal setting and reviewing the goal worksheets. For new group members, at-home practice assignments can be introduced in the following way:

> "It is important that you participate in this class regularly in order to achieve your goals. If you listen carefully, work hard, and practice the skills at home, you will reach your goals and improve the quality of your life. I will be here to help you learn skills and take steps toward your goals, but you will have to work at it too, both here and at home."

Summarize the Session

The key points to summarize for this session are:

- One of the best ways to improve the quality of our lives is to set goals. We can break big goals down into small steps we can do each week to eventually accomplish big goals.
- Unhelpful thoughts can prevent us from working on our goals and make us feel bad. Unhelpful thoughts are just mistakes in thinking that can be corrected by testing them out and gathering all the facts.
- In CBSST, we learn how to achieve our personal goals by thinking about our thoughts and learning new skills.

Ask for Consumer Feedback

Providers should ask consumers for feedback about the session. Possible questions include:

"How am I doing today? Am I explaining things clearly?"
"What did you find most helpful and least helpful?"
"What do you think about the way we were setting goals?"
(For newcomers) "What do you think about your first day in class? Do you think it will help you achieve your goals?"

PROVIDER TIP

Session Reminders

- Setting a meaningful recovery goal is essential to a successful outcome in CBSST. The goal motivates engagement, homework completion and behavior change.

- Identify functioning goals (living, learning, working, and socializing). Avoid goals to eliminate symptoms, feelings, and behaviors that do not pass the Dead Person Goal Test.

- The consumer must really WANT the goal (establish personal meaning), think he or she can do what is necessary to achieve the goal (self-efficacy), and believe the CBSST program will help him or her achieve the goal (bridge the skill–goal gap).

- Collaborate with consumers to set SMART goal steps.

- Use the 7–7–7 Goal Jackpot! Worksheet and timeline to set goals, and use the worksheet to guide treatment in the CBSST modules.

CHAPTER 6

Cognitive Skills Module

MODULE OBJECTIVES

1. Teach how thoughts are related to feelings and behaviors, and how recovery goals can be achieved by changing unhelpful thoughts.

2. Teach how to change unhelpful thoughts by using the 3C's (Catch It, Check It, Change It) skill, identifying mistakes in thinking and conducting behavioral experiments.

3. Practice using the 3C's to challenge thoughts that interfere with recovery goal achievement.

MODULE OVERVIEW

Cognitive therapy is the focus of this module, but cognitive therapy techniques are also used throughout the other two modules. Session 1 of this module, like the other two modules, is the Introduction and Goal-Setting session, in which new consumers can enter the class and recovery goals are set and reviewed using the 7–7–7 Goal Jackpot! Worksheet (see Chapter 5). In Session 2, consumers are introduced to the general concepts of cognitive therapy, including the relationship among thoughts, feelings, and behaviors (generic cognitive model), and are taught skills to challenge and change thoughts that interfere with recovery goal achievement in Sessions 3–6. The primary thoughts targeted are dysfunctional attitudes that contribute to negative symptoms and poor functioning, such as negative expectations about activities ("It won't be fun") and low self-efficacy beliefs ("I can't do it"), but psychosis-related beliefs are also addressed if they interfere with functioning ("I will be harmed by spirits if I go out"). By challenging and changing dysfunctional thoughts, consumers are more likely to engage in effortful, goal-directed functioning behaviors. The specific session content associated with module objectives is shown in Table 6.1.

The primary thought-challenging skill trained is the 3C's: Catch It, Check It, Change It; the "it" is the unhelpful thought. Using a series of increasingly complex thought record sheets, the 3C's steps are systematically taught. In Session 2, consumers identify and write down thoughts and label them as helpful or unhelpful. In Session 3 (Catch It), situational antecedents are linked to the unwanted feelings and behaviors that arise in them. This is done to emphasize that consumers need to use these feelings and behaviors as an alert or "red flag" reminder to examine their thinking (Catch It). In Session 4, (Check It), consumers are taught to examine evidence about the accuracy of thoughts and identify common mistakes in thinking (e.g., jumping to conclusions; all-or-none thinking). In Session 5 (Change It), alternatives therapy, Socratic questioning, and thought chaining are used to help consumers examine the logic of beliefs and generate more adaptive alternatives to mistakes in thinking or thoughts without sufficient evidence (see Chapter 3 for an overview of these techniques). In Session 6, behavioral experiments are introduced as a means of testing the accuracy of thoughts (Chapter 3 also describes this technique). The session then puts it all together as consumers practice using the 3C's skill by filling out 3C's Worksheets to challenge thoughts that interfere with goals. Table

TABLE 6.1. Cognitive Skills Module Objectives and Related Session Content

Cognitive Skills Module objectives	Session content
Introduce the general concepts of CBT, including the relationship between thoughts, feelings and actions, and how thoughts are related to recovery goals.	Discussion and at-home practice (homework) addressing relationships between thoughts, feelings and behaviors, identifying unhelpful thoughts, the difference between thoughts and feelings, and how different thoughts can lead to pleasant or unpleasant feelings and helpful or unhelpful goal-directed behaviors (Session 2).
Challenge and change unhelpful beliefs that lead to unpleasant feelings or interfere with real-world functioning and goal-directed action.	Teach and practice the 3C's thought-challenging skill: Catch it, Check it, Change it (Sessions 3–6), including Catching unhelpful thoughts (Session 3), Checking evidence for the accuracy of beliefs (Session 4), identifying common mistakes in thinking (e.g., jumping to conclusions, mind reading, all-or-none thinking, in Session 4), Changing to helpful thoughts (Session 5), and conducting behavioral experiments to test out thoughts (Session 6).
Increase self-efficacy and confidence in using thought challenging skills in the real world to achieve recovery goals.	Practice using the 3C's in session and at home to reduce conviction in defeatist beliefs, low self-efficacy beliefs, delusion-related beliefs and beliefs about voices that interfere with recovery goals (Sessions 4–6).

TABLE 6.2. 3C's Examples for Employment and Socialization

Situation/goal	Feelings/behaviors ("red flags")	Catch It	Check It	Change It
Sitting at home thinking about money *Goal:* Employment	Frustrated; sad; pessimistic Did nothing; did not fill out job application	"They will never hire me." "I'm not good enough." "It's too hard."	*Mistakes in thinking:* All-or-nothing thinking; fortune telling *Evidence for:* "I haven't worked in a long time. I will have to work long hours." *Evidence against:* "How do I know they won't hire me? I used to do a job like that. I can work hard."	"Maybe I can get an interview if I fill out the application." "Maybe I can succeed if I keep trying."
See a pretty girl and want to talk to her *Goal:* To have a relationship; increase social interaction	Scared; nervous; anxious Stayed quiet; did nothing	"She will laugh and reject me." "I'm flawed." "I will have nothing to say."	*Mistakes in thinking:* Jumping to conclusions; fortune telling *Evidence for:* "The last girl said no. I've been tongue-tied before." *Evidence against:* "Even movie stars don't get all girls to say yes. I've had girlfriends before. Everyone has weaknesses and strengths."	"Everyone doesn't have to like me; I only need to find one girl who does." "We can talk about something I know."

6.2 shows examples of how the 3C's can be used to challenge thoughts that interfere with specific recovery goals (e.g., employment and socialization) that were set in Session 1, the Introduction and Goal-Setting session. Table 6.2 provides examples that can be used to teach consumers how to fill out the 3C's Worksheets in the Cognitive Skills Module Consumer Workbook. Sessions 5 and 6 of the Consumer Workbook have additional examples of completed 3C's Worksheets.

USING THE COMMON THOUGHTS CHECKLIST

The Common Thoughts Checklist (see Appendix C) is a multiple-choice list of possible self-defeating thoughts for particular situations, with more hopeful, alternative thoughts listed to their right. When consumers are having difficulty identifying thoughts (starting in Session 2, but throughout the module), the checklist is a tool that can help them identify self-defeating thoughts that may interfere with goal attainment. The list can also be used to illustrate the link among thoughts, feelings, and behaviors (introduced in Session 2). To do so, ask consumers to iden-tify feelings and behaviors for defeatist thoughts, then ask what different feelings and behaviors might stem from the more helpful alternative thoughts on the right. In this way, you can emphasize that people can change their lives if they consider alternative ways of thinking. As you go through the Automatic Thoughts Check-list, try to identify the thoughts consumers have previously mentioned, and nor-malize the fact that automatic thoughts occur for everyone. It is not necessary to review the entire list at one time; instead, pick a situation that is most relevant to the personalized goals of the consumer and review the thoughts for that situation (e.g., introducing yourself to others for someone who has a goal to make a friend; or taking a class for someone who wants to complete his or her degree). The Com-mon Thoughts Checklist can be used anytime consumers are having difficulty identifying unhelpful thoughts or generating more helpful alternative thoughts in Sessions 2–6.

Session 1: Introduction and Goal Setting

In Session 1 (see Chapter 5), new members may join the group, and consumers iden-tify long- and short-term goals and the goal steps they will take to achieve them, and write them on their 7–7–7 Goal Jackpot! Worksheet. When introducing CBSST, it is helpful to call on experienced members to begin teaching the concept that thoughts can influence feelings and behaviors (e.g., by describing examples from their own lives that they have identified in previous sessions). This can boost self-efficacy about mastering the content in the experienced members, and new members learn that oth-ers with similar problems are making important progress.

Given that cognitive skills will be trained in this module, goal-setting work in Session 1 should include adding goal steps about "check out thoughts about . . ." to the 7–7–7 Goal Jackpot! Worksheet. For example, if someone has a goal to work but is troubled by hallucinations (e.g., voices threatening harm if he or she leaves home), include the goal step "Check out thoughts about voices" or "Test whether voices can harm me," or "Learn ways to ignore the voices." In the case of Juan, described in Chapter 5, the provider noted several thoughts that could interfere with his two short-term goals of managing money for a new apartment (e.g., "I'm bad with han-dling money") and learning to communicate with a roommate (e.g., "He'll never listen to me"), so goal steps to check these thoughts were added to the Juan's 7–7–7 Goal Jackpot! Worksheet (see Figure 5.3).

Each of the following sessions specific to cognitive skills (Sessions 2–6), begins with the provider writing the session's agenda on a whiteboard or pad and inviting consumers to add their own agenda items. This simplified agenda is also listed in the Consumer Workbook. Providers, however, should follow the more detailed plans that begin each session below.

Session 2: The Thoughts–Feelings–Behaviors Link

PROVIDER PLAN FOR THIS SESSION

- Set the Agenda Collaboratively
- Review At-Home Practice
- Introduce the Thoughts–Feelings–Behaviors Link
  - Thoughts Are Not Always Accurate
- In-Session Skill Practice: Thoughts versus Feelings
  - Labeling Thoughts as Helpful or Unhelpful
- Assign At-Home Practice: Identifying Thoughts
- Summarize the Session
- Ask for Consumer Feedback

CONDUCTING THE SESSION

Set the Agenda Collaboratively

- Review At-Home Practice: Setting Goals
- What is the Thoughts–Feelings–Behaviors Link?
- Thoughts versus Feelings
- Assign At-Home Practice: Identifying Thoughts
- Additional Agenda Items?

Consumers often add nothing to the agenda but may bring up concerns or crises. Here is an opportunity to say, "I'm glad you brought that up; it fits well with what we are going to work on today." Issues raised by consumers do not have to distract from skills learning, because all of the skills can be used to help resolve or cope with concerns or crises. In this session, consumers learn about how thoughts impact feelings and actions, so providers can use the concerns raised by consumers as personally relevant examples to illustrate the impact of thoughts on potential feelings and actions in the situations raised by consumers. For example, if a crisis about imminent eviction from housing is raised, providers can write the issue on the agenda, then when teaching about how thoughts impact and feelings and actions, can ask questions to try to elicit thoughts about the crisis (fortune telling and catastrophizing thinking mistakes; e.g., "I'm going to be homeless" or "There's nothing I can do about it") by writing these thoughts on the board and drawing arrows to unpleasant feelings (fear, anger, hopelessness) and unhelpful actions (lashing out at landlord, doing nothing). Some group time might be also allocated to problem-solving about the crisis if the problem cannot be deferred to a case manager or other provider. In this way, items raised by consumers during collaborative agenda setting can be integrated into the specific skills training content planned for the session.

Review At-Home Practice: Setting Goals

The 7–7–7 Goal Jackpot! Worksheets are reviewed. Ask for volunteers to describe their long-term goal and any progress made in completing short-term goals and goal steps on their worksheet. Celebrate and applaud volunteers to reinforce any effort. Then, if working in a group format, go around the room and call on members until everyone has had an opportunity to speak. Problem-solve with consumers who did not complete their homework about how to be more successful in future sessions (e.g., use SCALE as described in Chapter 8). The most common difficulty with this homework assignment involves the goal-setting challenges discussed in Chapter 5. It is important that consumers set a motivating long-term goal as soon as possible. During homework review, help consumers break down goals into manageable goal steps written on the goal worksheet using the 7–7–7 Goal Jackpot! timeline (see Chapter 5). Session 1 of each module and this homework review period in Session 2 is the primary time allocated to goal setting during the intervention. If this is not sufficient to elicit meaningful goals and several goal steps, consider adding an additional individual goal-setting session for consumers who are struggling.

Introduce the Thoughts–Feelings–Behaviors Link

Following the review of the goal-setting session's assignment, introduce the concept that our feelings and actions are influenced by our thoughts. It is important to use the words "our" and "we" when discussing the model, because thoughts influence actions and feelings in everyone, not just in people with serious psychopathology. Normalize how moods and behaviors are influenced by thinking for everyone (see the Provider Tip on page 105). The groundwork for future cognitive work is laid by illustrating how our thoughts can sometimes lead to unwanted feelings and actions that can interfere with our recovery goals. This can be overwhelming at first, so use the triangular diagram in Figure 6.1 (also in Session 2 of the Consumer Workbook for this module). Draw the triangle on a whiteboard or pad and point to the components as you describe them. For example:

> "Thoughts are all of the things we tell ourselves—for example, 'I think I can achieve my goals,' 'I hope I remembered to lock the door.' Actions or behaviors are what we do, for example, watching TV, talking to someone, or taking a walk. Feelings are the many emotions and moods we experience. Feelings can usually be described using one word such as 'happy,' 'sad,' and 'afraid,' but thoughts are usually more than one word. Our thoughts, feelings, and actions affect each other."

You versus We and Yours versus Ours: Choose Your Words Wisely to Normalize Mistakes in Thinking

The words you choose can pathologize or normalize. Everyone's thoughts influence his or her feelings and behaviors. This is not just true for people with mental illness.

Nobody is perfect, and we all make mistakes in thinking.

Using "we" or "our," rather than "you" or "your" implies that mistakes are a normal part of being human. Avoid saying "*Your* thoughts are mistaken" or "*You* have incorrect thinking." This can be experienced as blaming or attributed to illness and can compromise rapport and working alliance. Say "*We* all make mistakes in thinking" and "If *we* correct *our* thoughts, *we* can achieve *our* goals."

If possible, use an example of a thought from a consumer's own life and experience, and write that down in quotes on the triangle diagram (see Figure 6.1). Ask the consumer what feelings that thought leads to, then ask how those feelings influence his or her actions. If the consumer is unsure, suggest some options to choose from, or ask group members to make some suggestions. Write the specific feelings and actions on the diagram. For example, the thought, "Nobody likes me," can lead to feeling "sad, pessimistic." Those feelings can lead to "staying home, doing nothing." Draw arrows from the thought to the feelings and behaviors that stem from it, as shown in Figure 6.1.

Providers next use the triangle diagram to introduce the power of changing thoughts. Generate a different thought that the consumer might have in response to the same situation. If in a group, ask group members to help generate an alternative thought. If the initial thought was "Nobody likes me," an alternative thought might be "Someone likes me." Ask what feelings and actions the new thought would produce (e.g., hopeful, optimistic feelings, which in turn could lead to going out and talking to people). Contrast the negative feelings and behaviors from the first

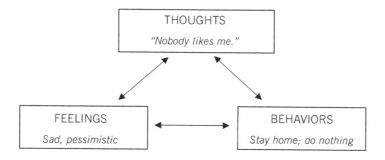

FIGURE 6.1. The thoughts–feelings–actions triangle.

thought with the more positive feelings and behaviors from the alternative thought. Draw similar diagrams on the board and go through several examples. This helps to illustrate the model, and the repetition compensates for cognitive impairment. The "triangle" (as consumers often label it) is often identified as one of the topics best recalled from CBSST sessions. If needed, consult the Common Thoughts Checklist (Appendix C) for further examples of self-defeating thoughts and more optimistic, alternative thoughts.

Thoughts Are Not Always Accurate

Begin to introduce the idea that thoughts are not always correct, but mistakes in thinking can be corrected. The corrected thought (a more accurate thought) might lead to more desirable feelings and behaviors. Normalize the idea that our thoughts are not always correct.

> "We all make mistakes in thinking. If these incorrect thoughts are leading to unwanted behaviors or feelings, we can learn to change our thinking. Changing thoughts can also change how we feel and what we do. Our thoughts can either help us do things to achieve our goals or prevent us from achieving our goals. We can correct them to improve our quality of life."

Some people need more help accepting the concept of making mistakes. Talk about how nobody is perfect and have consumers describe a strength and a weakness. Emphasize that everyone has different strengths and weaknesses. Providers can also describe a personal mistake in their own thinking and how it resulted in negative feelings and behaviors. Mistakes in thinking are part of being human, not part of mental illness. We control our own thoughts. It is empowering to learn that we can change our thinking and that doing so can help us achieve our goals and feel better.

In-Session Skill Practice: Thoughts versus Feelings

Distinguishing thoughts and feelings can be challenging for some consumers. Many of us were never taught how to differentiate between thoughts and feelings, or that there is a wide array of emotions. For some, the range of emotions is limited to "happy," "sad," or "angry," or simply feeling "good" versus feeling "bad." Helping consumers label emotions will help them differentiate between thoughts and feelings and, subsequently, challenge their thoughts. There may be some confusion stemming from common English language usage of "I think" and "I feel" synonymously. For example, people often say, "I *feel* like he doesn't like me," when they mean "I *think* he doesn't like me."

Ask consumers who have difficulty with labeling feelings and thoughts to pick from the list of "Common Pleasant and Unpleasant Feelings" in Appendix C (also in Session 2 of the Consumer Workbook for this module). The "Common Thoughts Checklist" in Appendix C may also be helpful. An easy way to help consumers distinguish between feelings and thoughts is to point out that feelings can be described with one word; thoughts usually require more than one word, such as a phrase or sentence. Any one of the following exercises can also help consumers learn to distinguish thoughts from feelings and label them.

- There are several experiential learning games in Appendix B that very effectively illustrate these concepts (e.g., Ball Toss Game, Funny Videos Activity, and Spinner Game). The Ball Toss Game, in particular, is a very effective and fun way to teach about the link between thoughts and goal-directed actions, and that thoughts need to be tested out, because they are not always accurate. To teach the distinction between thoughts and feelings, play the Thoughts versus Feelings Flash Card Game.
- Ask: "What were you feeling this week? Which pleasant feelings did you have in the past week? Where were you? Do you remember what you were doing? What were you thinking? What unpleasant feelings did you have in the past week? Where were you? What were you doing? What were you thinking?"
- To practice linking thoughts to feelings, write two thoughts on the board that would be associated with contrasting feelings and ask consumers to label the feelings they might feel if they had the thoughts. Draw an arrow from each thought and write the feelings at the end. For ideas, refer to the list of Common Pleasant and Unpleasant Feelings and the list of contrasting thoughts in the Common Thoughts Checklist, both in Appendix C.

Labeling Thoughts as Helpful or Unhelpful

Often the best way for providers to categorize thoughts is as helpful or unhelpful, especially when struggling to agree with consumers on the accuracy of thoughts. Thoughts are helpful if they help people achieve their goals and unhelpful if they interfere with achieving goals. Other common approaches to labeling thoughts (positive vs. negative or accurate vs. inaccurate) have important limitations. Thoughts are not inherently positive or negative or good or bad; rather, thoughts have positive or negative consequences. Labeling thoughts as positive versus negative may also imply a value judgment on thoughts (e.g., right vs. wrong or good vs. bad thoughts). The

PROVIDER TIP

Remember This

Feelings are one word.

and

Thoughts are (usually) more than one word.

terms "accurate" versus "inaccurate" can be useful, and we do include this in our education about thoughts. However, providers may find themselves in detailed and lengthy discussions bordering on arguments about the accuracy of beliefs. Arguing is not likely to be productive, and if discussion of accuracy leads in that direction, it is important to shift away from arguing. If you find yourself in a hole, stop digging. The reason we emphasize helpful versus unhelpful thoughts is that even when consumers disagree about the accuracy of thoughts, they can usually acknowledge when thoughts are unhelpful and likely to interfere with goal-directed activities. We have found that focusing on whether thoughts are helpful or unhelpful keeps treatment moving and also keeps the focus on goals the consumer has set.

Assign At-Home Practice: Identifying Thoughts

The purpose of the At-Home Practice assignment is for consumers to try to do one of the goal steps on their goal worksheet, and to catch and write down one thought when they try to do it. Give consumers the choice of which goal step to attempt and help them develop a plan to accomplish the step. They also have to decide whether the thought is helpful (e.g., "I can do this") or unhelpful (e.g., "Why bother, this will never work out") with regard to making it easier or harder to do the goal step. Try to help consumers identify thoughts in the context of attempting a goal step. For example, during the goal-setting session with Juan, the provider asked Juan whether he was more or less likely to manage his money successfully if he thinks, "I will mess it up." The provider can refer back to this discussion at this point in the session and ask Juan to write down one of his money management goal steps (e.g., "complete a budget worksheet") in the "Practice Right Now" row of his At-Home Practice Worksheet in Session 2 of the Consumer Workbook, then write the thought, "I will mess it up" in the next column, and ask Juan to circle "Helpful" or "Unhelpful." Juan can then be instructed to identify another thought related to a goal step (it can be the same goal step) and decide whether the thought is helpful or unhelpful for homework. Help other consumers to similarly fill out the "Practice Right Now" row with guidance during the session, before completing the next row on their own at home.

Summarize the Session

The key points to summarize for this session are:

- Our thoughts influence how we feel and what we do.
- Thoughts can be accurate or inaccurate, helpful or unhelpful.
- If you correct inaccurate, unhelpful thoughts, then you can feel better and do the things you want to do.
- Feelings may be expressed with one word; thoughts require more than one word.

Ask for Consumer Feedback

Check to make sure consumers understand the session content and the At-Home Practice assignment. Ask, for example, "What are the main things you got out of this session? What did you find most helpful and least helpful? Do you think you will use this skill to start checking out what you are thinking when you work on your goals? How did I do today; did I explain things well or did I go too fast?" If in a group, try to check in with everyone. If the feedback suggests that the basic idea that thoughts can impact feelings and behaviors is not clear, spend some extra time during homework review in the next session to review the thoughts–feelings–actions link and "the triangle."

Session 3: The 3C's—Catch It, Check It, Change It

PROVIDER PLAN FOR THIS SESSION

- Set the Agenda Collaboratively
- Review At-Home Practice: Identifying Thoughts
- Introduce the 3C's (Catch It, Check It, Change It)
- In-Session Skill Practice: Catch It—Recognizing Unhelpful Thoughts
  o Using Feelings as a "Red Flag" to Catch Thoughts
- Assign At-Home Practice: Catch the Thought
- Summarize the Session
- Ask for Consumer Feedback

CONDUCTING THE SESSION

Set the Agenda Collaboratively

- Review At-Home Practice: Identifying Thoughts
- The 3C's: Catch It, Check It, Change It
- Catch It: Recognizing Unhelpful Thoughts
- Assign At-Home Practice: Catch the Thought
- Additional Agenda Items?

Most consumers do not add anything to the agenda. If concerns or crises are raised, say, "I'm glad you brought that up; it fits well with what we are going to learn today." Use the issues raised by consumers as personally relevant content to teach the 3C's. For example, if an issue about conflict with a roommate is raised, write "disagreement with roommate" on the agenda. Then, later in the session, when teaching Catch It, briefly discuss the situation with the consumer, write down some of the identified thoughts, and use one of them to complete an in-session 3C's Worksheet. In this way, items raised by consumers during collaborative agenda setting can be integrated into the specific skills training content planned for the session.

Review At-Home Practice: Identifying Thoughts

Review the thoughts that consumers identified, with a focus on whether they facilitated or hindered performance of goal steps. It is important that consumers identify their thoughts, regardless of whether they achieved the goal step. Celebrate all goal step accomplishments, but it can be more difficult to perform goal steps than to identify the thoughts that come up while attempting to perform them, so celebrate when thoughts are identified, regardless of whether goal steps were achieved. This homework review provides an opportunity to continue teaching how changing thoughts that interfere with goal steps might help consumers try goal steps again and be more successful. For example, pointing out to Carol (see Chapter 5 and Figure 5.4) that changing the thought "I will get lost if I take the bus" to "I'm confident I know the route to my provider's office" or "If I get lost, I can ask the driver for help" might help Carol accomplish her short-term goal of using the public transportation system. Providers may also have to help consumers revise their plans to accomplish the goal step (e.g., help Carol brainstorm other ways to find the bus route to the provider's office, if she could not find it). It may be necessary to review other factors that may have interfered with goal steps (e.g., resources needed, such as people, places, and things, or skills deficits, such as not knowing what to say to someone). Problem-solving about accomplishing goal steps can become very time-consuming, however, so focus on using this homework review time to teach how thoughts impact goal-directed actions rather than problem-solving extensively about other factors that interfered with goal progress. The CBSST program will provide many opportunities to teach skills and solve problems relevant to accomplishing goal steps. Some consumers have difficulty identifying thoughts, which can be a brief opportunity to link this skill to the current session content, which is teaching consumers to Catch It (e.g., "This is an important skill that takes practice to learn, and we are going to talk more about how to catch our thoughts during today's class").

Introduce the 3C's (Catch It, Check It, Change It)

Begin this part of the session by giving consumers an overview of the 3C's thought-challenging skill. For example:

> "The primary skill we will be using to help change our unhelpful thinking is the 3C's: Catch It, Check It, Change It. What's 'it'? 'It' is a thought. The thought

might be accurate or it might be a mistake. Changing mistakes in thinking is a skill that takes practice, like learning to ride a bike. The first C is Catch It. We will learn how to recognize and catch thoughts and write them down. The second C is Check It. We will learn to decide whether the thought is accurate or inaccurate, helpful or unhelpful. The third C is Change It. If a thought is inaccurate or unhelpful, changing it can help you feel better and do things to achieve your goals. Let's start by learning how to Catch It."

In-Session Skill Practice: Catch It—Recognizing Unhelpful Thoughts

Providers can use one of the games (e.g., "Catch a Thought Game") in Appendix B to help consumers learn how to catch and identify thoughts. Alternatively, write, then discuss, the following unhelpful thoughts on the whiteboard or pad:

> "There's no point in trying. Things will never get better."
> "I can't trust anyone."
> "People won't like me, because I have a mental illness."
> "I can't change the way I am. I was born this way."
> "I'm too sick to do what I need to do to have fun."

Ask, "What do you notice about all these thoughts?"

> "Would these thoughts help you reach your goals?"
> "If you had these thoughts, how would you feel?"
> "If you had these thoughts and feelings, what would you do or not do?"

In the discussion, try to use consumers' own thoughts verbalized in the session or from the At-Home Practice. Ask the consumer if the specific thought might be helpful or unhelpful in achieving his or her goal. Ask, "Why do you think this?" For example, both of Carol's short-term goals (see Figure 5.4) require her to go out into the community and interact with others. The provider had made note of several thoughts Carol had verbalized, such as "I won't be able to cope with the voices," "I'll be embarrassed," "I guess I've been able to do it before," and "People will laugh at me." For each thought, the provider can ask, "Do you think this thought would help you achieve your goal of riding the bus or get in the way?" Also, "How does this thought make you feel?" Focus the discussion on the importance of catching thoughts that might be interfering with achieving goals and enjoying activities in daily life.

Using Feelings as a "Red Flag" to Catch Thoughts

Explain that unhelpful thoughts can sometimes be hard to catch, but they can often leave a trail of unpleasant feelings such as fear, sadness, or anger. Bad feelings are an

PROVIDER TIP

Red-Flag Catch It Technique

This strategy can help consumers learn when to catch unhelpful thoughts. An unpleasant feeling (e.g., sad, angry, afraid) or lack of goal-directed behavior (e.g., staying home to avoid people, missing an appointment) is a "red flag" to signal when to examine thoughts. Some providers wave an actual red flag in session when these signals come up, which makes the lesson more memorable.

important signal telling us to look for the thoughts we just had. Use feelings as red flags to tell you when to catch your thoughts. Ask yourself, "What went through my mind just before I had that feeling?" There are also games described in Appendix B to help teach about catching "red flag" feelings.

Helping Consumers Identify Thoughts

Identifying unhelpful thoughts is a critical first step in the 3C's process. If the thought is not articulated well, the 3C's will not work as effectively. When writing thoughts on the board or a pad, try to rephrase them, if possible, into thoughts that have obvious implications for goal achievement and, especially in the beginning, thoughts that are more easily challenged (e.g., using terms such as "never" or "always" to create all-or-none mistakes in thinking that are easy to identify). Common problems include consumers describing a situation or feeling rather than a thought. Praise these attempts, then correct them by returning to discussions about the differences between thoughts and feelings (Session 2). Another common problem is describing thoughts that do not have obvious implications for goal achievement. Initially, this can be useful to teach the 3C's skills, but the focus should soon shift to thoughts that interfere with recovery goal achievement. Again, praise the attempt, then ask questions (or start over) until you get to a thought that has implications for goals. Another challenge is when someone states a thought as a question, for example, "How can a girl like that ever date a guy like me?" It can be helpful to ask consumers to answer their own questions, then challenge the response: "She could never date a guy like me."

See the Provider Tip on page 113 for other strategies to help consumers identify thoughts. For example, a consumer with a goal of making a friend identifies the following thought about a social situation: "I don't want to go." The provider can ask follow-up questions to determine what that thought means to the consumer: "Why not?"; "What do you expect to happen if you go?" In this example, the provider and consumer determine that the consumer expects to be ignored because he or she believes "I am unlikable" and "Nobody likes me." This is the unhelpful automatic thought that they can use for the 3C's skills. Pick a thought that interferes with the consumer's goal(s) and is easy to dispute. This thought is an all-or-none thought that will be easy to dispute in the next session when discussing the Check It skill. All you have to do is produce an example of someone who likes the consumer (e.g., you or anyone in the group, or in the consumer's life) to prove the thought inaccurate.

You can also use the Common Thoughts Checklist (see Appendix C) to identify defeatist beliefs. The thoughts in the checklist are organized according to specific situations related to recovery goals. Select situations related to a consumer's goal and ask the person to pick thoughts he or she has in that situation. Put key defeatist beliefs on an index card to refer to in later sessions and give a card like this to consumers.

Assign At-Home Practice: Catch the Thought

The assignment is to catch a thought before the next session. Consumers can choose to do a goal step from their 7–7–7 Goal Jackpot! Worksheet and catch a thought when they try to do it, or they can catch a thought when they are experiencing an unpleasant feeling (a "red flag" feeling). In addition to catching the thought, the situation, feeling, and action linked to it are also noted on the At-Home Practice Worksheet for Session 3. This assignment begins the process of learning about the types of situations that give rise to specific thoughts, as well as the emotional and behavioral consequences of thoughts. Ask consumers to practice filling out the worksheet in session. For example, you can use the group itself as the situation (e.g., consumers write "sitting in class" in the situation box) and ask about a thought consumers

---

PROVIDER TIP

Helping Consumers Identify Thoughts

- **Ask about the meaning of the situation.** For example, if someone recently lost a friend and can only identify feeling sad, you could ask, "What does it mean that your friend is gone?" This may prompt the consumer to say something like, "No one else will want to be friends with me."

- **Assume the opposite.** For example, if someone isolates, you could say, "Do you like being with other people?" The response might be, "No! I'm afraid of looking stupid around people."

- **Use guided imagery.** Ask the consumer to imagine the sights, sensations, sounds, and smells of a specific situation in the recent past and ask, "OK, now that you are back there, what is going through your mind?" or "What are you saying to yourself?"

- **Identify key words that signal mistakes in thinking.** Key words such as "always," "never," "every," nobody," or "can't" signal mistakes in thinking, like all-or-none thoughts. Ask consumers to use the whiteboard or a pad of paper to write down their thought and then circle and highlight these key words.

- **Use the Common Thoughts Checklist.** The common thoughts checklist (see Appendix B) is a multiple-choice list from which consumers can select thoughts they may have been thinking.

had during group, such as "I'm never going to get this" or "This is not too hard for me," and link the thought to feelings (e.g., frustrated or confident), and actions (e.g., zoning out or talking and asking questions). Be sure to link achievement of consumers' goals to the skill of catching unhelpful thoughts. Bridging this skill–goal gap is easier if consumers agree to try a goal step and check out their thoughts when they do it. For example, one of Juan's goal steps was to open a savings account at a bank (see Figure 5.3), so while he was still in class, he would write "going to the bank to open a savings account" in the situation box of the At-Home Practice form, and at home when he attempts the goal step (or thought about doing it), he might catch the thought, "It will be too complicated to use" or "The bank won't let someone like me open an account," which may interfere with accomplishing this goal step. Once these thoughts are identified, they can be addressed in a subsequent session.

Summarize the Session

The key points to summarize for this session are:

- The 3C's is a skill for changing inaccurate or unhelpful thoughts that interfere with achieving your goals.
- Use feelings as red flags to tell you when to catch your thoughts.

Ask for Consumer Feedback

Remember to ask consumers for feedback about the session and the key points just summarized. One way to ask for feedback, as explained in Chapter 3, is to draw a horizontal line with one end marked "0"—"Unlikely to use this skill" and the other marked "10"—"Definitely will use this skill." Ask consumers to come up and mark an X on the line to indicate whether they will use the skill. Troubleshoot with consumers who are not close to "10." For example, if someone is a "6," ask why he or she is a "6" and not an "8." If the consumer says that he or she thinks he or she will forget, brainstorm ways to remember (e.g., reminder notes, putting the workbook in an obvious place, setting an alarm, asking someone to remind him or her). If the consumer doubts whether he or she can do it or that it will work, use the 3C's to challenge this defeatist belief, or ask, "Are you willing to try it and test out whether you can do it?"

Session 4: The 3C's—Check It

PROVIDER PLAN FOR THIS SESSION

- Set the Agenda Collaboratively
- Review At-Home Practice: Catch the Thought
- Introduce the Check It Step
- Mistakes in Thinking
- In-Session Skill Practice: Mistakes in Thinking
  - Game or Other Activity and Discussion
  - Thinking Mistakes as Habits
  - Checking Evidence
- Assign At-Home Practice: Catch and Check the Thought
- Summarize the Session
- Ask for Consumer Feedback

CONDUCTING THE SESSION

Set the Agenda Collaboratively

- Review At-Home Practice
- Check It: What's the Evidence for That Thought?
- Mistakes in Thinking
- Assign At-Home Practice: Catch and Check the Thought
- Additional Agenda Items?

Additional items raised by consumers should be discussed in the context of catching and checking the thoughts associated with the situation or problem added to the agenda. For example, if Mary says, "I'm stressed about an argument with my boyfriend," say, "I'm glad you brought that up. Today we are going to talk about how the thoughts you have about that are related to how stressed you are and what you might do about it." Then write "Mary's argument" on the agenda and use this situation as an example when practicing catching and checking thoughts later in the session.

Review At-Home Practice: Catch the Thought

Reviewing the Catch It homework is an excellent opportunity to identify dysfunctional thinking that might be a barrier to goal achievement in the real world. If consumers have attempted a goal step, review the impact of their thought on their success or failure to complete the step. If someone was successful, what thought did he or she have that facilitated performing the behavior (e.g., "It's worth a try"), and if unsuccessful, was a defeatist belief in the way (e.g., "I can't")? Even if the consumer did not catch a thought, review the situation and ask questions in an attempt to identify what might have been going through his or her mind in the situation. A thought is not always in the way, so review the attempt and help problem-solve a solution to try in the next attempt. Of course, applaud and celebrate all homework completion and goal step successes, and be sure to check off the step on the goal worksheet and place a gold star on it or give the consumer a raffle ticket (see Chapter 3).

Introduce the Check It Step

In Session 4 ("Check It"), consumers practice listing "evidence for" and "evidence against" the thought (see the At-Home Practice Worksheet for this session). We previously described this to consumers as "evidence that *supports* or *disputes* the thought," but this was confusing to group members, who sometimes thought they were supporting the person or having a dispute with him or her. Consumers want to support each other in groups. The discussion should focus on whether the *thought* is accurate, not whether the *consumer* is accurate, which minimizes interpersonal aspects. Mistakes in thinking are also taught, and participants practice identifying whether thoughts represent one of these common mistakes. The Check It skill can be introduced as follows:

> "Today we will learn about the second of the 3C's: Check It. The purpose of this step is to help you check out all of the evidence to decide whether a thought about a situation is accurate or helpful. One way to *Check It* is to act like a scientist or a detective. Look at the evidence, the facts for and against a thought. How do we find *evidence for* a thought? Often this will be the easy step, since we pay more attention to things that confirm the thoughts we have. How do we find *evidence against* a thought? Sometimes this can be very difficult. Try asking yourself:
>
>> 'Are there any alternative explanations?'
>> 'If someone else had this thought, what would I tell him or her?'
>> 'Am I missing any facts that contradict my thought?'
>> 'Is the thought helping me reach my goals or feel better?' "

Mistakes in Thinking

In traditional cognitive therapy, the term "cognitive errors" is often used. We prefer the term "mistakes in thinking" to reduce the stigma attached to these common errors. Remember to emphasize that anyone can make a mistake, and everyone makes them. We all make assumptions to help us interpret events in our lives. However, our assumptions can be mistaken. And they can also be damaging when they keep us from trying new things or making changes. Mistakes in thinking can be introduced as follows:

> "There are several common mistakes in thinking that we all tend to make. These thinking mistakes can lead to unhelpful or inaccurate thoughts that make us feel bad and keep us from our goals."

Then review and explain the following six common mistakes, using the examples in the Consumer Workbook:

1. All-or-nothing thinking
2. Mind reading
3. Fortune telling
4. Jumping to conclusions
5. Catastrophizing
6. Emotional reasoning

In-Session Skill Practice: Mistakes in Thinking

Providers can also conduct the activity in the Consumer Workbook that asks, "What is the common mistake in thinking in the following thoughts?" These examples of mistakes can be written in a column on the whiteboard or pad, with a column of names of mistakes to the right in a different order, so the mistakes do not match up with the examples on the left. Then, consumers can come up one at a time and draw lines from the example on the left to the mistake on the right. A clear understanding of these mistakes will facilitate the Check It step on the 3C's Worksheets, where consumers check off the mistakes they identify in their own thinking. Several games in Appendix B can facilitate learning the definitions of mistakes in thinking, for example, the Jumping to Conclusions Game, the Headbands Game, and the Jeopardy Game.

Thinking of Mistakes as Habits

Emphasize that mistakes in thinking have usually become habits, so it will take time to catch them and change them. For example,

> "Thinking mistakes can become habits. Is there a particular thinking mistake you make most of the time? What is your 'favorite' mistake in thinking? We all have a favorite mistake in thinking."

In general, most people engage in one mistake in thinking more frequently than in others—their "favorite" mistake. This can be very helpful in thought challenging, in which we have found that consumers often say, "There I go again, making my favorite mistake!" If you are comfortable with disclosure, normalize mistakes by sharing your favorite mistake in thinking. For example, "I like fortune telling the best. I'm always predicting what can go wrong in the future and trying to prevent it or overprepare for it. This makes me worry too much, so I have to watch out." This can help normalize mistakes. In a group format, you can ask members to guess each other's favorite mistake and promote "me, too" experiences based on shared common mistakes. This process of labeling a "favorite" mistake can also help to normalize mistakes. Ask people to write down their favorite mistake with its definition and an example on an index card, so they can have this as a reminder when challenging thoughts using the 3C's skill.

Sometimes consumers focus on the fact that common mistakes "feel" comfortable, and that alternative thoughts do not "feel" true or accurate, even in the face of evidence. We want to validate their statements and point out that these are common

TABLE 6.3. Common Mistakes in Thinking

Mistake in thinking	Definition
All-or-nothing thinking (or all-or-none or black-and-white thinking)	Viewing situations in terms of absolutes: "I am a complete failure."
Mind reading	Making assumptions about other's perceptions: "They think I'm stupid."
Fortune telling (or predicting the future and probability estimation errors)	Overestimating the likelihood of a negative event: "I know she will laugh at me if I try to talk to her."
Jumping to conclusions	Not gathering enough evidence before making a decision: "He is going to hurt me, because he is looking at me."
Catastrophizing	When we jump to conclusions, we often predict the worst possible situation that can occur; for example, one person turns you down for a date, so you think: "I will never get a date and be alone forever."
Emotional reasoning	Judging a situation based on one's emotional response rather than objective evidence: "I was feeling anxious, so I must have looked foolish."
Selective attention (or ignoring the positive)	Attending mostly to negative information and/or ignoring positive information; for example, noticing conflict with a sibling and ignoring other supportive family members: "There's no use in visiting family; my sister just argues with me."
Shoulds	Holding rigid rules and expectations; refusing to accept realities outside one's control: "I should be able to do all the things I used to do."
Overresponsibility	Feeling guilt for situations outside of one's control: "It is my fault my parents are unhappy."

experiences when changing a habit. Encourage consumers as much as possible when they are learning this new skill, and acknowledge and validate the difficulty. Some common types of mistakes in thinking are defined in Table 6.3. Not all of these are included in the Consumer Workbook, but they may be useful when helping consumers identify the ones they tend to use more.

Checking Evidence

Practice the Check It step in session. Select (catch) a thought from a consumer to be checked (e.g., "Does anyone remember a thought they caught this week when they were trying a goal step or having a 'red flag' feeling?") or select a thought from the Catch It homework review at the start of this session, or elicit a thought related to an agenda item. For example, this is an opportunity to explore "Mary's argument," which she added to the agenda at the start of the session. Ask what the argument was about and what was going through Mary's mind during or after the argument. Additional guidance on helping consumers catch thoughts was presented in Session 3. This questioning might lead to the thought, "He never does anything to help me." Write the thought in quotes on a notepad or on the whiteboard and draw two columns below it—one labeled "Evidence for" and the other, "Evidence against." Ask for evidence that supports the thought first, which is typically easier to generate, then ask for evidence against. In a group, ask all the consumers, not just the consumer with the thought being examined. Providers can add pieces of evidence that the consumers do not generate. After all the evidence has been generated, ask the group or consumer to decide whether the thought is accurate or inaccurate based on which column has stronger evidence, and ask whether they can identify a mistake in thinking (in this example, All-or-Nothing Thinking).

To help consumers generate evidence, suggest they think like a detective, lawyer, or scientist to generate facts and observations. Use Socratic questioning (see Chapter 3) to help consumers consider evidence. Ask for more detail or for clarification to identify mistakes in thinking. For example,

> "What exactly does this mean?"
> "What do we already know about this?"
> "Can you give me an example?"

Probe assumptions that are helpful in checking a thought for accuracy:

> "You seem to be assuming. . . . Is that right?"
> "What else could we assume?"
> "How did you decide that was true?"
> "How can we verify or disprove that assumption?"
> "If _____ is true, what does that mean about _____?"
> "If _____ is not true, what does that mean?"

Probe rationale, reasons, and evidence:

> "Why is that happening?"
> "How do you know this?"
> "What do you think causes . . . ?"
> "How might it be refuted?"
> "Why?" (Keep asking why.)
> "What evidence is there to support what you are saying?"

Assign At-Home Practice: Catch and Check the Thought

Consumers are asked to fill out the At-Home Practice Worksheet to catch and check a thought. Go over the worksheet in session with consumers and help each identify a likely situation that is related in some way to his or her goals. For example, ask consumers to select a goal step from their 7–7–7 Goal Jackpot! Worksheet that they want to attempt before the next session. This goal step can be translated into the "situation" on the worksheet. One of Carol's goal steps was to practice taking the bus to the provider's office (see Figure 5.4). This goal step can be translated into a situation written on the 3C's Worksheet as "riding the bus to my provider's office" or "waiting for the bus to the office." Then, Carol would try to catch a thought (e.g., "The cartels will hurt me") when she was in this situation. Another option is to help consumers look for "red flags," situations in which the consumer feels angry, sad, or frightened, or did not act but perhaps could have during the week, especially when emotion or inaction interferes with goal achievement. A red flag for Juan might be feeling angry when his roommate plays loud music at night when he is trying to sleep. Discuss what evidence for and against thoughts might look like.

Summarize the Session

The key points to summarize for this session are:

- Check It means to decide whether a thought is accurate by examining the evidence for and against it.
- We all make mistakes in thinking, and we usually have a favorite mistake we make more often.
- If we check and correct mistakes in thinking that lead to unpleasant feelings and that interfere with our goals, we can improve our lives.

Ask for Consumer Feedback

Remember to ask consumers how you are doing: "Am I explaining things clearly?" There is a lot of content in this session, so you may get feedback that you went too fast, or that there is too much to remember. Normalize this and mention that this is common feedback about this session, and it is unusual for people to think they understand it all after the first try. You will be reviewing this again in the next couple sessions, and these skills take practice. This is why At-Home Practice is so important. Suggest that consumers reread the session material in their workbooks this week (e.g., while on the bus), especially the definitions of mistakes in thinking. You can suggest that consumers play another mistakes in thinking game from Appendix B at the beginning of the next session, so it would help to review the definitions if they want to win the game.

Session 5: The 3C's—Change It

PROVIDER PLAN FOR THIS SESSION

- Set the Agenda Collaboratively
- Review At-Home Practice: Catch and Check the Thought
- Introduce the Change It Step
- In Session Skill Practice: Generating Alternative Thoughts
  - Alternatives Therapy Exercise
- Assign At-Home Practice: Catch, Check, and Change the Thought
- Summarize the Session
- Ask for Consumer Feedback

CONDUCTING THE SESSION

Set the Agenda Collaboratively

- Review At-Home Practice: Catch and Check the Thought
- Change It
- Assign At-Home Practice: Catch, Check, and Change the Thought
- Additional Agenda Items?

Review At-Home Practice: Catch and Check the Thought

As in Session 3, reviewing the homework in Session 4 is an excellent opportunity to identify dysfunctional thinking that might be a barrier to goal achievement in the real world. If a consumer attempted a goal step, review the impact of his or her thoughts on the success or failure to complete the step, and stress the importance of checking whether the thought is accurate, if it is interfering with goal progress. If a consumer caught a thought in a "red flag" situation, review the impact of thoughts on emotions or inaction. Write thoughts on the board and draw arrows to feelings and actions. The evidence for and against the thought is then reviewed, including whether the thought was a common mistake in thinking. Ask the consumer, "Was this your favorite mistake? Who else in group has this favorite mistake?" Try to engage the group in brainstorming about evidence for and against the thought. Applaud and celebrate all goal step successes, and be sure to check off completed steps on the goal worksheet and place a gold star on the sheet.

There will be times when a consumer is not making progress and completing goal steps. This may be because a thought (defeatist attitude) is in the way. In Juan's case, he did not accomplish the goal steps of negotiating quiet hours with his roommate. Juan's prediction that his roommate would get angry if he attempted to negotiate quiet hours in their room continued to be a barrier to accomplishing that goal step. The provider made a note to encourage Juan to challenge this thought as part of a 3C's exercise during the session or as an At-Home Practice assignment.

Introduce the Change It Step

In this session, consumers learn to replace thoughts that are judged to be inaccurate and unhelpful with more accurate, helpful thoughts. The skill can be introduced as follows:

> "The final step of the 3C's is 'Change It.' In the Change It skill, you develop a more helpful, accurate thought that better matches the evidence you found in the Check It step. The *new* thought you develop needs to be realistic, helpful, and make sense to you. It is helpful to ask yourself:
>
> > 'What alternative conclusion is a better match with the evidence?'
> > 'What alternative thought might help me achieve my goals?'
>
> "For any unhelpful, inaccurate thoughts you might have, there are many other thoughts that may be more accurate and helpful."

By asking these questions, the consumer can often generate a new thought that is more accurate. You can help brainstorm together with the consumer (or with the group) about how to transform the thought. This might involve only minor insertion of a word or two into the thought (e.g., change "Nobody likes me" to "Someone likes me" to transform an all-or-nothing mistake into a more accurate thought) or a completely new thought. Write possible new thoughts on the board, then erase them and generate others until the consumer agrees that the new thought is more consistent with the evidence. If consumers still struggle with confirming whether a new thought is accurate, we have found it helpful to focus on whether the new thought is *more* accurate than the old one. It is most important to generate a thought that is less likely, even if only a little less likely, to interfere with goal-directed actions.

For example, Carol reported thinking, "I will get lost if I take the bus." Having previously agreed that this thought will not help Carol accomplish her short-term goal, Carol and the provider examined the evidence for and against the thought. Carol stated that there were two times when she got lost while riding the bus but acknowledged that she had not spent time identifying the proper route beforehand. Carol also recalled numerous times she rode the bus and did not get lost. Given the evidence, Carol identified the thought as the common mistake of fortune telling, and changed the thought to "I don't always get lost when riding the bus." After further discussion, she agreed that an even more helpful thought was "I won't get lost on the bus if I plan the route before I leave." This thought allowed Carol to move on to the next step of solving the problem of how to plan the route (e.g., using the SCALE problem-solving skill) so she could take action toward achieving her short-term goal of using the transit system.

In-Session Skill Practice: Generating Alternative Thoughts

Conduct an alternatives therapy exercise with consumers. Refer consumers to the worksheet, "Generating Alternative Thoughts" activity in the Consumer Workbook for this session. This is an exercise to practice generating alternative thoughts in the Change It step. "Alternatives therapy" is a technique used to help consumers brainstorm alternative thoughts or alternative explanations for events and situations. Begin with relatively benign situations, which are typically easier, then progress to more personal and emotionally charged situations, which are more challenging. Several situations previously identified by consumers are presented in this session. After describing the first situation, "Why would someone look at me at the mall?," identify the potential thought ("They think I am strange and will laugh at me"), and explain that this is an automatic thought that can interfere with accomplishing a goal step, such as going to the mall to buy a shirt for a job interview, but the thought can be challenged by generating possible alternatives. Then list alternative explanations for the situation, including ones that are often considered by consumers to be humorous, such as "They may think I look attractive." Then guide consumers to identify some additional explanations.

> **Situation:** "Why would someone look at me at the mall?"
>
> **Thought:** "He thinks I am strange and will laugh at me."
>
> **Alternative Explanations:**
> 1. He may think I look like someone he knows and want to say "hi."
> 2. He may not be looking at me at all and is just looking in the store windows behind me.
> 3. He may think I look attractive.
>
> 4. _____
> 5. _____

The goal is to help consumers stop accepting or perseverating on the first or most obvious explanation and instead entertain as many alternatives as possible. Providers should repeat the basic axiom "For every event there is more than one possible explanation." Ideally, providers should try to create examples relevant to individual consumers. For example, if a consumer introduces himself to someone at the clubhouse because his goal is to make a friend and the other person does not respond positively or just looks at the floor, this might be interpreted as evidence that supports the thought "They won't think I'm interesting" or "They won't like me." The provider can write this situation and thought down as an example and try to identify alternative explanations for why the person did not respond positively.

> **Situation:** "Why wouldn't someone talk to me when I introduce myself?"
>
> **Thought:** "He doesn't think I am interesting."
>
> **Alternative Explanations:**
> 1. The person was having a bad day and didn't feel like talking to anyone.
> 2. He didn't hear me because the room was too loud.
> 3. He feels anxious when talking to new people.
>
> 4. _____
> 5. _____

If you identify defeatist beliefs in consumers, the more helpful beliefs in the right-hand column on the "Common Thoughts Checklist" (Appendix C) can supply possible alternatives. The Provider Tip on page 125 summarizes the uses of the Common Thoughts Checklist for identifying and correcting defeatist beliefs.

Assign At-Home Practice: Catch, Check, and Change the Thought

As in Session 4, consumers are asked to fill out the At-Home Practice Worksheet for at least one thought that interfered with their goals during the week. Discuss with consumers what goal steps they might take over the next week and how they can use the 3C's to examine their thinking as they attempt goal steps. They can also use the 3C's Worksheet to examine their thinking when they experience "red flag," unpleasant emotions. Review the worksheet in session to help consumers begin to identify what thoughts might come up and how they might complete the homework.

Summarize the Session

The key points to summarize for this session are:

- If we change inaccurate thoughts to more accurate, helpful thoughts, we can feel better and achieve our goals.
- Practice makes it easier to generate alternative thoughts.

PROVIDER TIP

Use the Common Thoughts Checklist to Identify and Correct Defeatist Beliefs

- The thoughts in the checklist are organized according to specific situations related to recovery goals. It is not necessary to cover them all. Select situations related to a consumer's long-term goal (e.g., introducing him- or herself to others for someone with a goal of making a friend) and ask the consumer to pick thoughts he or she might have in that situation.
- Take note of the unhelpful thoughts endorsed, because you can use these thoughts in 3C's exercises.
- Put key defeatist performance beliefs on an index card to refer to in later sessions, and give a card like this to consumers.
- Refer to the more helpful alternative beliefs in the columns on the right when doing alternatives therapy and the 3C's Change It step of generating more helpful thoughts.
- To teach how changing thoughts can change feelings and behaviors, ask consumers what feelings and behaviors could stem from a defeatist thought on the left, then what feelings and behaviors might stem from the more helpful thought on the right.
- Ask which selected thoughts are helpful and which are unhelpful with reference to personal goal(s). Why are they helpful–unhelpful?

Example: When you are trying to meet new people, do you think, "People won't like me because I have schizophrenia?" Is it hard to meet new people when you have this thought? Why? Are you more or less likely to go out and try to meet someone if you have this thought? How does this thought make you feel? How do you feel when you avoid meeting people?

Ask for Consumer Feedback

Now that you have put it all together and consumers have had some experience using the 3C's, ask whether they think the 3C's might be a helpful skill to check out their thoughts. Some consumers enjoy these sessions and are very satisfied with changing dysfunctional thoughts. It can be an uplifting experience to be told that you are much better at doing things and more likable than you thought you were. Many people with schizophrenia have very few opportunities for success experiences and positive feedback to nurture self-efficacy and positive beliefs about the self. Other consumers may voice some resistance, especially with regard to firmly held beliefs. Normalize this and remember your neutral stance with regard to accuracy of beliefs. Some beliefs are accurate and others are inaccurate; the important thing is to gather evidence to figure out which beliefs are accurate and change thoughts that do not have sufficient evidence to support them. You can foreshadow that in the next session, they will learn how to do experiments to test out beliefs, and you can ask, "Are you willing to keep coming back to learn more about how to test them out? Together we can try to figure it out."

Session 6: 3C's Practice

PROVIDER PLAN FOR THIS SESSION

- Set the Agenda Collaboratively
- Review At-Home Practice: Catch, Check, and Change the Thought
- Introduce Behavioral Experiments to Check It
- In-Session Skill Practice: The 3C's with Behavioral Experiments
- Assign At-Home Practice: Catch, Check, and Change the Thought
- Summarize the Session
- Ask for Consumer Feedback

CONDUCTING THE SESSION

Set the Agenda Collaboratively

- Review At-Home Practice
- Doing Experiments to Check-It
- Practice the 3C's to Achieve Goals
- Assign At-Home Practice: Catch, Check, and Change the Thought
- Additional Agenda Items?

Note agenda items presented by consumers and try to use them in the session as content for teaching about behavioral experiments. For example, if someone raises an issue about voices, say, "I'm glad you brought that up, because we are going to talk today about how to design experiments to test out whether it is possible to control voices."

Review At-Home Practice: Catch, Check, and Change the Thought

Review of the 3C's worksheets will provide valuable information about which consumers are understanding and able to use the skill in the real world outside group, and which consumers are still struggling to understand the skill. Session 6 provides an opportunity to further practice the 3C's, so consumers who have a better understanding can be called upon as experts to help teach the skills to others who might be struggling. For example, you could pair highly skilled consumers to work on 3C's sheets with less-skilled consumers, while providers go around the room and coach. Consumers who need a bit more practice can also be the focus of 3C's practice later in the session. Even consumers who understand the skill well often do not use it appropriately in the real world when firmly held beliefs come up and interfere with functioning; they use it instead in more benign situations. When assigning homework later in this session, try to remind these consumers to use the skill when they are attempting a goal step (or when they are avoiding action, which is more difficult to catch). For example, when it became apparent that Juan was avoiding completion of the goal step of negotiating quiet hours with his roommate, he was encouraged to catch the thoughts that he had immediately preceding the planned conversation with his roommate. Juan had previously expressed concern that his roommate might react negatively to the conversation, so he was encouraged to use the 3C's to modify these thoughts to help him accomplish the goal step.

Introduce Behavioral Experiments to Check It

As described in Chapter 3, behavioral experiments are planned activities performed by consumers to test out beliefs either in session or for homework. They are a powerful way to challenge maladaptive cognitions and increase productive behaviors in the community. When someone is hesitant to try a new activity due to an interfering cognition (e.g., "It will never work"), say, "Are you willing to do something to test that belief out?" You can introduce behavioral experiments as follows:

> "One way to gather evidence on whether thoughts are accurate is to design an experiment. Just like any scientific experiment, it means figuring out a way to test the accuracy of a thought or hypothesis."

In this session and in the Consumer Workbook, the behavioral experiment process is simplified into three steps. However, providers should follow the five-step process of planning behavioral experiments described in Chapter 3 and Table 3.2.
Explain the steps for a behavioral experiment:

1. What's the thought or belief you want to test? Write it down. That's your hypothesis. For example: "Someone's stealing my mail."
2. Design an experiment to test the belief. For example: "Send myself a letter. If the letter comes, nobody is stealing my mail."
3. Record the results and draw conclusions about the belief. For example: "The letter arrived, so mail was not stolen. My belief is not accurate."

In-Session Skill Practice: The 3C's with Behavioral Experiments

The skill practice for this session involves completing additional 3C's Worksheets in session to test out thoughts that came up during the session or in recent weeks in situations related to goal-directed activities or unpleasant emotions. The Provider Tip on page 129 presents several suggestions for practicing the 3C's. For this session, the 3C's Worksheet also includes additional space for describing a behavioral experiment that can be used to test out the belief. Thus, in addition to identifying evidence for and against a thought and mistakes in thinking, consumers are encouraged to try to come up with an experiment to test out beliefs. Several examples of experiments to test out specific types of beliefs are presented in the Consumer Workbook, but personally relevant examples from agenda items presented by consumers at the beginning of the session or, by now, dysfunctional belief themes or psychotic beliefs that interfere with functioning that have become apparent, should be the focus of skills practice.

For example, Carol and her provider designed an experiment to test out her thought, "The cartels will harm me if I ride the bus." She agreed to ride the bus one stop from her home, then cross the street and ride another bus back home one stop, while observing other passengers for potential signs of danger. She was willing to try riding the bus for this short time even though she believed there were *always* cartel gang members who wanted to harm her on the bus. Since this is an all-or-nothing thought (i.e., there is *always* danger on the bus), the experiment was likely to succeed by demonstrating that she was not *always* harmed on the bus. After riding the bus and not being harmed, Carol concluded she would not *always* be harmed on the bus. This opened the door to riding the bus sometimes, rather than never, and started a discussion about determining *when* it is safe to ride the bus, rather than never traveling away from home. Changing the all-or-nothing thought to a thought that permitted some bus travel opened the door to more goal-directed activities away from home.

Thoughts and Behaviors: Chickens and Eggs

Although the skills in CBSST can generally be divided into predominantly cognitive or behavioral interventions, most skills have both cognitive and behavioral aspects. Behavioral interventions, like behavioral experiments, can lead to changes in cognition (e.g., doing an activity and finding out whether it is more enjoyable than predicted provides evidence to dispute low expectations), and cognitive interventions can lead to behavior change (e.g., challenging the belief that one has to "feel" like doing something before doing it). Research has shown that both cognitive and behavioral exercises can lead to change in both cognition and behavior.

Although this module focuses on changing thoughts to change both feelings and behaviors, remember also to discuss how changing behaviors can change feelings and thoughts. The arrows in the cognitive model go in both directions. When sad, we are more likely to think hopeless and pessimistic thoughts. Also, isolation and avoidance behaviors will not provide successful and pleasurable social experiences to contradict defeatist attitudes and loneliness. It is important to remember these

PROVIDER TIP

Developing the 3C's Skills

Catch It

- Try to phrase the thought as one that interferes with recovery goals. Ask, "Does the thought help you reach your goal?"

- Try to phrase the thought as a mistake in thinking, if possible, or exaggerate the thought to make it easier to challenge (e.g., use words such as "always," "never," "everyone," and "nobody" to create an all-or-none thought that is easy to challenge).

- Use the "red flag" technique: Unwanted feelings and behaviors are "red flags" that signal the need to examine thoughts.

- Make sure the consumer has caught a thought, and not an emotion or behavior. If it is not a thought, reinforce the effort and correct it.

Check It

- Mistakes in thinking

  o Ask if the thought is a mistake in thinking (maybe the consumer's favorite mistake) and why the particular mistake in thinking was chosen.
  o Praise the effort, and prompt for other mistakes that may have been missed. Sometimes more than one mistake applies.

- Evidence for the thought

  o It is usually easier to generate evidence for beliefs.

- Evidence against the thought

  o This is more difficult, so normalize this if consumers have trouble. People tend to have a bias against noticing disconfirmatory evidence.

- Help consumers discover evidence against the thought by asking questions: What conclusion would a judge or a detective make based on the evidence? Have I had any experiences that show that this thought is not completely true all the time? If someone else had this thought, what would I tell him or her?

- Use the other members of the group to brainstorm. It is usually easier for people to generate evidence against other people's beliefs rather than their own.

Change It

- Use the alternatives therapy exercises to help consumers become more flexible in their thinking.

- It is often possible to slightly modify the original thought to interfere less with goal achievement (e.g., change "never" to "sometimes I succeed" and "nobody" to "some people like me").

- Ask, "Does the new thought help you reach your goal?"

reciprocal interactions if consumers are having difficulties working on thoughts. For example, consumers with concrete cognitive styles may have difficulty identifying thoughts or how thoughts can affect emotions and behaviors abstractly. Learning, in this case, can be facilitated by asking consumers to generate thoughts "in the moment." That is, people sometimes have an easier time generating thoughts shortly after they *do* something, so try taking a walk, facilitating an in-session game or activity, or doing a role play with the consumer and ask about thoughts in the moment. This is a behavioral experiment.

It is not necessary first to change defeatist beliefs, delusional beliefs, or other goal-interfering thoughts before taking action to achieve goals. If you find yourself in endless debate about evidence to support or disconfirm beliefs, turn your attention to behavior change. Encourage behaviors related to goals (e.g., "experiment" by going out, taking a class, talking to someone). These activities will present evidence (success or failure experiences) that can be used to challenge unhelpful beliefs. Get people behaving differently, and deal with the thoughts and data that come up as a result of the behavior change. This is often difficult. Automatic thoughts are often so ingrained (this is why they are automatic) that people accept them as truth. Elicit these thoughts when people take action, then examine them. This can demonstrate that many undesirable feelings and behaviors are linked to these unquestioned thoughts. One way to increase the likelihood that someone will try a behavioral experiment or take action to test out an automatic thought is to plan a reward afterward, regardless of the outcome. For additional guidance on addressing resistance to conducting behavioral experiments, see the Provider Tip on page 131.

Assign At-Home Practice: Catch, Check, and Change the Thought

Ask consumers to use the 3C's to correct thinking and work toward goals at least once during the week. They should fill out the At-Home Practice Worksheet in the Consumer Workbook for Session 6. The worksheet includes a space for planning a behavioral experiment to test out the accuracy of the thought. In some cases, the plan for this experiment will have been generated during the session. For example, a consumer with a belief that command hallucinations have power to harm or control might have generated an experiment during the session to test it out by not

PROVIDER TIP

"I Can't"

The suggestion of a behavioral experiment is sometimes met with resistance:

> CONSUMER: I can't.
> PROVIDER: That sounds like an expectation. What might happen if you try?
> CONSUMER: I don't know.
> PROVIDER: Would you be willing to try or test it out?

Or:

> PROVIDER: What thoughts are you having about trying that out? What goes through your mind when you think about trying?

Or: If that doesn't work, you may want to try reflections to discover the source of resistance.

> PROVIDER: Sounds like you are frustrated with this or hopeless; can we try to figure out why?

complying once during the week and see whether the voice follows through on a threat. Others may need to generate an idea for an experiment during the homework assignment part of group, which may require additional time in this session.

For example, Juan had not yet completed the goal step of finding ways to be more independent at his board-and-care facility. The provider had identified a thought that seemed to be impeding Juan's progress on this goal step: "There is no way the manager will let me do anything." The provider proposed that Juan test it out despite Juan's prediction that it would not work. Juan and the provider designed an experiment in which Juan would request to speak with manager to ask about just one way he could be more active in his own care at the home. Juan agreed that even if the manager suggested a task that Juan was not interested in doing, the experiment would still provide evidence against the thought that the manager would not let him do anything independently at the home.

Summarize the Session

The key points to summarize for this session are:

- One way to check the accuracy of our thoughts is to design experiments to test them out.
- Doing experiments and correcting mistakes in thinking with the 3C's get easier with practice.

Ask for Consumer Feedback

Generating experiments requires creativity and can be quite challenging. The feedback from consumers may reflect this. Even if this is not reported, it is important to set up consumers for success rather than failure, by letting them know that it is difficult and they may not always be able to design an experiment on their own. Even if they are not able to conduct an experiment to test a belief, they can use the 3C's skill to examine a belief that is in the way of their goals.

PROVIDER TIP

Module Reminders

- Give consumers the skills handout for each session or give them the entire Cognitive Skills Module Consumer Workbook, as well as a small laminated card that contains the Cognitive Triangle, the 3C's, and Mistakes in Thinking for reference in and out of sessions.

- Use a whiteboard or notepad to write down the Cognitive Triangle and put thoughts on the board in quotes, with an arrow from thoughts to feelings or behaviors. Use experiences from consumers to highlight each point.

- Emphasize the 3C's and take time to make sure consumers understand and practice each step of the 3C's. Get consumers curious about their thoughts and help them examine evidence for and against the accuracy of unhelpful beliefs.

- Relate thoughts to personalized recovery goal(s) and focus on using the 3C's and behavioral experiments to address thoughts that are interfering with goals.

- Give lots of praise, especially for completing at-home practice (homework).

- Get feedback about the sessions:
  - What did they like? Dislike?
  - What was the most difficult part?
  - Was it helpful?

CHAPTER 7

Social Skills Module

1. Explain how communication skills can help consumers achieve personal recovery goals and practice applying basic communication skills to goal-directed social interactions in the community.

2. Teach nonverbal communication skills and use role plays to teach four basic communication skills.

3. Improve self-efficacy for social communication and reduce defeatist performance beliefs about interacting with others.

MODULE OVERVIEW

Social interactions require that individuals *perceive* social situation cues, *process* that social information, and *respond effectively* (Bellack, 2002). Social perception involves accurately detecting social situation cues such as facial expressions, gestures, body posture, and other contextual cues, as well as verbal content. Social cognition involves the processing or analysis of social situation cues such as recognizing and labeling emotions in others, interpreting the intentions of others, and planning an appropriate response. Behavioral response involves choosing and expressing the right words along with nonverbal behaviors such as eye contact, gestures, and body posture. Effective social interaction integrates all three of these abilities. An extensive body of research indicates that these abilities and skills can be trained (see Chapter 2).

The emphasis of this module is on expressive social skills, with some focus on perceiving and interpreting social cues. No systematic social cognition training is provided, although there is some training in recognizing and expressing affect in facial expressions and speech prosody. Social problem solving is addressed to some extent in this module and again in the Problem-Solving Skills Module (see Chapter 8).

Four basic communication skills are trained in this module: Active Listening (Session 2); Expressing Pleasant Feelings (Session 3); Making Positive Requests (Sessions 4 and 5); and Expressing Unpleasant Feelings (Session 6). Starting with Session 3, the communication skills trained in this module follow a similar structure:

When you DO _____, I FEEL _____.

Consumers are taught to describe what other people do, or what they want them to do, and how other people's actions make them feel, or would make them feel if the requested action is performed. This structure emphasizes the impact of observable behavior in others (what people DO) on the speaker (how the speaker FEELS). In Session 3, Expressing Pleasant Feelings, the speaker identifies a specific target behavior performed by another that made the speaker feel good. In Session 4, Making Positive Requests, the speaker identifies a behavior he or she would like the other person to DO, because it would make the speaker FEEL good. Because the making positive requests skill can be so helpful when applied to recovery goal achievement, the skill is the focus of two sessions (Sessions 4 and 5). Session 4 primarily focuses on learning the skill and Session 5 focuses on identifying support persons and asking them for help with goal-related tasks. In Session 6, the speaker targets a behavior he or she would like the other person to stop doing, because it makes the speaker FEEL bad. To perform the skills well, speakers must clearly describe how specific behaviors cause pleasant and unpleasant feelings. To make this easier for consumers to remember, point out that all these communication skills involve saying, "When you DO _____, I FEEL _____."

This structure increases the likelihood that others will do what we ask. Describing the specific behavior of another makes it clear to the other person exactly what you want him or her to do (or not do). Actions are observable and measurable, so it is difficult to argue about whether the action was performed. For example, if we say, "Don't be rude," or worse, use name-calling and say, "Don't be a jerk," it is not clear what behavior we want the other person to change. It is more effective to say, "When you interrupt me when I'm talking, it makes me angry, so please wait until I'm done." The behavior the speaker wants the other person to DO is clear. It is also difficult to argue with someone about his or her feelings; only you know how you feel. If someone says that something you did made him or her angry or sad, it is difficult to respond, "No, you're not." Focusing on what others DO and how we FEEL is an effective way to get our needs met with minimal conflict or and arguing. Also, if the listener cares about the person making the request, he or she will want to make the person feel good, not bad, so expressing how we feel can motivate the listener to do (or stop doing) the action.

The primary therapeutic technique in this module is behavioral rehearsal or role play of simulated conversations, as described in more detail below. The goal is to improve assertive, clear, and comfortable communication in social interactions. Consumers and providers simulate interactions with roommates, friends and family, teachers, bosses, coworkers, and case managers and other service providers to teach consumers, for example, how to ask for a ride, make new friends, be assertive with parents or roommates, ask for help with classes, interview for jobs, or manage their own health care.

The group therapy format is ideal for role-play training. Group members who have previously received the Social Skills Module and members with better communication skills can be encouraged to help teach new members about the communication and social skills. This contributes both to a sense of mastery for the skilled group member and increased perception that the skill is learnable for the new or unskilled group member. Consumers can also sometimes accept feedback better from peers than from providers, and role-play scenarios between group members are more similar to real-world experiences than role plays with providers. The specific session content associated with module objectives is shown in Table 7.1.

ROLE-PLAY TRAINING

In this module, skill learning occurs through role plays and experiential learning, not discussion or lecture. In role-play training, complex social interactions, such as

TABLE 7.1. Social Skills Module Objectives and Related Session Content

Social Skills Module objectives	Content
Improve communication skills	Role plays using shaping, repeated practice, and reinforcement to train verbal and nonverbal elements of communication skills involving active listening (Session 2), expressing pleasant feelings (Session 3), making positive requests (Sessions 4 and 5), and expressing unpleasant feelings (Session 6).
Apply communication skills to personal recovery goal achievement	Role plays of simulated interactions with roommates, housing staff, friends, family, bosses, coworkers, teachers, classmates, doctors, case managers, and other service providers on topics related to personal living, learning, working, and socializing goals (Sessions 2–6).
Improve self-efficacy and reduce defeatist performance beliefs	Self-efficacy and performance beliefs are elicited (e.g., 0–10 ratings of how successful you think you were/will be), and role plays are used as behavioral experiments to test out self-defeating beliefs in session and at home (Sessions 2–6).

asking for a favor, are broken down into simple steps that include nonverbal communication (e.g., maintain eye contact, nod, smile) and specific verbal content (e.g., "When you DO _____, I FEEL _____"). Providers teach the steps of each skill and model the skill to demonstrate how to do it, then consumers practice the skill—ideally three times—and learn to perform it smoothly through shaping and reinforcement of successive approximations. "Shaping" means picking one component of the skill at a time to improve (e.g., eye contact, saying how you feel, or keeping it short), and practicing the skill until that component improves, before introducing another component to practice, until all components of a complex skill are performed well. Reinforcement (e.g., positive feedback, praise, applause, gold stars) of each attempt to improve a component is crucial to learning the skill. Role-play training involves a systematic, multiple-step process, as outline in Table 7.2.

Step 1: Bridge the Skill–Goal Gap

When introducing the skill, it is crucial to link the skill to personal recovery goals. Consumers will be more motivated to learn skills if they are associated with achieving personally meaningful goals. Avoid a generic rationale such as "It is important

TABLE 7.2. The Steps of Role-Play Training

1. *Bridge the skill–goal gap.* Discuss how the skill can help consumers achieve their personal recovery goals.

2. *Describe the skill.* Providers teach the steps of the skill and discuss the rationale for each step.

3. *Model the skill.* Providers perform the skill in a role play.

4. *Elicit thoughts.* Ask about expectations ("How well do you think you will do it?"; 0, "I will fail/do badly," to 10, "I will succeed/do great!").

5. *Role play.* Engage the consumer in a role play related to his or her recovery goal.

6. *Reinforce.* Provide a lot of positive feedback and reinforcement, such as applause and verbal praise. Ask, "What did he or she do well?"

7. *Shape.* Provide corrective feedback. Ask, "What can he or she do to improve?" Pick just one behavior to improve in the next role play.

8. *Practice.* Engage the consumer in the same role play again.

9. *Reinforce and shape.* Provide additional positive and corrective feedback.

10. *Practice.* Engage the consumer in a third and final role play using the same skill and situation (practicing each role play three times is ideal).

11. *Be positive.* Provide reinforcement but no corrective feedback. Identify what the consumer did well and celebrate success.

12. *Correct dysfunctional thoughts.* Ask the consumer to rate his or her success ("How well do you think you did?"; 0, "I failed/did badly," to 10, "I succeeded/did great!") and compare this rating with the initial expectations rating from Step 4. Discuss how expectations can impact actions.

13. *Assign at-home practice.* Assign the role play as homework to be reviewed in the next session.

to learn good communication skills" or "Communication skills can help you reach your goals." The more specific the link to personal goals, the more motivation to learn. In a group setting, providers can ask members how they think the skill might help with their goals, and provide some examples and guidance, until each member has a clear skill–goal link, in the following way:

> "Today we are going to learn how to make a positive request. This is a skill we can use to ask others to do things we want them to do. This is a very useful communication skill to help us reach our goals, because all goals involve asking others to do things. For example, Jim, your goal is to get a girlfriend, so you could use this skill to ask someone to go on a date with you, and Mary, you could use the skill to ask for help finding a job. Joe, can you think of a way you could use the skill to ask someone to do something to help you get your own apartment?"

Step 2: Describe the Skill

Teach the steps of the skill. Read the steps from the handouts in the Consumer Workbook, or ask consumers to read them, and discuss the rationale for each step. It is helpful to display them on a whiteboard or a poster for reference while reviewing the steps and later when practicing the skills in role plays. After describing each step, ask, "Why do you think it is important to do [or say] that?"

Step 3: Model the Skill

Provider(s) perform a role play to model the skill. Set up two chairs in front of the room. With two providers in a group, one provider sits in one chair and models the skill, while the other sits in the other chair and plays the other role. With one provider, the provider models the skill, while a consumer plays the other role. It is sometimes helpful for providers to model making mistakes during the role play to normalize mistakes and model accepting corrective feedback appropriately, as long as the skill is ultimately modeled correctly. Keep role plays "short and sweet," typically, less than 15 seconds.

Step 4: Elicit Thoughts

Once consumers understand the requirements of the specific role play, ask about their performance expectations: "What thoughts do you have about the role play?"; "How well do you think you will do on a 0 to 10 scale?" (0 = "I will do badly"; 10 = "I will do great!"). Different consumers have different types of dysfunctional beliefs that may interfere with skill performance in the community. For some consumers, expectations about their ability to perform the skill (self-efficacy) may get in their way. For others, expectations about the skill's outcome will get in their way (e.g., a request will be refused). Providers can decide which type of success expectation rating to use, based on the nature of each consumer's individual beliefs, or have consumers rate both ability and outcome success. For example, bolstering beliefs about performance ability may be more relevant for consumers with low self-efficacy; bolstering beliefs about outcome success may be more relevant for consumers who expect to be treated poorly by others, even if they perform the skill well. Emphasize that mastering these skills will give them the best chance of getting their needs met; however, this does not guarantee that other people will do what they ask every time. Asking consumers to rate both ability and outcome success provides an opportunity to discuss how expectations about both types of success can impact emotions and the willingness to engage in goal-directed actions in the community. See the Provider Tip on this page. The Consumer Workbook for Sessions 3–6 contain forms for recording before and after role-play thoughts and ratings.

Step 5: Role Play

The consumer then attempts the skill in a role play, while a provider plays the other role or, if in a group, another consumer comes up to the chairs and takes the role as listener. In deciding the content for the role play, providers should

---

PROVIDER TIP

Elicit Thoughts about Role Plays

1. Before the role play, ask, "What do you think about doing this role play? How well do you think you will do it?"

2. Rate how well you think you will perform the skill (0–10).
      0 = "I will do badly."
      5 = "I'm not sure."
      10 = "I will do great!"

3. For Making Positive Requests and Expressing Unpleasant Feelings, ask, "Do you think they will do it? Rate your prediction about the outcome of the skill, that is, the other person's response (0–10)."
      0 = "Definitely will not do it."
      5 = "Not sure."
      10 = "Definitely will do it."

4. After practicing the role play three times, ask, "Now that you have had a chance to try the role play, what do you think about it? Did it turn out better or worse than you thought it would? Rate how well you did it (0–10). Rate your prediction about the outcome again (0–10)."

5. Post-role-play ratings are rarely below the earlier expectations, so providers can point out that consumers did better than they thought they would. You can then have a brief discussion to challenge low expectations to increase the likelihood that consumers will try the skill in the community.

select content relevant to each consumer's goals. For example, if several members in a group have socialization goals, the role plays for these members can involve starting a conversation with a compliment for Expressing Pleasant Feelings (e.g., "Hi, I'm Eric. When you told your story at the meeting, it was inspiring and made me feel hopeful about my situation"), or asking someone to join them for coffee for Making a Positive Request ("I would be so happy if you would meet me for coffee"). Modify the role-play scenario for each person, so it will generalize to real-world situations related to each person's recovery goals. Someone with a work goal should not practice a role play asking someone for a date; asking for help filling out a job application would be more relevant to his or her work goal. The goal steps on the consumer's 7–7–7 Goal Jackpot! Worksheet can provide ideas for personalized goal-related role plays. In this way, individual role plays can be tailored to the unique needs of each consumer. If the Active Listening skill has been trained, one consumer can practice active listening, while the other consumer practices the new skill being trained.

As in modeling the skill, keep consumer role plays "short and sweet," less than 30 seconds. Direct, simple, brief communications are more clear and effective. In groups, there will not be sufficient time for all members to practice longer role plays. If the consumer goes off topic or takes too long, place your hand on the consumer's shoulder and give him or her a brief phrase to use that captures what he or she is trying to say (e.g., "Just say this, . . ."). This hand-on-the-shoulder coaching technique is a way to shape the performance without stopping the role play. See also the Provider Tip on this page.

After the role play everyone applauds. Some providers use hand signals or say something to mark the end of a role play. We use applause because it feels good and is reinforcing. Clap at the end of every role play. Reinforce and reassure consumers that better communication skills can help people achieve just about any social functioning goal, and there is room for improvement for everyone (normalization)—this is why you ask for feedback at the end of each role play.

PROVIDER TIP

Hand-on-the-Shoulder Coaching to Keep It "Short and Sweet"

Role plays are "short and sweet" (less than 30 seconds). When role plays go off topic or are too long, shape performance by placing your hand on the consumer's shoulder during a role play and saying (modeling) a brief phrase into his or her ear to capture what he or she is trying to say: "Just say this. . . ." This hand-on-the-shoulder coaching technique is a way to shape performance quickly, in the moment, without having to stop the role play. Nonverbal coaching can also be helpful, in which the provider points to skill steps or a script on the board to focus the consumer during a role play.

Steps 6 and 7: Reinforcement and Shaping

The provider then asks for positive feedback from the group and from the consumer.

> "What did she or he do well?"
> "What did you do well?"

Provide any positive feedback that wasn't observed by others. Praise well-performed elements. Then, ask if anything could be added or improved to make the skill even better: "What could he or she do to make it even better?"

Shaping involves successive reinforcement of one element at a time. Select *only one* component to focus on in a second role play, and be specific. For example, ask the consumer to make more eye contact *or* speak louder *or* be more specific about what the consumer wants the other person to do. For the latter, suggest specific sentences (e.g., "Would you drive me to the store on Saturday right after lunch?") or how it would make the consumer feel (e.g., "It would make me happy"). Asking for improvement in more than one element can be overwhelming.

Steps 8, 9, and 10: Practice, Practice, Practice

The skill is then practiced in the same role play again, with a focus on correcting one element. This is followed by applause, positive feedback for well-performed elements, and corrective feedback for one additional element or the same element, if it was still not performed well. Repeated practice is the key component of social skills training (see the Provider Tip on this page). Ideally, with sufficient session time, each consumer will practice each role play three times, although sometimes there is only time for two role plays per consumer.

If the skill is performed perfectly (even if it is the first try), you can celebrate and move on to the next consumer, or you can make the role play more challenging (e.g., by having the listener refuse the request) and coach the consumer through a response as needed. This will prepare consumers for scenarios that do not work out perfectly when they attempt the skill in the community. We have found it helpful to provide a warning when you make a role play more difficult, so that the consumer is prepared

---

PROVIDER TIP

If Providers Talk Too Much, They Are Wasting Everyone's Time

Social skills training is a behavioral intervention in which skills practice is the key element. While providers must verbally explain the rationale for skills and address expectations and self-efficacy beliefs, lecturing or talking too much about issues in the community takes time away from skills practice. The focus is on role-play practice of communication skills.

to problem-solve. For example, "I'm going to make it a little tougher on you now; I might throw you a curve ball on this one." Providing a warning that you are going to make it particularly difficult can also make it less disappointing if the performance is not perfect. Minimizing failure protects self-efficacy.

Step 11: Be Positive

After the last role play, ideally the third, nothing is corrected, and only positive feedback is given for well-performed elements, because there will be no additional role-play opportunities to correct any elements. Focus on the positive, and keep role plays fun for both consumers and yourself. If someone overcomes some real challenges and performs an excellent role play, give him or her a standing ovation and ask the group to join you or give out awards (e.g., gold star stickers or plastic Oscar trophies), or ask the consumers to circle the group getting high fives from all the members. Use your sense of humor and playfulness. Doing so will make role plays more engaging and reduce anxiety about attempting a new skill. Encourage consumers to laugh, and appreciate the inevitable mistakes made while attempting something new. This can normalize mistakes in the learning process. Dr. Alan Bellack, a master social skills trainer (Bellack, personal communication, 2011), has said, "If you walk by a group room at the clinic and everyone is laughing inside, you know there is a social skills training group going on." SST groups are fun for consumers and providers, because they focus on the positive (reinforcing what consumers are doing well), on learning to laugh at our mistakes, and on increasing success and self-efficacy. See also the Provider Tip on this page.

Step 12: Elicit and Challenge Dysfunctional Thoughts

The next step is to ask the consumer about his or her thoughts about performance in the role plays. How does the person rate ability and outcome now? Using the same scaling technique, ask for a rating of success versus failure. Compare this appraisal

---

PROVIDER TIP

Stay Positive

One of the pitfalls for providers is forgetting to stay positive and focusing too much on what consumers did not do well in role plays. To make it easy, so consumers can do well, skills are broken down into simple elements, and shaping involves gradually increasing skill performance a little bit at a time. Small steps ensure success. Consumers may not do well the first time, but celebrate elements performed well with applause and plenty of reinforcement, before focusing on only one element to improve during the next role play. Too much focus on the end product can make a consumer feel like a failure.

to expectations for performance before the role play. The post-role-play rating is rarely below the earlier expectations, so providers can point out that consumers did better than they thought they would. You can then have a brief discussion about how low expectations could be raised. For example,

> "You rated yourself a 4 before you tried it and an 8 after; your score doubled! Maybe you are too hard on yourself. You did a lot better than you thought you would. I think you did a terrific job and should have higher expectations for yourself. Do you think you are more likely to try asking for a ride to the store now when you're an 8 and think you're likely to succeed than when you thought you were a 4 and more likely to fail?"

Consumers may become very skillful at engaging with providers during role plays, then do not attempt the skills in the community. This is often because a thought is in the way (e.g., "He won't want to talk to me" or "I'll make a fool of myself"). Role plays can be used as behavioral experiments to test out these beliefs that can interfere with social interactions in the community. Defeatist expectations such as "It will be too hard for me" or "I will make mistakes and look stupid" can be corrected by encouraging consumers to try out a role play and evaluate the evidence for and against their thoughts (e.g., ask group members if they thought the person looked stupid). Role plays in session can provide clues about the thoughts that are likely to be interfering with skilled performance in the community (e.g., ask, "What were you thinking when you made that request in the role play?"). These thoughts can then be targeted for change using the 3C's or by encouraging performance of an experiment to test them out. Listen for possible changes in beliefs after role plays (e.g., "I didn't think I could do it" or "That wasn't so bad"). Draw attention to how expectations are usually worse than reality, and how this might prevent them from engaging in helpful social interactions related to their recovery goals. It may be useful to identify common mistakes in thinking, such as fortune telling or jumping to conclusions. Encourage people to test things to find out whether they might do better than they thought they would. See also the Provider Tip on this page.

PROVIDER TIP

Catch It, Check It, Change It during Role Plays

Elicit and examine thoughts (especially about success or failure) before and after each role play. If someone expects to fail, he or she may not even try. Role plays are behavioral experiments that provide data to challenge low self-efficacy beliefs ("I can't do it well") and change them to more accurate, helpful thoughts ("I'm actually pretty good at this") to bolster self-confidence.

Step 13: Assign At-Home Practice

The final step of the role-play sequence is to assign the skill for at-home practice. Collaborate with consumers before they leave the role-play chairs to decide how they could use the skill in the community. If the role-play situation was tailored to the individual consumer's needs and goals at the beginning of role-play practice, the At-Home Practice situation will naturally unfold (e.g., "Now that you practiced in class asking Joe for a ride to the store, are you willing to try to ask him at home sometime this week? What day will you see him?"). Time permitting, you could also ask for the consumers' rating of how successful they think they might be at performing the skill in the community and begin to fill out the at-home practice sheet together. Alternatively, the consumer can return to his or her seat and begin to fill out the At-Home Practice Sheet as the next consumer starts a role play.

When one consumer is finished practicing the skill, a new consumer comes up to the chairs, and the 13-step role-play training procedure is repeated with the new consumer. If one consumer was practicing active listening skills while another consumer was practicing the new skill, the active listening consumer switches to learn the new skill, and another group member takes on the active listening role. The rest of a group proceeds in this way, rotating through the role-play chairs, with the same 13 steps followed with each consumer.

ENGAGING RELUCTANT CONSUMERS IN ROLE PLAYS

Occasionally, consumers are reluctant to participate in role plays. Of course, many people feel uncomfortable or anxious about talking in front of others or giving a speech, so it can help to acknowledge and normalize this. You might comment on how you felt the first time you tried a role play in a group. Then suggest that it is worth it to try role plays even if they are uncomfortable, because role-play practice can produce better communication skills to help consumers achieve their goals. Mention the specific long-term goals of reluctant participants and link role-play practice to learning the communication skills needed to achieve those goals. In the case example of Juan, discussed in Chapter 5 (see Figure 5.3), a provider could describe how learning to express negative feelings (frustration) with his current roommates could help Juan with his goal of living comfortably with roommates in his own apartment (e.g., "If you have to have roommates to get an apartment, it will help to learn how to get along with them better and get them to stop doing things that bother you"). Providers can also emphasize that by role playing in class, which is a safe and fun place to learn, people usually feel more comfortable and confident when they need to use the skills to communicate in the real world.

Observing others in role plays also helps consumers realize that people are not criticized, embarrassed, or otherwise treated badly. In fact, there will typically be laughter, fun, applause, and celebration. The consumer can also gradually become engaged in the process by being asked to provide specific feedback to others about their role-play performance (e.g., check for eye contact or mentioning a feeling). After participating in feedback discussions and observing others in role plays, providers can invite reluctant consumers to try it out, maybe with a briefer role play or only one step of the skill. Praise any participation (e.g., "I really like the way spoke loud enough for me to hear you" or "You made really good eye contact; that's an important first step of the skill"). In this way, providers can shape and reinforce successive approximations of skill performance, building up to more confident participation in role-play practice.

Another strategy to facilitate engagement of consumers who are still reluctant to engage in role plays or are having trouble thinking of something to say in a role play is to write out a script to follow during a role play. Some examples are provided in the Provider Tip on this page. These scripts allow consumers to participate in simple

---

PROVIDER TIP

Scripted Role Plays Promote Engagement of Reluctant Consumers

Role Play: Expressing Pleasant Feelings

You

When you gave me a ride to the store, I was so relieved that I didn't have to bring my groceries on the bus. Thank you so much.

Friend

You're welcome. Anytime.

Role Play: Making a Positive Request

You

Hello. How are you doing today?

I am fine. Thanks for asking. I would really like to have lunch with you. It would make me happy to catch up.

Yes, tomorrow is a good day. How about noon?

Family Member

I am doing very well, thank you. How about you?

That sounds like a great idea. Are you available tomorrow?

Great. I will come by at noon.

Role Play: Expressing Unpleasant Feelings

You

When you play your music loud after 10:00 P.M., it makes me angry and frustrated because I cannot sleep. Would you please turn it down or use headphones after 10:00 P.M.?

Thank you. I really appreciate it.

Roommate

OK. I didn't know it bothered you.

No problem.

conversations that are less threatening or emotionally charged, because they are not necessarily related to any person's particular needs. Ask consumers to identify thoughts they may have before reading through the lines ("I can't do it" or "I will be embarrassed"). These can be challenged and changed to more helpful thoughts after practicing with the script. After some practice, providers can decrease the use of the scripted role plays and use personalized content from the consumer's life that is more directly relevant to recovery goal achievement.

Session 1: Introduction and Goal Setting

In Session 1 (see Chapter 5), new members may join the group, the CBSST program is introduced, and new and previous members both identify long-term and short-term goals, and add goal steps to their 7–7–7 Goal Jackpot! Worksheet. The At-Home Practice Review for previous members who have been in the group (there is no homework to review for new members) is typically the homework from Session 6 of the Cognitive Skills Module (using the 3C's and behavioral experiments to challenge thoughts that interfere with goal steps), unless the Problem-Solving Module was the last module delivered, in which case the homework was from Session 6 of that module (using SCALE to solve problems related to goal steps). In either case, reviewing homework provides an opportunity to review the skills from the prior module with previous members, and provides an opportunity to explain to new members that At-Home Practice is a key component of the CBSST program (see Chapter 5).

When describing CBSST to new members in Session 1 of this module, focus on the importance of learning communication skills to achieve recovery goals, and how thoughts might interfere with using these skills. This will be introduced in greater detail in Session 2, but this is part of the orientation to CBSST in general in Session 1. In particular, it is helpful to call on experienced members (e.g., members who are repeating the Social Skills Module) to begin teaching the benefits of good communication and how thoughts can impact interpersonal interactions (e.g., by describing examples from their own lives, identified in previous sessions).

The majority of this session is then devoted to setting goals and adding to the 7–7–7 Goal Jackpot! Worksheet. For new members, this work begins with establishing a motivating long-term goal and at least one short-term goal with at least a couple of goal steps (see Chapter 5), and for existing members, a new short-term goal and/or goal steps that will contribute to achievement of the long-term goal can be developed and added to the goal worksheet. Given that communication skills will be trained in this module, this goal-setting work should include adding a short-term goal and/or goal steps related to learning communication skills (if not already included). The goal-setting case examples of Juan and Carol described in Chapter 5 (see Figures 5.3 and 5.4) both include goal steps to practice communication skills. For example, Juan has goal steps to learn to express frustration and negotiate quiet hours with his roommate, and Carol has goals steps to role-play asking about positions and practice interviewing.

Each of the following sessions specific to communication skills (Sessions 2–6) begins with the provider writing the session's agenda on a whiteboard or pad and inviting consumers to add their own agenda items. This simplified agenda is also listed in the Consumer Workbook. Providers, however, should follow the more detailed plans that begin each session below.

Session 2: Communicate Effectively to Achieve Our Goals

PROVIDER PLAN FOR THIS SESSION

- Set the Agenda Collaboratively
- Review At-Home Practice: Goal Setting
- Introduce the Rationale for Communication Skills
- Describe and Model Nonverbal Communication Skills
  - Discuss Cultural Differences
- Introduce Role Plays
- Describe and Model the Active Listening Skill
- In-Session Skill Practice: Role Plays of Active Listening
  - Elicit Thoughts before Role Play
  - Role Play Practice, Reinforcement, and Coaching
  - Elicit Thoughts after Role Play
- Assign At-Home Practice: Active Listening
- Summarize the Session
- Ask for Consumer Feedback

CONDUCTING THE SESSION

Set the Agenda Collaboratively

- Review At-Home Practice: Goal Setting
- Why Learn to Communicate Well with Others?
- Learn Nonverbal Communication Skills
- Assign At-Home Practice: Active Listening
- Additional Agenda Items?

Review At-Home Practice: Goal Setting

Review and celebrate any goal steps added to the 7–7–7 Goal Jackpot! Worksheet. This homework review time in Session 2 provides an additional opportunity to add goal steps related to learning communication skills, as described earlier. Also, this additional goal-setting time can be used to help consumers who are new to the CBSST program identify a meaningful long-term recovery goal, if they are still struggling to do so (see Chapter 5 for tips on how to help consumers do this).

Introduce the Rationale for Communication Skills

At the beginning of the module, the rationale for learning communication skills is discussed. As emphasized in both of the other modules, it is crucial to link communication skills to personal recovery goals. The skill–goal link is more obvious in this module, because it is easy to understand how effective interpersonal communication can help someone achieve social functioning goals. For example, making friends, renewing relationships with family, interviewing for jobs, asking for help from teachers, negotiating chores with roommates, and seeking help from health care providers can obviously be facilitated by effective communication skills. Explaining this rationale can be accomplished through group discussion, which is more engaging than teaching or lecturing. A provider might start a discussion about the benefits of improving one's social skills by asking:

> "Why is being able to talk to other people important?"
> "How does talking with people help us reach our goals?"
> "What makes it hard to ask for things you need?"
> "Are there particular times, places, or people where asking for something is hard?"
> "What feelings are easy to share? What feelings are hard to share? Why?"
> "When you don't feel understood, what feelings do you have?"
> "What communication skills would you like to improve in yourself?"
> "Do you feel better when someone understands you or does what you ask?"

The benefits of good communication can flow naturally from these discussions. It may also be possible to elicit from consumers examples in which improved communication positively changed their lives, helped them accomplish a task or achieve a goal, or could have made a bad situation better. Highlight the following key benefits by writing them on the board:

- Effective communication is how we get our needs met.
- People are more likely to understand us and help us.
- We can ask others to do things for us so we can get what we need to achieve our goals.

- When we feel upset, it usually helps to talk to someone.
- Checking out our negative thoughts with others can make us feel better, because these thoughts may not be accurate.

Learning to ask for support from trusted others when one is feeling hopeless provides an opportunity to challenge the inaccurate thoughts that led to hopelessness and distress. Although this module focuses on learning new social communication behaviors, there are multiple opportunities to address cognitions and teach how thoughts can impact emotions and goal-directed actions.

Describe and Model Nonverbal Communication Skills

After the rationale for learning communication skills is discussed, introduce nonverbal communication skills and their rationale. For example:

> "To communicate well, we need to learn the best words to say, but that's not all. We also need to know how to act when we are talking and when we listen to others. Nonverbal communication skills are the things we do to convey information in conversations. Also, by paying attention to nonverbal communication in other people, we can gather more information about what the other person wants to say."

Providers next describe how specific nonverbal communication skills convey information and model different examples. Table 7.3 lists specific nonverbal elements, along with how they facilitate communication and modeling suggestions. Consumers can try performing variations of each one to experience its impact on meaning in conversation. The purpose of these exercises is to explore how nonverbal elements provide useful cues about what people are trying to communicate and to practice perceiving, processing, and expressing these cues in interpersonal interactions.

Teaching nonverbal communication skills can be fun and engaging, if you use your sense of humor. Ask a consumer to read the explanation of a nonverbal skill in the Consumer Workbook, then model how *not* to do the skill in a playful or exaggerated way, before modeling effective communication. For example, while discussing posture, slouch down in the chair to the point of nearly sliding off and ask, "What does this say about my attitude about the conversation?" There are also experiential learning games in Appendix B (e.g., Facial Emotion Drawing Game, and Emotional Charades) that can be used to teach facial affect recognition and emotional prosody components of nonverbal communication.

After describing each of the nonverbal communication skills, ask consumers to identify their own strong and weak skills (see the Provider Tip on page 150). Asking about strengths is a way to stay positive and emphasize that we all have skills we are good at and all have room for improvement. The weak skill will be a priority skill

TABLE 7.3. Have Fun Teaching Nonverbal Communication Skills

Eye contact: Look people in the eyes; don't stare.

Communication: Connects the speaker with the listener; shows the speaker you are paying attention and shows the listener you are talking to him or her.

Modeling: Briefly stare at one or two people and ask how it feels. Look at the ground while talking or while someone talks to you and ask what impact this has on them. Contrast this with effective eye contact. If someone says it is uncomfortable to look people in the eyes, suggest that he or she can look at the forehead or nose.

Posture: Stand or sit up straight, facing the other person. Look relaxed but upright.

Communication: Shows engagement and expresses feelings.

Modeling: Try sitting in your chair different ways (e.g., lounging like you're bored; leaning forward in a threatening way) and ask consumers to guess what emotion or message you are trying to convey. Contrast this with sitting up in an engaged posture.

Gestures: Use movements of the hands or body that emphasize what is being said.

Communication: Emphasizes the point or message.

Modeling: Use your hands to make a point or send a message (e.g., thumbs up; OK; raised fist) and ask consumers to make a gesture that conveys or emphasizes a message. Watch out for inappropriate gestures; laugh along but discuss their potential negative consequences.

Facial expressions: Facial expressions of feelings should match the discussion. Smiling and head nods tell people you are listening.

Communication: Expresses feelings.

Modeling: Model different emotions and ask consumers to make different facial expressions. This is a great opportunity to have fun in group. Play a guess-the-emotion game (see Appendix B). Point out how key features (eyes, mouth) differ between different emotions (happy vs. sad; surprise vs. fear; anger vs. disgust). Use mirrors to show consumers what feelings, if any, their own expressions communicate to others.

Voice volume and tone: Voice volume should be pleasant, not too loud or soft, and the pitch of your voice should go up and down naturally with emotions and emphasis (avoid monotone).

Communication: Makes sure you are heard and expresses feelings.

Modeling: Ask someone to say something using soft speech or mumbling, then speaking too loud, then just right. Ask which volume is likely to be most effective. Ask what people were thinking about the person at each volume. Also, say the same sentence using different emotional tones (e.g., say "You're a good communicator," sounding encouraging vs. sarcastic; or "I'll go with you to the movies," sounding excited vs. bored). Discuss how tone, energy level, and volume change the meaning, even though the content was the same. Ask consumers to try it, too.

Speech pace and duration: Don't talk too fast or slow, and pause to let others speak. Be "short and sweet."

Communication: Maintains engagement and clarity.

Modeling: Have someone ask you a question, then model rambling speech in which there is no opportunity to interject, or model very slow responses. Ask about the impact on the listener. Emphasize the importance of short-and-sweet responses that give others a chance to speak. Model "go" and "no-go" cues (e.g., pauses to signal when to start talking, and rolling the eyes or looking away to signal when to stop talking).

What Are Your Strong and Weak Nonverbal Skills?

Ask consumers to try to identify one nonverbal communication skill they do well and one they can improve upon. Build links between strengths that can help with goal attainment and weaker skills that can hinder goal attainment activities. Focus on improving performance of weaker skills during future role-play practice in this module.

to practice during role plays. If the consumer has difficulty identifying strong and weak skills, you can ask questions to guide his or her choice, or you can ask other group members for feedback about their skills. For example, notice and celebrate what people are doing well (e.g., "I can hear everything you say, you speak slowly and clearly, you get right to the point "short and sweet" when you talk to me; just terrific"). However, if the same person looks away or at the floor while talking, ask, "When you were talking, did you notice what you were looking at? Was it my eyes?" The person may notice that he or she was not looking at you, so you can suggest a focus on this as a priority communication skill. Or you could ask the group whether everyone could hear what that person was saying. If the person has tangential or disorganized speech, you can ask whether he or she has ever notice people getting confused when he or she speaks, or even walking away or saying something about not understanding him or her. Often people do not notice this, so you could also comment that sometimes you get confused when people include a lot of details in stories, and that this is common. This can lead to a suggestion that this is an issue with speech pace or duration and not being "short and sweet," and set this as the priority. If someone does not smile when talking about something pleasant, you could say, "I notice you didn't smile when you were talking about how fun that was; maybe we could work on smiling more. You have a great smile which would tell people when you are happy. Do you think people like to be with people who look happy?"

Discuss Cultural Differences

As described in Chapter 3, cultural awareness is particularly important when teaching social skills. For example, several nonverbal skills (eye contact, gestures, etc.) have different meanings in different cultures. One way to determine the meaning of nonverbal behaviors and beliefs about appropriate and inappropriate verbal communication in the context of an individual consumer's cultural background is to ask. We have found it very informative to ask, "In your family or the community where you grew up, how would this be perceived (or would it be OK to do/say this)?" A good time to initiate a conversation about cultural differences and how the various forms of nonverbal communication might be perceived differently in different cultures is at this point in Session 2.

Introduce Role Plays

A useful way to introduce the concept of role plays is to explain that communication skills are behaviors, and like all behavioral skills, people need to practice them to do them well. For example, after nonverbal communication behaviors are described, role plays can be introduced in the following way:

> "Role plays are a way to practice communication skills. Talking with others involves *doing* the nonverbal communication behaviors we just learned about, as well as *saying* the right words. These are all actions or behaviors, and like all behavioral skills they take practice, just like riding a bike or playing the piano are behavioral skills that take practice. You have to practice to become skillful."

Describe and Model the Active Listening Skill

Learning to listen to others is a useful skill to teach first for several reasons. First, the skill is easier to learn than the other skills, so the chances of success during potentially stressful first-time role plays is greater. Successful first-time role plays will increase self-efficacy and comfort in the more difficult role plays to come. Second, if active listening is taught first, the skill can be practiced by one consumer while another consumer practices a new communication skill (e.g., expressing a pleasant feeling). Third, if the consumer becomes an effective listener, then he or she reinforces the people around him or her (by listening), and is likely in turn to experience more positive interactions. The rationale for the skill can be explained as follows:

> "When we hold conversations with others, it's very important that we pay attention and understand what the other person means and how he or she feels. Doing this is called 'active listening.' It can improve our relationships."

The following are the steps of the Active Listening Skill (with the rationale for each step in parentheses):

1. Maintain eye contact. (Shows the other person that you are paying attention.)
2. Nod your head. (Shows that you are maintaining attention.)
3. Say, "Uh-huh," "OK," or "I see." (Shows you understand what the other person is saying.)
4. Repeat what the other person said in your own words. (You need to check out what you heard to see if you got it right.)

Point out that the first three steps involve nonverbal communication skills (eye contact; nodding; and brief, low-content verbalizations) that were just introduced and can now be practiced. These nonverbal communication steps help the listener focus attention on the speaker, and they inform the speaker that the listener is paying attention. People often just "wait to speak," are distracted by their own thoughts or other internal stimuli, or interrupt or talk over the speaker rather than focusing attention on what the speaker is saying. Explain the rationale for each step (shown in parentheses in the previous list). This is best accomplished by asking, "Why do you think this step is important? What message do you think this sends to the other person?"

Consumers need to identify an appropriate pause in the conversation, when they can offer a brief ("short and sweet") summary of what they heard. Step 4 of the skill is the most difficult. It requires the listener to have paid attention to the speaker. This step involves rephrasing or paraphrasing what the speaker said, in the listener's own words. For example, "Sounds like you had fun at the baseball game," or "So, he really made you mad." This can be phrased as a clarifying question to check out what was heard and avoid assumptions of accuracy (e.g., "Are you saying that . . ." or "I'm not sure I understand . . . ?" or "What did he do that made you mad?").

Providers then model the Active Listening Skill.

In-Session Skill Practice: Role Plays of Active Listening

Explain that consumers will now role-play a conversation in which one person talks about something, while the other person practices active listening and nonverbal communication skills. The goal is for the listener to do all four steps of the active listening skills and to practice his or her "priority" (weakest) nonverbal communication skill identified earlier. Rather than talk about just anything, it is most helpful to link the conversation to the consumer's goals. For example, the provider working with Carol might select a scenario related to Carol's short-term goal of learning to use the public transit system, such as giving Carol instructions about how to take a bus from her residence to a shopping center.

Elicit Thoughts before Role Play

Remember to ask the listener, "What is going through your mind just now about the role play?" and "How do you think you'll do on a 1- to 10-point scale?"

Role Plays, Reinforcement, and Coaching

Additional coaching is often needed to help with remembering, rethinking, and solving the problem of how to rephrase or check out what you heard. Use the hand-on-the-shoulder coaching technique, if people are struggling to find the words (see the

Provider Tip on page 139). One way to identify an appropriate time to perform Step 4 is to teach "go/no-go" cues. These include don't go (interrupt) while the speaker is talking; go when you get eye contact and hear a longer pause or when the speaker asks you a question. There are also several games in Appendix B (e.g., One-Minute Interview Activity; Send a Message Game; A What? Game) that make practicing listening skills fun and engaging.

Try to provide feedback (positive or corrective) about the specific nonverbal communication skill on which the consumer has chosen to work. One powerful way to do this is to make a video recording of consumers performing role plays and ask them to watch the recording and critique their own performance. This is often a surprising and memorable experience. They may notice, for example, that they cannot hear themselves or that they are looking at the ground for the entire role play.

Remember to stay positive and reinforce the practice, then offer one piece of corrective feedback. The consumer repeats the role play, ideally twice more. However, there is a lot of content in this session, so with larger groups, it may not be possible to practice three role plays with each consumer. Following each consumer's final role play, praise the effort and any effective use of the skills. Do not offer corrective feedback.

Elicit Thoughts after Role Play

Ask the consumer, "What's going through your mind right now about the role plays?" and "How do you think you did?" Compare the consumer's post-role-play rating with the pre-role-play rating and discuss this with the consumer, with a focus on challenging defeatist performance beliefs.

Assign At-Home Practice: Active Listening

Because the active listening role play was linked to the consumer's goals, the homework assignment will follow naturally. For example, if the person practiced listening to a boss or friend, assign homework to practice the active listening skill with a boss or friend in the real world. Since Carol practiced listening to instructions on how to go somewhere on the bus, she and the provider created an At-Home Practice assignment to visit the transit office near her home and use the active listening skill to ensure that she got complete instructions about how to travel to her provider's office. Homework can be assigned immediately after practicing the role plays by asking the consumer to return to his or her own seat and start to fill out the first three boxes of the Active Listening At-Home Practice Worksheet in Session 2 of the Consumer Workbook (with whom, when and where they will practice; how well they think they will do it; and what nonverbal communication skill they will practice). Then at the end of the session, the providers can go around the room and help consumers who may be struggling.

Summarize the Session

The key points to summarize in this session are:

- Much communication is nonverbal, involving our facial expressions, eye contact, posture, gestures, and voice volume, pace, and tone.
- Active listening can help people in our lives feel understood, which improves relationships.

Ask for Consumer Feedback

This session includes a significant amount of content, including additional work on goal setting during homework review, introducing the importance of communication skills for goal achievement, and teaching nonverbal communication skills and active listening role plays. For some consumers, the pace may be too fast. Normalize this and ask, "Did I go too fast today? We certainly covered a lot in a short period of time. Most people don't get it all the first time." Reassure consumers that one of the reasons we have homework assignments is so they can review the session in the workbook to practice the skill more at home. Modules are also often repeated, so there will be additional learning opportunities. There will also be additional review during the At-Home Practice Review at the start of the next session, so consumers can write down questions that may come up at home.

Session 3: Expressing Pleasant Feelings

PROVIDER PLAN FOR THIS SESSION

- Set the Agenda Collaboratively
- Review At-Home Practice: Active Listening
- Describe and Model Expressing Pleasant Feelings
- In-Session Skill Practice: Role Plays of Expressing Pleasant Feelings
  o Elicit Thoughts before Role Play
  o Role Plays, Reinforcement, and Coaching
  o Elicit Thoughts after Role Play
- Assign At-Home Practice: Expressing Pleasant Feelings
- Summarize the Session
- Ask for Consumer Feedback

CONDUCTING THE SESSION

Set the Agenda Collaboratively

- Review At-Home Practice: Active Listening
- Learn Expressing Pleasant Feelings Skill
- Assign At-Home Practice: Expressing Pleasant Feelings
- Additional Agenda Items?

Review At-Home Practice: Active Listening

This is not a particularly challenging homework assignment, and most consumers find an opportunity to listen to someone between the sessions. Celebrate and reinforce all homework attempts with applause, stickers, gold stars, or other reinforcers. Address any homework adherence problems, as described in Chapter 3.

Describe and Model Expressing Pleasant Feelings

This is typically an easier and more enjoyable session. The skill provides a structure for consumers and providers to give compliments and positive feedback to each other. The following is a general rationale for this skill:

> "Expressing pleasant feelings means telling someone that something he or she did made you feel good. This skill helps us start and maintain friendships and good relationships. If we want to keep our friends, we need to tell them how important they are to us, and how they make us happy. If we tell someone that we appreciate him or her, and feel happy because of what he or she does, that person is more likely to keep doing what makes us happy, again and again."

Explain the rationale for each step. This is best accomplished by asking, "Why do you think this step is important? What message do you think this sends to the other person?" Explain that the key to this skill is saying how the things people *do* make us *feel*. The steps for the Expressing Pleasant Feelings Skill (with the rationale for each step in parentheses) are:

1. Maintain eye contact. (To get and keep the person's attention.)
2. Say exactly what the person did that pleased you. (So the person knows exactly what to do more of.)
3. Say how it made you feel. (So the other person knows you liked what he or she did; positive feedback can get him or her to do it more.)

First, get the attention of the other person by making eye contact, and if necessary by saying "Hi" or "Excuse me." The next steps follow the "When you DO _____, I FEEL _____" structure that all the subsequent skills in this module will also follow. The speaker describes what the other person DID (clear, specific behavior) and how this made him or her feel.

Providers then model the skill. For example, they might express a pleasant feeling to a consumer about one of his or her strengths or a goal step he or she accomplished (e.g., "When you did your at-home practice last week, I felt proud of you and glad you were making progress toward your goal of making a new friend" or "When you laugh at my jokes in group, it makes group fun and I feel happy").

In-Session Skill Practice:
Role Plays of Expressing Pleasant Feelings

Explain that consumers will now role-play a conversation in which one person expresses a pleasant feeling, while the other practices the active listening skill from Session 2. In this way, consumers in both roles have an opportunity to practice communication skills.

In groups, this skill can provide an opportunity to increase pleasant interactions among group members by requiring them to tell each other about things other group members have done that made them feel good. For example, "When you gave me a ride to group, I was relieved to not have to ride the bus" or "When you helped me with my homework, I felt more confident about being able to do it." To help consumers generate these examples of behaviors, offer examples such as helping with rides, or homework, or saying funny things, offering their phone numbers, or other positive things you may have observed members do for each other. This provides an opportunity to practice giving compliments to peers.

The content of this role play should also be personalized to the consumers' specific goals. For consumers with socialization goals, giving compliments can facilitate dating or meeting new friends. Juan practiced this skill when thanking the board-and-care manager for assisting him with his goal step of identifying ways to be more independent at his residence. Explicitly discuss with consumers how using this skill can be beneficial when completing goal steps. For example, ask Juan, "Is your board-and-care manager going to be more or less likely to help you increase your independence at home if you express your appreciation when he helps you?"

The goals of role play in this session are:

- Practice nonverbal communications skills.
- Do all three steps of the expressing pleasant feelings skill.
- Remember to say what the person DID.
- Use the List of Pleasant Feelings to label your feelings.

Elicit Thoughts before Role Play

Remember to elicit each consumer's thoughts before beginning the role play. Ask, "How well do you think you will do it?" and ask consumers to rate how they think they will do on a scale of 1 to 10. It can be helpful to normalize but still challenge some of the thoughts that might get in the way of consumer practice of this skill. For example,

> "It can sometimes feel uncomfortable to express how we really feel to someone else. We may not know how to say it or we may be concerned about how someone will react. We may have thoughts such as "He doesn't want to know how I'm feeling" or "She might get mad." The only way to find out if these thoughts are correct is to express pleasant feelings and test it out. We will learn how to express pleasant feelings and how to correct these unhelpful thoughts that get in the way expressing them."

Role Plays, Reinforcement, and Coaching

Additional coaching is often needed to help consumers describe behaviors in specific, observable terms. For example, "When you tell jokes in class" is more specific than "When you are funny," and "When you showed me where the pharmacy was" is more specific than "When you helped me." If consumers are having difficulty labeling pleasant feelings (e.g., always defaulting to "good" or "happy"), offer more choices from the list of pleasant feelings to improve their skills in identifying and labeling feelings (see Appendix C). Write specific behaviors or feeling words on the board as cues about what to say. Use the hand-on-the-shoulder coaching technique if people are struggling to find the words (see the Provider Tip on page 139). Try to provide feedback (positive or corrective) about the specific nonverbal communication skill on which the consumer has chosen to work. Remember to stay positive and offer only one piece of corrective feedback to change for each role play, and try to practice the role play three times.

Elicit Thoughts after Role Play

Interactions around this skill are typically rewarding and pleasant. People generally like to be told that their actions make others feel good. However, occasionally a thought such as "They won't care if I'm happy or not" or "They will get mad" might be identified. If so, use Socratic questioning (see Chapter 3) to explore the evidence for these thoughts (e.g., "Why would they be mad if you tell them you liked what they did?") and keep asking "Why?" to try to understand the underlying reasoning for this expectation (e.g., a more general core belief such as "People don't care about me" or "I am unlovable"). You could ask whether this might be a common mistake in thinking (e.g., fortune telling). It is also possible that the thought about the other person being mad might be accurate, so ask whether the person is always irritable with others and, if so, suggest doing the skill with someone else with whom success is more likely. You can also try a behavioral experiment by asking whether the consumer is willing to test out the thought by trying the role play for homework to check out how the person responds.

Assign At-Home Practice: Expressing Pleasant Feelings

If the role-play content is linked to the consumer's goals, the homework assignment will follow naturally. The homework is to perform the same role play again for at-home practice (e.g., if the role play was to compliment an imagined roommate, the homework is to compliment the real roommate at home). Homework can be assigned immediately after practicing the role plays by asking the consumer to return to his or her own seat and start to fill out the first three boxes of the Expressing Pleasant Feelings At-Home Practice worksheet in Session 3 of Consumer Workbook (with whom, when, and where he or she will practice; how well the consumer thinks he or she will do it; and what nonverbal communication skill he or she will practice). If the role-play content involved complimenting one of the other group members, then brainstorm to help the consumer to identify someone in the community to be complimented for homework. At the end of the session, the providers can offer additional help to consumers who may be still struggling to plan the assignment.

Summarize the Session

The key points to summarize in this session are:

- Expressing pleasant feelings means telling people about the things they do that make us feel good.
- This skill will help keep people doing things that make us feel good.

Ask for Consumer Feedback

This is typically an enjoyable session, and since the role plays are generally positive and fun, the feedback is generally positive. However, some consumers may still be reluctant to participate in role plays. The Provider Tip on page 144 includes some scripted role plays that may help engage reluctant consumers. Also, eliciting and challenging unhelpful thoughts about role plays (see Provider Tip on page 138) can also help with engagement. On the other hand, some consumers may report that this skill was too simple. If they performed well, compliment them on their skills and suggest that they will be learning several communication skills, so they may find skills in the next couple of sessions more helpful and relevant to achieving their goals.

Session 4: Making Positive Requests

PROVIDER PLAN FOR THIS SESSION

- Set the Agenda Collaboratively
- Review At-Home Practice: Expressing Pleasant Feelings
- Describe and Model Making a Positive Request
- In-Session Skill Practice: Role Plays of Making a Positive Request
  - Elicit Thoughts before Role Play
  - Role Plays, Reinforcement, and Coaching
  - Elicit Thoughts after Role Play
- Assign At-Home Practice: Making Positive Requests
- Summarize the Session
- Ask for Consumer Feedback

CONDUCTING THE SESSION

Set the Agenda Collaboratively

- Review At-Home Practice
- Learn the Making a Positive Request Skill
- Assign At-Home Practice: Making Positive Requests
- Additional Agenda Items?

Review At-Home Practice: Expressing Pleasant Feelings

Typically, consumers who complete this homework report that it went well, because the reaction in the other person is usually positive. Use these real-world success examples to emphasize how this skill can enhance a relationship and make other people want to interact more with the consumer. This can be linked to interpersonal goals by pointing out how expressing pleasant feelings enhances relationships. Ask, "How did you feel and what were you thinking when he smiled after you expressed your pleasant feeling? What do you think the other person was thinking?" Write all the pleasant feelings and positive thoughts on the board to illustrate for the group the many reasons to use the skill. If consumers report that they forgot the steps or stumbled, practice a role play of the skill again and suggest that they try to use the skill at home in the coming week. Celebrate and reinforce all homework attempts with applause, stickers, gold stars, or other reinforcers. Address any homework adherence problems, as described in Chapter 3.

Describe and Model Making a Positive Request

The Making a Positive Request Skill provides an effective way to ask for help with recovery goals. For example, the skill can be used to ask for a date or ask for help with navigating an online school registration website. The skill can be introduced as follows:

> "Making a positive request is asking someone to do something that would help us achieve our goals and feel good! Everyone needs to ask others for help, and sometimes we just want to ask someone to do something fun with us to make us feel good. If we learn how to make positive requests effectively, we are more likely to get others to help us and do fun activities with us."

While generally helpful for everyone, this skill may be particularly useful for people who appear blunt or demanding, as well as for passive, unassertive people. Emphasize that asking for things assertively but nicely, with a focus on very specific desired behaviors and resulting feelings, increases the likelihood that consumers will get what they want and achieve their goals.

The skill follows the same "When you DO _____ , I FEEL _____ " structure. The following skill steps are almost the same as the steps for Expressing Pleasant Feelings, but the focus of Making Positive Requests is on what we want others to do in the future, not commenting on what they did in the past. The steps of the skill (with the rationale for each step in parentheses) are:

1. Maintain eye contact. (Gets and keeps the person's attention.)
2. Say exactly what you would like the other person to do. (The other person knows what to do.)
3. Say how it would make you feel. (The other person knows it will help you feel better and succeed.)

Explain the rationale for each step by focusing on what we want others to *do* and how it would make us *feel*. For example:

PROVIDER: The first step is the same as the Expressing Pleasant Feelings skill. Why do we look people in the eyes?

CONSUMER: So they know we are talking to them.

PROVIDER: Right, good, and it helps us get them to pay attention to us. The second step is to tell the other person what you want them to *do*. Why is this step important?

CONSUMER: If you don't tell them what to do, they won't know what to do.

PROVIDER: Right! It helps to be as specific as possible to make it very clear to the other person what you want. If they don't know exactly what you want, they might do the wrong thing or just not know what to do. The next step is to say how it would make you feel. Why do you think it could be helpful to tell the person how you would feel, like that you would feel happy, if they do what you want?

CONSUMER: They might want to make you happy.

PROVIDER: Right! If people care about you, they will want to do it for you because they want you to be happy. That is a great reason to say how it would make you feel.

It can be helpful to write the following choices of phrases to use when making requests on the whiteboard. These phrases are also provided in the Consumer Workbook.

"I would like you to _____."
"I would really appreciate it if you would do _____."
"It's very important to me that you help me with the _____."

Next, providers should model the skill. If there are two providers, for example, one could say, "I would really appreciate it if you would meet me for coffee. It would make me so happy, and you'd make my day."

In-Session Skill Practice: Role Plays of Making a Positive Request

Explain that consumers will now role-play a conversation in which one person Makes a Positive Request, while the other practices the Active Listening skill from Session 2. In this way, consumers in both roles have an opportunity to practice communication skills.

The content of this role play should be personalized to each consumer's specific goals. Consumer goal steps from their goal worksheet frequently include tasks that require the help of others. For example, Carol (see Figure 5.4) could role-play Making a Positive Request of her case manager or a transit office employee, in identifying the bus route to a specific location. Juan (see Figure 5.3) could role-play Making a Positive Request of a bank employee for help opening a savings account or role-play asking his case manager for information about getting off payee status. When selecting role-play content, it is important to remember that the At-Home Practice assignment for this session will be to use the communication skill in the community before the next session, so select a role play that would be feasible for the consumer to perform by the next session, given his or her personal strengths and limitations. For example, if Juan or Carol cannot transport him- or herself to the bank or transit store by the next session, then the role play should not involve talking to bank employees or transit workers. Instead, select a role play that would not require transportation.

Elicit Thoughts before Role Play

Ask, "How well do you think you will do it?" and ask consumers to rate how they think they will do on a scale of 1 to 10. Providers could also ask, "What's going through your mind right now as you are about to try the skill?" As in the previous session, ask consumers what they think of the pending role play and ask whether they are willing to try the role play to test whether their expectations are accurate. Encourage them to try the skill to gather data to test these thoughts, and ask whether they notice any mistakes in thinking (e.g., fortune telling, mind reading), as they do (see the Provider Tip on this page). As mentioned at the start of this chapter, one strategy to engage reluctant consumers in role plays is to provide a script. This allows participation in simple conversations unrelated to the consumer's need and therefore less emotionally charged. See the Provider Tip on page 144 for an example of a role-play script for making a positive request.

Role Plays, Reinforcement, and Coaching

Each consumer practices the role play three times using personalized content that is tailored to his or her own recovery goals, as described earlier. Applaud after each role play, solicit positive and corrective feedback, praise all verbal and nonverbal components performed well, and assign one component to improve in the next practice role play. As in the previous session, additional coaching is often needed to help consumers describe behaviors in specific, observable terms and label feelings. Be sure to provide feedback (positive or corrective) about the specific nonverbal communication skill on which the consumer has chosen to work. Remember to stay positive and applaud, praise, and pass out stickers and other reinforcers often.

The goals of role play in this session are:

- Practice nonverbal communication skills.
- Do all three steps of the making a positive request skill.

PROVIDER TIP

"It won't work. They won't do it."

A frequent concern among our consumers is that the skill won't produce the desired outcome. We cannot promise that the communication skills will work; we cannot control what other people will do. The skills, however, have been proven to have the greatest likelihood of success. They may not work every time, but they get other people to do what we want more often than other ways of asking. The only way to find out if they will work is to try. Ask, "Are you willing to test it out?" People feel better having tried, even if they don't get the results they want.

- Remember to say what you want the other person to DO (his or her actions).
- Use the List of Pleasant Feelings to label your feelings.

Occasionally, consumers take a passive approach and do not follow-up on requests. A consumer may say, "I asked the person to do it, so I'm sure he will" or "He said he would do it," but the consumer becomes increasingly frustrated waiting for the person to complete the request. In these situations, it can be helpful to include a deadline in the specific behavior requested (e.g., "Would you please return my iPod by Tuesday? I need my music to relax"). The consumer can also practice a role play in which he or she follows up with the person and inquires about the timing of the requested task.

Elicit Thoughts after Role Play

Following the role play, ask for a rating of how successful it was and compare these ratings with ratings made before the role play. Ratings typically increase, so point out how people perform better than they think they will, and how these low expectations for success can interfere with skill performance in the real world. If the thought that the other person won't do what is asked or might get mad still persist after practice, reiterate that the only way to find out is to try the skill and see what happens. Developing a planned response (e.g., leaving the situation; role-playing a response) for possible negative outcomes can also increase the likelihood that the skill will be performed.

Assign At-Home Practice: Making Positive Requests

Homework that involves trying out the skill in the community can be assigned following the third practice role play, while the person is still in the front of the room. If the role play content was linked to recovery goals, as described earlier, the homework assignment will follow naturally (e.g., "Now that you have done so well practicing the skill here, you are ready to try it out at home. When can you ask _____ to do this for you before our next session?"). The place and time can be written on the homework form provided in Session 4 of the Consumer Workbook in the "Situation" box. After practicing in session, most consumers are ready and willing to try the skill in the community. Some consumers, however, are still reluctant to perform this skill. This is most often because a thought is in the way (e.g., "If I ask my son to pay rent, he will move out of my home and I'll never see him again" or "I don't deserve the help"). Try to elicit such thoughts when assigning homework and use the cognitive therapy tools described in Chapters 3 and 6 to challenge them. Again, remind people that the only way to determine whether these thoughts are accurate is to try out the skill and see what happens.

Summarize the Session

The key point to summarize in this session is:

- People may not do what you ask, but by using the Making a Positive Request skill, you will have the greatest chance of getting people to do things to help you reach your goals.

Ask for Consumer Feedback

This skill is particularly helpful when applied to consumer goals. Ask, "What do you think of this skill? Do you think you will use it to ask people to help you do things related to your goals? Do you think people will be more likely to help you if you use this skill?" These questions may reveal a clear understanding and willingness to use the skills or they may uncover thoughts that are barriers to skill performance that need to be challenged. In a group format, try to elicit feedback from every group member.

Session 5: Asking for Help with Your Goals

PROVIDER PLAN FOR THIS SESSION

- Set the Agenda Collaboratively
- Review At-Home Practice: Making Positive Requests
- Introduce Asking for Help with Your Goals
  - o Identifying Support Persons
  - o Identifying What Help You Need
- In-Session Skill Practice: Role Plays of Asking for Help with Goals
  - o Elicit Thoughts before Role Play
  - o Role Plays, Reinforcement, and Coaching
  - o Elicit Thoughts after Role Play
- Assign At-Home Practice: Making Positive Requests
- Summarize the Session
- Ask for Consumer Feedback

CONDUCTING THE SESSION

Set the Agenda Collaboratively

- Review At-Home Practice: Making Positive Requests
- Introduce Asking for Help with Your Goals
- Assign At-Home Practice: Making Positive Requests
- Additional Agenda Items?

Review At-Home Practice: Making Positive Requests

Homework review allows additional time to teach steps of the making positive requests skill and to elicit and challenge thoughts about performing the skill. In particular, reviewing this homework often provides an excellent opportunity to examine whether the outcome of the skill provides evidence to challenge defeatist attitudes about the skill that may have been uncovered in the prior session. If other people agreed to do what was requested, this positive outcome provides evidence against any negative predictions. If people did not laugh or get mad, this outcome provides data to contradict these predictions. Listen carefully for any evidence that contradicts defeatist or low self-efficacy predictions and ask, "What does that tell you about your thought that this would not work at all?"

Introduce Asking for Help with Your Goals

In this session, support persons are identified who can assist with illness management, daily needs, and recovery goal attainment. Consumers then practice using the making positive requests skill to ask these support persons for help with goals. Possible support persons may include family, friends, residential facility staff, clergy, health care professionals, case managers, fellow group members, and even the CBSST provider(s). If there is limited time for this activity, ask consumers to identify at least one person in session, and fill in as many others as possible for At-Home Practice. Providers may need to assist consumers in locating phone numbers or other contact information for support persons, or use SCALE to problem-solve how to obtain this information. It is also helpful to ask which support person is most helpful, and which ones are difficult to talk to (make note of this for possible role-play scenarios). Expanding social support systems and increasing contact with support persons can have a significant impact on functioning. This can be introduced as follows:

> "There are many people who might be able to help us achieve our goals. Sometimes these support persons are professionals (doctors, case managers, work counselors, teachers, bosses). Other times support persons are family members, spouses, and friends. Some of these support persons can help with professional matters, like getting a job, taking a class, or moving to a new place to live.

Others may know us well enough to be able to notice changes in our moods, behaviors, and thinking (sometimes even before we can notice it ourselves). These support persons can be very helpful to us when we don't realize we are becoming overwhelmed by stress in our lives or if our illness gets worse. Different support persons are helpful for different concerns."

Identifying Support Persons

Ask consumers to identify their support persons. They can use the following guidelines, also listed in the Consumer Workbook:

- Think of people who know you well, whom you can trust, and who are willing to help you without being critical.
- Think of people who are open-minded and understanding about your illness and able to give you accurate and positive feedback.
- At least one of these people should be someone you can see often and is available to help you.
- These people can be friends, spouses, other relatives, health-team members, or other professionals in the community; anyone you can think of who you can ask for help with your goals.

Identifying What Help You Need

Next, ask consumers to consider what they need help with and which support persons might be able to give them that help. Consumers can review the goal steps on their Goal-Setting Worksheet and consult the following list of possible needs in the workbook:

- Help with finding better housing
- Help with transportation to appointments (e.g., taking bus rides, getting directions)
- Help with sobriety
- Writing letters or making phone calls to keep communication open
- Making time for weekly outings (e.g., beach, dinner)
- Filling your time with fun activities (working, volunteering, school, leisure activities)
- Finding a job
- Help with finances or problems with benefits
- Registering for a class
- Helping you notice illness warning signs

In-Session Skill Practice: Role Plays of Asking for Help with Goals

The in-session skill practice follows the same structure as that in the previous session. Assuming that consumers have identified at least one support person, ask them to decide what kind of help to ask for from this person. This becomes the role-play scenario practiced in the session. For example, Juan identified his brother as a trusted support person and practiced a role play asking his brother to show him how to do his laundry at a laundromat, which would help him achieve his goal of learning to do everyday living activities in his own apartment. Carol said her case manager was a trusted support person, and she elected to role-play asking her case manager to practice a mock job interview with her, so she would be prepared for an interview at an animal shelter.

Elicit Thoughts before Role Play

Elicit thoughts and follow the same suggestions for addressing thoughts that may come up, as described in the previous session.

Role Plays, Reinforcement, and Coaching

Each consumer practices the role play three times using personalized content tailored to the support person and specific help the consumer needs. Include a timeline to perform the task, if needed (see description of prior session). Applaud after each role play, solicit positive and corrective feedback, praise all verbal and nonverbal components performed well, and assign one component to improve in the next practice role play. Remember to stay positive and applaud, praise, and pass out stickers and other reinforcers often. The Provider Tip on page 144 contains examples of scripted role plays asking support persons for help. These can be used with consumers who have difficulty thinking of what to say or are otherwise reluctant.

The goals of role play in this session are:

- Practice nonverbal communication skills.
- Do all three steps of the making a positive request skill.
- Remember to say what you want the other person to DO (his or her actions).
- Use the List of Pleasant Feelings to label your feelings.

Elicit Thoughts after Role Play

Following the role play, ask for a rating of how successful it was and compare these ratings with ratings made before the role play to challenge defeatist predictions and low self-efficacy ratings, as in the prior session.

Assign At-Home Practice: Making Positive Requests

Homework to try the skill in the community can be assigned following the third practice role play, while the person is still in the front of the room. Since the role-play content was linked to the consumer's specific support person and personalized recovery task, the homework assignment follows naturally (e.g., "When can you ask [support person] to help you before our next session?"). The place and time can be written on the homework form in the Consumer Workbook in the "Situation" box, provided in Session 5. After practice in session, most consumers are ready and willing to try the skill in the community. If not, address any thoughts that are in the way, as described for the prior session.

Summarize the Session

The key point to summarize in this session is:

- If we make positive requests of the support persons in our lives, we will make progress toward our goals.

Ask for Consumer Feedback

This skill is particularly helpful when applied to consumer goals. Ask, "Now that we have practiced this skill a lot, what do you think about it? Do you think you will use it to ask support people in your life to help you do things related to your goals?"

Session 6: Expressing Unpleasant Feelings

PROVIDER PLAN FOR THIS SESSION

- Set the Agenda Collaboratively
- Review At-Home Practice: Making Positive Requests
- Describe and Model Expressing Unpleasant Feelings
- In-Session Skill Practice: Role Plays of Expressing Unpleasant Feelings
  - Elicit Thoughts before Role Play
  - Role Plays, Reinforcement, and Coaching
  - Elicit Thoughts after Role Play
- Assign At-Home Practice: Expressing Unpleasant Feelings
- Summarize the Session
- Ask for Consumer Feedback

CONDUCTING THE SESSION

Set the Agenda Collaboratively

- Review At-Home Practice: Making Positive Requests
- Learn the Expressing Unpleasant Feelings Skill
- Assign At-Home Practice: Expressing Unpleasant Feelings
- Additional Agenda Items?

Review At-Home Practice: Making Positive Requests

Homework review allows time to add additional support people or social contacts to the list started in the previous session, as well as additional time to elicit and challenge thoughts about asking for help. As described in the prior session, reviewing this homework often provides an excellent opportunity to examine whether the outcome of the skill provides evidence to challenge defeatist attitudes about the skill or about asking others for help in general. If other people agreed to do what was requested, this positive outcome provides evidence against any negative predictions. Ask, "What does that tell you about your thought that this would not work at all?"

Describe and Model Expressing Unpleasant Feelings

The expressing unpleasant feelings skill provides an effective way to ask someone to change behaviors that interfere with goals or cause distress. While generally helpful for everyone, this skill may be particularly useful for people who become angry or aggressive when they are unhappy with another person's behavior, as well as for passive or unassertive people. This skill provides a nonthreatening approach to asking others to change, without escalating into an argument. The skill follows the same "When you DO _____, I FEEL _____" structure, which, as noted earlier, helps avoid arguments. Actions are observable, so arguments about whether the action was performed are less likely, as are arguments about how someone feels. The skill can be introduced as follows:

> "Expressing unpleasant feelings is telling someone that something he or she did made us feel bad, like sad or angry. It is important to do this, because it may get them to stop doing things we don't like. If we never ask people to stop and never suggest that they do something more helpful for us, how would they know that we want them to do something different?"

The key to the skill is saying what the other person DID that made us FEEL bad, and what they could DO to make us FEEL better. Remember, all the communication skills we are learning follow similar "When you DO _____, I

FEEL _____" steps, although this skill focuses on what the other person *did* in the past and what they could *do* better in the future. The following are the skill steps (with the rationale for each step in parentheses):

1. Maintain eye contact. Speak firmly but calmly. (Gets the other person's attention and shows you are determined to make your point.)
2. Say exactly what the other person did that upset you. (It is clear exactly what you don't want the other person to do anymore.)
3. Say how it made you feel. (The other person knows that he or she made you feel bad, and saying how you feel can make you feel better.)
4. Suggest what the other person should do to prevent this from happening again. (The other person knows exactly what to do to make the situation better.)

The first three steps are similar to the other communication skills. After making eye contact, the speaker describes what the other person DID (clear, specific behavior) and how this made him or her feel. The fourth step is to suggest an alternative, more desirable behavior. Without this, the listener is left wondering what to do differently. The more specific the description of behavior, the more the listener will understand exactly what to do and what not to do. For example, providers can model the skill as follows: "When you left your dirty dishes in the sink, I had to wash them, which made me angry. Would you please wash the dishes after you eat?"

Review the rationale for each step of the skill. This is best accomplished by asking consumers why they think each step is important (see the Provider Tip on page 140). The rationale for maintaining eye contact and describing behaviors and feelings in specific terms has been discussed when describing communication skills in previous sessions. Speaking firmly but calmly is a new element introduced in this skill to emphasize the importance of making your point without seeming too passive or too aggressive. The negative consequences of each of these extremes can be illustrated by modeling very quiet requests and almost yelling in an angry voice and asking for the listener's impression about these nonverbal aspects of communication (e.g., "Did that make you want to do what I was asking?"). Then, model it with a calm and firm tone and ask about the relative impact on the listener.

Expressing unpleasant feelings is a difficult skill, and it is not uncommon for people to be reluctant to try it. In particular, this skill often involves the difficult task of addressing conflict with others. In emotionally charged conflicts, people can be reluctant to share feelings and often doubt that the other person will change his or her behavior. Therefore, a lengthy discussion of the rationale and potential benefits of expressing unpleasant feelings is worthwhile. This can be initiated as follows:

PROVIDER: How can it be helpful to tell others about your unpleasant feelings?

CONSUMER: Letting the other person know how you feel can make you feel better.

PROVIDER: Right! Saying it and getting it off your chest can make you feel better, so it doesn't build up and make you explode or feel worse. Why else is it helpful to say how you feel?

CONSUMER: If you don't tell them, they will never know.

PROVIDER: Right! They might be able to guess or figure out how you feel, but they might not. If you don't tell them they will never know for sure that they made you feel bad. If you want the person to make a change, you need to tell them they are making you feel bad and suggest a better way to behave.

CONSUMER: But, if you say how you feel, then you will seem weak.

PROVIDER: Possibly, but saying the feeling can make you feel calmer, and the person doesn't have to guess about how his or her actions make you feel. Saying the feeling can actually make you stronger, rather than weaker, because you are taking more control of changing the actions in others that make you feel bad.

CONSUMER: Yeah, but just because you tell people to stop doing things doesn't mean they will.

PROVIDER: You're right, asking them to change is not a guarantee they will change, but it maximizes your chances of getting them to change. This skill is the best way to do both: Get unpleasant feelings off your chest so you feel better and also try to change the situation.

It may also be helpful to point out that it is difficult to argue with your feelings:

"If you say you are sad or mad, it is hard for people to say, 'No you're not.' They are your feelings, and only you know how you feel. Saying how you feel about what they did helps prevent them from arguing with you."

In-Session Skill Practice: Role Plays of Expressing Unpleasant Feelings

Explain that consumers will now role-play a conversation in which one person expresses a negative feeling, while the other practices the active listening skill from Session 2. In this way, consumers in both roles have an opportunity to practice communication skills. The content of this role play should be personalized to each consumer's specific goals. For example, Juan's short-term goal of improving communication with his roommate and the housing manager includes goal steps of negotiating quiet hours and expressing frustrations with the roommate (see Figure 5.3). Both of these goal steps can be accomplished using the expressing unpleasant feelings skill, beginning with expressing frustration with his roommate about playing loud music late at night and negotiating a less frustrating behavior (e.g., "Please don't play music after 9:00 P.M."). While it has not been added as a goal step yet, Juan also mentioned during the initial goal setting session that his board-and-care manager is intrusive. Juan could role-play establishing clear, specific boundaries with his manager, using this communication skill.

The goals of role play in this session are:

- Practice basic nonverbal communication skills.
- Do all four steps of the expressing unpleasant feelings skill.
- Remember to say what the other person DID and what you want that person to DO differently (his or her actions).
- Use the List of Unpleasant Feelings to label your feelings.

Elicit Thoughts before Role Play

This can be a difficult skill to master, because practicing the skill can generate strong feelings (e.g., fear, anger, frustration). Take the opportunity to identify those feelings and elicit the thoughts that lead to them, including expectations about the potential success of the role play in the real world (e.g., "He won't do it"), the other person's reaction (e.g., "He will get mad and hit me"), and beliefs about expressing unpleasant feelings (e.g., "It would make me look weak and vulnerable"). Conviction in these thoughts may diminish after the skill is practiced, so wait until after role-play practice to challenge these thoughts.

Role Plays, Reinforcement, and Coaching

For most consumers, this is the most difficult skill, so three practice role plays (possibly more) are likely required to begin to master the skill. It is also more likely that providers will need to use the Hand-on-the-Shoulder technique to keep it "short-and-sweet" (see the Provider Tip on page 139), and possibly write specific dialogue on the whiteboard to guide consumers who are struggling. In addition to the consumer's priority nonverbal communication skill, listen to speech volume and prosody ("speak calmly but firmly") and provide positive reinforcement or corrective feedback about this after every role play. If consumers are having difficulty labeling unpleasant feelings (e.g., always defaulting to "bad" or "mad"), offer more choices from the List of Pleasant Feelings to help them learn to identify and label unpleasant feelings (Appendix C and Cognitive Skills Workbook Session 2).

Elicit Thoughts after Role Play

The 3C's and other thought-challenging skills can be used to correct inaccurate thoughts that interfere with performance of this skill. For example, the person may want to change the behavior of a roommate at an assisted living home (e.g., stop coming into the consumer's room uninvited) but may think, "He will get mad and get in a fight with me." The 3C's can be used to challenge this thought by writing the thought on the board (Catch It), examining the evidence for and against the thought in two columns (Check It), and identifying the mistake in thinking (fortune telling). Ask, "Has he ever hit you or someone else there before?" If it appears that the thought is not accurate (more evidence in the "against" column), emphasize that the evidence does not support the thought and rewrite the thought (Change It: "He might get mad but probably won't fight me, and he might actually do what I ask") and encourage the consumer to try the skill to test it out the thought. If the evidence suggests it is possible that the person might respond aggressively (more evidence in the "for" column), providers can help problem-solve about a safe place and time (e.g., in the presence of staff) to try the skill or suggest that the consumer use the skill with a staff member at the home (e.g., "When Jim comes in my room, I get scared. Would you please ask him not to go in my room?"). When it appears that a conflict might escalate, a coping plan can be established in this way to remove barriers to skill performance.

Assign At-Home Practice: Expressing Unpleasant Feelings

If the role-play content is linked to the consumer's goals as described earlier, then the homework assignment in the community will follow naturally and can be assigned following the third practice role play, while the person is still in the role-play chair (e.g., "When can you ask [person] to change this behavior before our next session?"). The consumer can then return to his or her seat and start filling out the homework form provided in Session 6 of the Consumer Workbook by writing the place and time to practice the skill in the "Situation" box, as well as the prediction for success and nonverbal communication behavior to practice, while providers move on to role-play practice with the next consumer (if using a group format). Then, at the end of the session, providers can review the homework forms and offer additional assistance to confirm understanding of the homework assignment for each consumer.

Summarize the Session

The key point to summarize for this session is:

- People may not do what you ask them, but if you use the expressing unpleasant feelings skill, you will have the greatest chance of getting people to stop doing the things that make you feel bad.

Ask for Consumer Feedback

Ask consumers what they think about the skill and whether they think it will help them achieve their goals. If any concerns are raised, they typically involve the thought that using the skill will cause or escalate conflict and/or that people will not change their behavior. These are realistic possibilities that should be acknowledged before reminding consumers again that the skill is not a guarantee that people will change, but that it has been found to have the best chance of getting people to change their behavior and help them feel better by getting unpleasant feelings off their chest. If feedback suggests that the skill is still poorly understood by some consumers, plan on practicing the skill again with them during the homework review at the start of Session 1 (Introduction and Goal Setting) of the next module.

PROVIDER TIP

Module Reminders

- At the beginning of each session, give consumers the skill handout for that session or give them the entire Social Skills Module Consumer Workbook.
- Provide small laminated cards that contain the steps of each of the four basic communication skills.
- Use a whiteboard or notepad to teach and write down the steps of each communication skills, or make a poster board displaying the steps.
- Relate each communication skill to personalized recovery goal(s), and guide consumers to select role plays that relate to goal achievement.
- Encourage consumers to take action to use skills in the community and give lots of praise, especially for completing At-Home Practice.
- Use the 3C's, mistakes in thinking, and behavioral experiments to challenge defeatist beliefs that are identified during role-play practice.
- Get feedback about the communication skills at the end of each session:
  o What did they like? Dislike?
  o What was the most difficult part?
  o Was it helpful?

CHAPTER 8

Problem-Solving Skills Module

1. Teach a structured, five-step problem-solving strategy (SCALE).

2. Relate problem-solving skills to the personal recovery goals of consumers.

3. Practice using SCALE to solve everyday problems and achieve goals.

MODULE OVERVIEW

In this module, standard problem-solving training (PST) is used to teach a five-step structured approach (SCALE) to solving real-world problems: "SCALE a mountain of problems to achieve your goals one step at a time." SCALE includes the following steps: Specify the problem, Consider all possible solutions, Assess the best solution, Lay out a plan, and Execute and Evaluate the outcome. The module targets problems that impede achievement of the consumer's personalized living, learning, working, and socializing goals. Challenging thoughts that might interfere with skills performance is also an essential component of this module. As in the other CBSST modules, it is crucial to elicit and discuss consumers' thoughts about the process of solving their own problems. Carrying out problem-solving plans typically involves performing new behaviors in the community and taking steps toward goals, and these activities can be used as behavioral experiments to challenge low self-efficacy beliefs and failure expectations. Thoughts about the expected success or failure of

175

possible solutions are elicited before the consumer tries the planned solution. After plans are carried out, evidence about the degree of success is reviewed, and the accuracy of defeatist beliefs is evaluated. Providers can increase self-efficacy and bolster consumers' confidence by helping them realize that they can be more successful than they might think at solving important problems and achieving goals. Finally, carrying out plans generated through the problem-solving skills also typically increases performance of new behaviors in the community. This can improve negative symptoms and reduce depression through behavioral activation. This module, in particular, can lead to a significant increase in activity level. The specific session content associated with module objectives are shown in Table 8.1.

THOUGHT CHALLENGING DURING PROBLEM-SOLVING TRAINING

The objective in CBSST is to train new skills, while simultaneously challenging the unhelpful thoughts that may be interfering with skills performance and goal-directed behavior in the real world. Although this module focuses on problem-solving skills, it is important to continue to assess thoughts and their impact on actions throughout the problem-solving process. As consumers identify and try out new solutions for long-standing problems, thoughts can interfere with the identification of novel alternative solutions and performance of new behaviors. Consumers who do not execute plans may have thoughts or expectations, such as defeatist beliefs, which discourage them from trying something new or reattempting a previously failed task. Interventions to address defeatist expectations during problem-solving training are described in several sessions of this module.

TABLE 8.1. Problem-Solving Module Objectives and Related Session Content

Problem-Solving Module objectives	Session content
Improve basic problem-solving skills.	Problem-solving skills are taught using the acronym SCALE: Specify the problem, Consider all possible solutions, Assess the best solution, Lay out a plan, and Execute and Evaluate the outcome.
Help consumers develop plans to solve real-world problems.	Practice using SCALE to address recovery goals, such as living situations, interpersonal conflict, finances, use of public transportation, finding a job, enrolling in school.
Develop self-efficacy and confidence in effective problem solving.	Challenge defeatist beliefs by eliciting ratings of expected success or failure before executing plans and review evidence about success after executing plans.
Improve negative symptoms and reduce depression.	Plan and schedule pleasant activities; use behavioral activation techniques.

BEHAVIORAL ACTIVATION

Behavioral activation may be an important factor contributing to change in mood and negative symptoms in this module, where most of the at-home practice assignments involve performing positive actions to solve problems. Positive behavior experiences can increase positive emotions and produce evidence to challenge unhelpful beliefs. Providers can strengthen these effects by suggesting "activity tracking," which is asking consumers to record all activities they do through the day, and "activity scheduling," which is identifying an activity that consumers may find rewarding and planning it into their day, as solutions to problems (e.g., related to depression, boredom, lack of leisure activities). Keys to successful activity planning include generating multiple options, working with consumers to identify choices they believe they can complete, and problem-solving potential obstacles to the activity. In addition, tracking mood before and after the activity can help consumers notice whether there is any benefit. Most consumers can manage some change in routine, if care is taken to focus on interfering cognitions (e.g., "But, I've been doing it this way for years") and problem-solve around limitations.

A variant on activity scheduling is pleasure predicting. This is a useful technique when consumers doubt they will enjoy an activity. Consumers with schizophrenia often anticipate less pleasure from future activities than they report experiencing when they are actually performing the activity. In addition to rating mood before and after the exercise, consumers can be asked to predict how much they will enjoy it. Comparing the predicted pleasure outcome with the actual pleasure outcome helps to challenge the belief "I won't enjoy it," and helps to highlight the tendency to underestimate the benefit of activities. The Funny Videos Activity described in Appendix B is a fun pleasure-predicting activity that can be used to illustrate this right in session. This activity involves showing a funny video and asking consumers to rate how funny they expect it to be before and after watching the video. A variation of this game involves watching Road Runner cartoons of Wile E. Coyote's failed solutions as a fun way to stimulate discussion about how solutions don't always work out the way we expect.

INCORPORATING OTHER MODULE CONTENT

If the 3C's and social communication skills have been trained in previous sessions, these skills can be incorporated into the SCALE process. For example, when unhelpful thoughts arise during a SCALE exercise, such as "My coworker won't help me do this" or "I can't go to the clubhouse, because people will laugh at me," write these thoughts on the board and encourage consumers to use the 3C's to challenge the thought and identify a mistake in thinking (mind reading or fortune telling). Similarly, for problems related to social skills, such as "My roommate won't do the dishes" or "I need a ride to the doctor," write "use the Expressing Unpleasant

Feelings skill" or "use the Make a Positive Request skill" in the list of possible solutions and/or as part of laying out a plan. It may also be helpful to practice the role play during the session.

If some consumers in a group have completed but others have not completed the Cognitive Skills Module or Social Skills Training Module (i.e., they entered the group at the start of the Problem-Solving Module), ask experienced members who have completed these other modules to teach new members briefly about the cognitive or social skills (e.g., review the generic cognitive model triangle, the 3C's, or the steps of a role play). This can bolster self-confidence in experienced members as they notice they have learned new skills well enough to explain them. Reinforce this by complimenting their explanations. The information in the Introductory Session (Session 1 of each module) or handouts from other sessions in the other modules can also be used to help the provider or experienced group members explain these concepts to new members.

SELECTING PROBLEMS TO SOLVE

Ideally, it will be possible to select problems linked to long-term functioning goals. Collaborate with consumers to help them identify problems that need to be solved in order to achieve the primary long-term recovery goal. One excellent way to identify problems related to recovery goals is to review the goal steps on consumers' 7–7–7 Goal Jackpot! Worksheet (see Chapter 5). Goal steps can be translated into problems to solve. In the case example of Carol (see Figure 5.4), her 7–7–7 Goal Jackpot! Worksheet included goal steps to find the bus route to her provider's office in order to learn to use the public transit system, which can be translated into a problem such as "How can I find the bus route to my provider's office at 1234 Broadway Street?" and to identify possible animal shelters to prepare for employment, which can be phrased as "How can I find an animal shelter where I can volunteer?" Barriers identified during at-home practice review (e.g., "I tried to execute the plan but couldn't find a way to get to the mall") or working on goals (e.g., "I don't have enough money to pay for the class") are also good sources of problems to solve. Concerns raised by consumers during collaborative agenda setting (e.g., "My mother is really stressing me out lately") can also be translated into problems to solve (e.g., "How do I get my mother to stop asking me about school?"). Using a relevant and salient current issue from a participant's life can be very effective and can help participants learn to identify daily life situations in which the SCALE skill can be applied. Problems related to illness might also be addressed, including coping with symptoms (e.g., "How can I concentrate in class when I hear voices?"), stress (e.g., "What can I do to relax around other people?"), and medication adherence (e.g., "How can I remember to take my morning medications?"). However, illness-related concerns are typically viewed as secondary targets in CBSST; obstacles to overcome if they are barriers to achieving recovery goals. Examples of problems to solve are printed in the Consumer Workbook in Part III to help consumers brainstorm about potential problems to solve, but providers are not required to use these specific examples if personally relevant problems can be identified.

SESSION FLOW AND SCALE WORKSHEETS

In each session of this module, providers help consumers select problems relevant to their long-term recovery goals and begin to fill out SCALE worksheets (see Part III), while working the SCALE steps together (as described in the session plans below). Consumers then finish working the SCALE steps and filling out worksheets as at-home practice assignments. In 50-minute individual sessions, there is typically more than enough time to complete the first four SCALE steps to address a problem (Specify, Consider, Assess, and Lay out a plan), culminating in a solution plan that can be Executed and Evaluated as an at-home practice assignment. In 60-minute group sessions, there is typically sufficient time in one session to complete these first four SCALE steps twice to address problems for two consumers. The at-home practice assignment for these two consumers is to Execute and Evaluate their solution plans before next session. The at-home practice assignment for all other consumers in a group is to begin to fill out as much of a SCALE worksheet as possible and, at a minimum, complete the first step to Specify a problem relevant to their long-term recovery goal. In the next session, consumers who executed plans for at-home practice discuss their evaluations of the outcomes, and two problems from consumers who began filling out SCALE worksheets for at-home practice are selected for in-session skills practice, when the first four SCALE steps are completed together. Then, the at-home practice assignment for these two consumers is to Execute and Evaluate the solution plans, and the at-home practice for everyone else is to continue filling out SCALE worksheets as much as possible. In this way, the at-home practice for every session in this module is either to execute and evaluate solution plans or to continue working SCALE steps and filling out SCALE worksheets to solve problems.

For example, in a group session with the case subjects Juan and Carol, described in Chapter 5, Juan might specify a problem related to his goal of learning to manage his money as "How can I find a bank to open a savings account?" and Carol might specify a problem related to her short-term goal of preparing for employment as "How can I find an animal shelter where I can volunteer?" After considering possible solutions and assessing the best solution (as described in the session plans below), the solution plan for Juan might be to "walk around my neighborhood to see if there is a bank," and the plan for Carol to "go to the library to search for animal shelters online." Executing and Evaluating these plans would be the at-home practice assignments for Juan and Carol. The at-home practice assignment for the other members of the group would be to begin filling out a SCALE worksheet relevant to their own recovery goals and, at a minimum, Specify a problem (the first SCALE step). For example, another group member might return to the next session with a problem specified as "Where can I practice having a conversation with someone?" This problem would then become the focus of group work in that session to complete the first four SCALE steps, possibly culminating in a plan to go to a clubhouse, and Executing and Evaluating that plan would be the at-home practice assignment for that group member. This process of working the SCALE steps is described in more detail in the session plans below.

Session 1: Introduction and Goal Setting

In Session 1 (see Chapter 5 for the session plan and agenda), new members may join a group, the CBSST program is introduced, and new and previous members both identify and review long-term and short-term goals, and add goal steps to their Goal-Setting Sheets. The At-Home Practice for previous members who have been in the group is typically from Session 6 of the Social Skills Module (Expressing Unpleasant Feelings). Reviewing this homework provides another opportunity to continue to improve this communication skill with previous members (e.g., by practicing additional role plays), as well as an opportunity to explain to new members that the CBSST program involves learning and practicing new skills, including At-Home Practice as a key component of the program (see Chapter 5).

When describing CBSST to new members in Session 1 of this module, focus on the importance of solving problems related to recovery goal steps (see the rationale in Session 2), and how thoughts might interfere with taking action to solve problems (e.g., "If we think, 'This solution will never work,' are we more or less likely to take action and try it out?"). Describing how thoughts can help or interfere with taking action to solve problems is part of the general orientation to CBSST in Session 1. In particular, it is helpful to call on experienced members (e.g., members who are repeating the Problem-Solving Skills Module for the second time) to begin teaching the benefits of following simple, structured steps to solve problems and how thoughts can impact action plans (e.g., by describing examples from their own lives in which they used SCALE to solve problems in previous sessions and how their expectations may not have matched the outcome).

The majority of this session is then devoted to setting goals and adding to the 7–7–7 Goal Jackpot! Worksheet. For new members, this work begins with establishing a motivating long-term goal and at least one short-term goal with at least a couple goal steps (see Chapter 5), and for existing members, a new short-term goal and/or goal steps that will contribute to achievement of the long-term goal can be developed and added to the 7–7–7 Goal Jackpot! Worksheet. Especially in this module, perhaps more than in the other two modules, providers and consumers will use goal steps to guide session content, because many goal steps are problems to solve. When adding goal steps to the 7–7–7 Goal Jackpot! Worksheet in Session 1, try to word them as specific problems that might be solved by using SCALE. For example, Juan could use SCALE to complete his goal steps of opening a savings account ("How can I open a savings account at the bank?"), learning how to obtain a money order ("How can I get a money order?"), and finding out what the steps are to get off payee status ("How can I find the paperwork to get off payee?").

Each of the following sessions specific to problem-solving skills (Sessions 2–6) begins with the provider writing the session's agenda on a whiteboard or pad and inviting consumers to add their own agenda items. This simplified agenda is also listed in the Consumer Workbook. Providers, however, should follow the more detailed Provider Session Plans that begin each session.

Session 2: Introduction to SCALE

PROVIDER PLAN FOR THIS SESSION

- Set the Agenda Collaboratively
- Review At-Home Practice: Goal Setting
- Introduce Problem-Solving Training
  - Rationale
  - Solicit and Address Consumer Concerns
- In-Session Skill Practice: SCALE Steps
  - Describe the SCALE Steps
  - Work the First Four SCALE Steps
  - Elicit Thoughts about the Plan
- Assign At-Home Practice: SCALE Worksheet
- Summarize the Session
- Ask for Consumer Feedback

CONDUCTING THE SESSION

Set the Agenda Collaboratively

- Review At-Home Practice: Goal Setting
- Learn Problem-Solving Skills: SCALE
- Assign At-Home Practice: SCALE Worksheet
- Additional Agenda Items?

Review At-Home Practice: Goal Setting

Review and celebrate any goal steps added to the 7–7–7 Goal Jackpot! Worksheet. This homework review time in Session 2 provides an additional opportunity to add goal steps that can be used as problems to solve, as described earlier. Also, this additional goal-setting time can be used to help consumers who are new to the CBSST program identify a meaningful long-term recovery goal, if they are still struggling to do so (see Chapter 5 for tips on how to help consumers do this).

Introduce Problem-Solving Training

Rationale

Discuss the importance of problem-solving skills and explain how problem-solving skills can help consumers achieve their long-term goals. Link specific consumer goals to these skills (see the Provider Tip on this page). Ask consumers to share some past attempts to solve problems that failed as well as succeeded. If possible, point out how better problem-solving skills could have made a bad situation better. Highlight skills that consumers already have. Consumers are participating in CBSST presumably because they have problems they would like to solve and treatment goals they would like to achieve, so the opportunity to learn skills to solve problems to achieve goals is typically intuitively appealing.

Solicit and Address Consumer Concerns

Some consumers, however, express concerns about problem-solving training, because they believe long-standing problems have no solution. It is important to solicit and address all of these concerns. You can stimulate discussion of these issues by asking:

> "Do you think you can change problems you've had for a long time?"
> "Would you be happier if you solved your problems or gave up on fixing them?"
> "How easy is it to change things? What makes change easy or hard?"
> "What has happened when you've tried to solve problems? What have you learned from those efforts?"

PROVIDER TIP

Solve Problems Related to Personal Recovery Goals

Goal Steps on the 7–7–7 Goal Jackpot! Worksheet completed in the Introduction and Goal-Setting Session can be specified as problems to solve. Relevant problems can also be derived from concerns raised by consumers during collaborative agenda setting and review of at-home practice assignments.

Listen for mistakes in thinking, such as "all-or-none thinking" (e.g., "Nothing helps," "I can't solve any problems") or "fortune telling" (e.g., "I've tried before; it won't work"). Challenge such thoughts by using the 3C's if consumers have completed the Cognitive Skills Module. Emphasize that learning new problem-solving skills can lead to future successes, despite past failures.

In-Session Skill Practice: SCALE Steps

Describe the SCALE Steps

Describe the steps of SCALE—to "SCALE a mountain of problems to achieve your goals one step at a time." SCALE is an acronym that stands for a standard five-step problem-solving approach that includes the following steps: (1) Specify the problem, (2) Consider all possible solutions, (3) Assess the best solution, (4) Lay out a plan, and (4) Execute and Evaluate the outcome (see Table 8.2). The acronym provides a mnemonic aid to help consumers remember the five steps. SCALE is introduced in Session 2 of the Problem-Solving Skills Consumer Workbook, with an example of a completed SCALE Worksheet using the problem of finding transportation. The SCALE approach breaks down the problem-solving process into these simple steps, so after practice, problem-solving can become easier and more successful.

Work the First Four SCALE Steps

Select a problem to solve and teach the steps of SCALE by working through the first four steps together (Specify, Consider, Assess, and Lay out a plan) and filling out the SCALE Worksheet in Session 2 of the Consumer Workbook. Providers write on the whiteboard, while consumers all write on the SCALE Worksheet in the workbook. If several consumers in a group have a similar goal (e.g., to make friends or find a partner), then select a problem relevant to as many people in the group as possible (e.g., "Where can I go to meet new people?"). If there are no overlapping goals, then ask for a volunteer with a problem or pick a problem

TABLE 8.2. SCALE

Scale a mountain of problems to achieve your goals one step at time:

Specify the problem.

Consider all possible solutions.

Assess the best solution.

Lay out a plan.

Execute and Evaluate the outcome.

relevant to one of the group members to use as an example for teaching the SCALE steps. To learn how to fill out the SCALE Worksheet in this session, everyone in a group writes the same thing in their Consumer Workbook, even if the problem is not relevant to everyone in the group. In subsequent sessions, consumers only fill out the SCALE Worksheet for a problem that is relevant to their own goals. The objective of the exercise is to teach the steps of SCALE and how to fill out SCALE Worksheet.

When working the SCALE steps in session, it is very important to keep in mind that consumer(s) who have the specific problem that is the focus of group work will be asked to Execute and Evaluate the solution plan for at-home practice. The problem, therefore, must be specified as a manageable problem with a potential plan that consumers could reasonably execute within a week, given their specific strengths and limitations. For example, if the problem is specified as "Where can I go to meet people?" and the plan generated is to "Go to the clubhouse," then providers should be certain the consumer has the transportation skills and means to execute the plan to go the clubhouse successfully before the next session. If not, the problem should be specified to address transportation barriers (e.g., "How can I get to places where I can meet people?" or "How do I take the bus?"), with a plan to arrange transportation before the next session.

After specifying the problem, ask consumers to generate at least six possible solutions and write them on the SCALE Worksheet, while providers write them on the board. Providers can also help to generate solutions. Encourage consumers not to judge or evaluate solutions during this brainstorming step. If someone comments that a solution will not work or was previously tried and failed, say "just generate, don't evaluate" solutions. Evaluating the pros and cons of each solution is the next step. For a fun way to teach consumers not to evaluate during the Consider step, see the Buzz the Evaluator game in Appendix B.

For the Assess step, the two best solutions are selected by the consumer(s) with the problem that is the focus of the exercise, and everyone generates the pros and cons of these two solutions. Consumers select only two solutions to assess, because there is not sufficient session time to review the pros and cons of all six solutions, and presumably, consumers select solutions that they would be more likely to try out. Based on these pros and cons, the best solution is selected by the consumer(s) who try out the solution, and a detailed step-by-step plan for executing the solution is generated and assigned as at-home practice for the consumer(s) with this problem.

More detailed guidance on completing each SCALE step is provided in Sessions 3–6, in which each session provides additional training for one of the SCALE steps. Since this is the first introduction to SCALE, it is unlikely that there will be sufficient session time to complete the steps for more than one problem during the session. The objective for this session is not to provide detailed training for each step or to solve problems for all group members. The only objective is to introduce the steps of SCALE using a relevant example for at least one consumer.

Elicit Thoughts about the Plan

In the CBSST program, cognitive therapy interventions are integrated into skills training practice, including problem-solving training. In this case, expectations about the possible success or failure of the solution plan can impact the likelihood that consumers will try to execute the plan. Consumers who expect to succeed are more likely to try harder to execute plans than consumers who expect to fail. Providers can elicit thoughts that might interfere with executing the plan in the following way (also see the Provider Tip on page 191):

> "After we lay out a plan, we check out our thoughts about the plan. On the SCALE worksheet, you mark the arrow line to indicate how successful you think the plan will be. If you think a plan will fail, you might not try it out. The only way to know for sure whether a plan will work is to execute it and evaluate whether it was successful or not. For SCALE to work well, we must check out our thoughts about each plan to make sure unhelpful thoughts do not stop us from trying out the plan. What do you think about our plan?"

Assign At-Home Practice: SCALE Worksheet

Consumer(s) who have the specific problem that was the focus of the in-session practice exercise will execute and evaluate the solution plan for at-home practice. For these consumers, the first four steps of the SCALE Worksheet were completed in session, so the at-home practice is to carry out the plan and fill out the Execute and Evaluate boxes of the worksheet. All other consumers fill out as much of the SCALE Worksheet as possible, at a minimum, completing the first step to Specify a problem. Some consumers may choose to complete all five SCALE steps on their own, but that is more common in Sessions 5 and 6 after further practice, and is not the expectation in this session. Assign only the first step, Specify, because this is easier to accomplish and increases the likelihood of a success, rather than failure, experience. Consumers can do more steps, if they want to exceed expectations, which can bolster self-efficacy. Remind consumers that they can use goal steps from their 7–7–7 Goal Jackpot! Worksheets to generate problems to solve (e.g., for the goal step, "Find apartments for rent downtown," for an independent housing goal, the problem could be specified as "How can I find apartments for rent downtown?").

Summarize the Session

The key points to summarize for this session are:

- The steps of SCALE are Specify the problem, Consider all possible solutions, Assess the best solution, Lay out a plan, and Execute and Evaluate the outcome.
- These five steps make it easier to solve problems and take steps toward achieving our goals.

Ask for Consumer Feedback

This session includes a significant amount of new content, and some consumers may report being overwhelmed by trying to learn all five steps of SCALE. The session can be taxing and may move slowly when consumers take time to write on their SCALE Worksheets. Normalize this and ask: "Did I go too fast today? We certainly covered a lot in a short period of time. Most people don't get it all the first time, but don't worry, we will practice the SCALE steps many times in session and for at-home practice, so it will get easier." Modules are also often repeated, so there will be additional learning opportunities.

Session 3: Specify the Problem

PROVIDER PLAN FOR THIS SESSION

- Set the Agenda Collaboratively
- Review At-Home Practice: SCALE Worksheet
- Teach How to Specify the Problem
  - Framing Problems as Questions
  - Problems to Be Solved in 1 Week
  - Break Big Problems into Smaller Ones
- Teach How Thoughts Impact Actions
- In-Session Skill Practice: SCALE Steps
- Assign At-Home Practice: SCALE Worksheet
- Summarize the Session
- Ask for Consumer Feedback

CONDUCTING THE SESSION

Set the Agenda Collaboratively

- Review At-Home Practice: SCALE Worksheet
- Learn to Specify Problems
- How Do Thoughts Impact Problems?
- Assign At-Home Practice: SCALE Worksheet
- Additional Agenda Items?

Review At-Home Practice: SCALE Worksheet

For at least one consumer, the at-home practice was to execute and evaluate a solution plan. Ask whether this consumer attempted to execute the plan and whether it was successful. Review his or her comments and success ratings in the Execute and Evaluate boxes of the SCALE worksheet (or his or her verbal account, if he or she did not complete the worksheet). Celebrate every attempt with applause and reinforcement, regardless of how successful. If the problem was not adequately solved, or an unexpected barrier was encountered, then work through the SCALE steps to address the new problem. For example, if a consumer asked someone for a ride, but the other person said "no," SCALE can be used to find another solution (e.g., Lay out a plan to execute the second-best solution, or Consider and Assess new solutions). For consumers who were assigned to complete as much of the SCALE worksheet as possible, review the problems specified and celebrate all attempts. Some problems may require shaping to modify them into manageable problems that are likely to lead to feasible plans that the specific consumer can execute before the next session. If consumers did not fill out any of the SCALE worksheet, help them specify a problem and write it down on their SCALE Worksheet during the at-home practice review. Identify problems during the at-home practice review that will be the focus of in-session SCALE practice later in this session.

Teach How to Specify the Problem

Additional training on how to specify the problem is provided in Session 3. The step may appear to be fairly straightforward, but it is actually quite challenging and crucial. Unless a clear, specific problem of manageable scope is identified, solving the problem can be overwhelming, and subsequent SCALE steps will be unnecessarily difficult and discouraging. Consumers need to learn to simplify problems and reframe them into specific, manageable problems or tasks that can be addressed with a high probability of success in a short period of time (i.e., before the next session). Providers can explain the step and its rationale as follows:

"Problems that are not specific are very difficult to solve:

> *Not specific:* 'I'm bored.'
> *Specific:* 'Where can I meet new people?'

"Being bored isn't a specific problem, so it is hard to solve. It is too big and too vague, so you don't know what to do to solve it. Why might people be bored? Maybe they don't go out and have fun with friends. So a more specific problem would be to find a place to meet new friends, so that they can go out and have fun with them. This is something you could do in one day to make yourself less bored. Here's another example:

Not specific: 'I need to keep my apartment clean.'
Specific: 'How can I make sure I wash the dishes every day?'

"Needing to keep the apartment clean is too big and too vague a problem, so it is difficult to solve. How would you know if the apartment is clean? Maybe the dishes in the sink are not dirty. If you find a way to be sure to wash the dishes every day, then you will be able to do something in one day that makes the apartment cleaner.

"To specify problems, consider your goals, the steps you have identified to achieve goals, and what obstacles stand in the way of your goals. These steps and obstacles are the problems to solve to achieve your goals. Sometimes, it helps to specify problems as questions that need to be answered, as we have done here."

Framing Problems as Questions

It is often helpful to phrase the problem in the form of a question (see Table 8.3). For example, the problem "I want to get the catalog of art classes at the community college" can be rephrased as "How can I get a catalog of art classes at the community college?" A question requires an answer, which naturally leads the consumer to the next step of considering (brainstorming) answers.

Problems to Be Solved in 1 Week

As a rule, providers should teach consumers to specify the problem as one that can be solved in 1 week, because by the end of each session, the SCALE process will culminate in a plan that will be assigned to the consumer as at-home practice to be completed by the next session (typically in 1 week). For example, "I want to go to the movies," can be simplified to "How can I find the closest movie theater?"— which is easier to accomplish in a week. The challenge for providers is to think through the SCALE steps for each problem to anticipate possible solutions that can be executed as homework assignments, given the specific strengths and limitations of each consumer. For example, Carol, described in Chapter 5, selected the problem

---

TABLE 8.3. Specify

Define the problem.
- Frame it as a question: "Where can I go to meet people?"
- Be specific and concrete.
- The problem must be solvable by next week (i.e., for homework).

Pitfalls—big, overwhelming problems (e.g., "I want to finish college").
- Break problems down into manageable steps.
- Use the consumer's 7–7–7 Goal Jackpot! Worksheet to find attainable steps.
- Be specific regarding what is needed and when it is needed.

PROVIDER TIP

Specify a Problem That Can Be Solved in a Week

By the end of each session, consumers will have worked through the first four steps of SCALE and laid out a plan to be Executed and Evaluated (the fifth step) as the at-home practice assignment to be completed by the next session, so specify manageable problems that will lead to plans that can be executed in a week.

of finding the bus route to her provider's office (see Figure 5.4). The provider knew that Carol did not have a bus pass and therefore could not execute any plan to ride a bus somewhere, so the provider suggested to Carol that it might be helpful to use SCALE first to solve the problem of how to purchase a bus pass. To bolster self-efficacy, consumers need to be successful, so providers must help consumers learn to break down problems and specify them as manageable tasks that can be solved with a high probability of success in 1 week (see the Provider Tip on this page).

Breaking Big Problems into Smaller Ones

Just as in goal setting, big problems must be broken down into smaller problems, which in turn are broken down into a sequence of goal-directed, attainable steps (e.g., getting a community college course catalog this week is a step toward ultimately getting a college degree some day). Sometimes consumers identify problems that are too broad or vague; for example, "I'm bored" is far too general. Ask questions using a Socratic approach to help the consumer be more specific, such as "What could you do that would reduce your boredom?"; "What things have you previously enjoyed?"; and "What is something you would like to try?" Such questions might arrive at something like "I want to take a pottery class." This is more specific, but it is not specific enough and probably not attainable in a week. For example, "I want to get a catalog with art classes at the community college," is even more specific and attainable as a homework assignment within a week. Even this problem may need to be broken down further for consumers who have problems with transportation (e.g., "How do I get to the community college?"). Learning to specify problems in this way can be challenging, but this is an essential skill to transform big, overwhelming problems into smaller achievable goals. The 7–7–7 Goal Jackpot! process of goal setting discussed in Chapter 5 is designed to help providers and consumers break down big goals into steps that can be accomplished in 7 days.

Teach How Thoughts Impact Actions

After providing additional training and practice specifying problems, Session 2 of this module reiterates that thoughts can interfere with actions such as trying out solutions. This concept was introduced in the Cognitive Skills Module, but consumers who enter the program at the start of the Problem-Solving Module have not been exposed to this idea. Consumers in groups who have been exposed to this material can be engaged as experts to help teach this to newcomers. This can be introduced in the following way:

> "How we think about our problems will influence how hard we work on solving them. Changing inaccurate, self-defeating thoughts about problems can help us try harder to solve problems, face challenges, and work toward our goals."

The provider then explains how defeatist thoughts, such as "Why bother, I'm just going to fail," can reduce the likelihood of trying a solution plan, whereas thoughts such as "I might do really well. I'll never know if I don't try" can increase the likelihood of trying. In this discussion, write these thoughts on the board and ask: Which thought is more accurate? Which is more helpful? Why? Which thought would make us try harder to solve problems? Examples of helpful and unhelpful thoughts are provided in the Consumer Workbook (Part III) to facilitate this discussion. During this discussion, draw an arrow from the thought to the actions that would logically stem from the thought (e.g., from defeatist thoughts to "Do nothing" or "Give up and stay home," and from helpful thoughts to "Work hard" or "Try new things"). In this way, the provider illustrates the connection between thoughts and actions directed at solving problems and taking steps toward recovery goal achievement. Emphasize the importance of checking out the accuracy of thoughts (e.g., "We should be sure that our thoughts are accurate if they prevent us from achieving our goals"). The only way to determine whether a plan will fail is to try it and Evaluate the outcome (e.g., "Are you willing to do an experiment and try out the plan to see if it fails?"). Problem-solving activities provide an excellent opportunity to use experiences to challenge defeatist thoughts.

Listen for failure expectations and defeatist attitudes during the SCALE process, and specifically ask consumers about their success expectations. On the SCALE Worksheet, for example, consumers are specifically asked to rate their confidence in their ability to successfully Execute the plan (see Provider Tip on page 191). Consumers mark a line corresponding to the extent to which they expect the plan to succeed or fail. Success ratings can focus on expectations about whether the plan will solve the problem (outcome) or on the consumer's ability to carry out the plan (self-efficacy). We have found it most helpful to emphasize whichever focus has the lower success expectation, because this is most likely to interfere with trying out the plan. For example, if someone is confident that he or she can execute a plan to ride a bus to a mall to meet people, but is doubtful that he or she will actually meet someone, it is better to focus on the low expectations about the outcome rather than on high self-efficacy expectations about getting there.

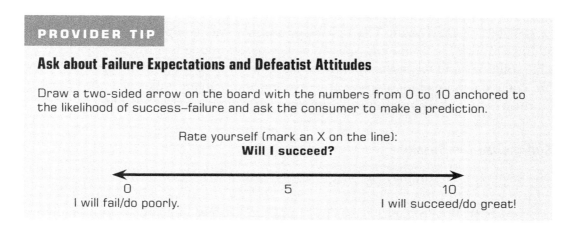

PROVIDER TIP

Ask about Failure Expectations and Defeatist Attitudes

Draw a two-sided arrow on the board with the numbers from 0 to 10 anchored to the likelihood of success–failure and ask the consumer to make a prediction.

Rate yourself (mark an X on the line):
Will I succeed?

0	5	10
I will fail/do poorly.		I will succeed/do great!

In-Session Skill Practice: SCALE Steps

The in-session skill practice follows the same procedures described in Session 2. Select a problem to solve, and teach the steps of SCALE by working through the first four steps together (Specify, Consider, Assess, and Lay out a plan). Providers write on the board while consumers start filling out the In-Session Practice SCALE Worksheet in Session 3 of the Consumer Workbook. Even though the problems solved during in-session skills practice are not relevant to everyone in group, everyone writes the same thing on the SCALE Worksheet to practice filling them out. For homework, the At-Home Practice SCALE Worksheet is used for personally relevant problems. The first part of this session focuses on learning how best to specify a problem, so the first step has already been completed and written in the box labeled "Exercise: Specify Problems" in Session 3 of the Consumer Workbook. Select a problem from someone who did not execute and evaluate a solution plan for homework after the last session and work the SCALE steps together for this problem. For at-home practice, the consumer with this problem will execute and evaluate the solution plan that grows out of the in-session practice. Typically, there is sufficient time to work through the first four steps for one or two problems during the session.

Assign At-Home Practice: SCALE Worksheet

The at-home practice for consumers who completed the first four steps of a SCALE Worksheet during the session is to execute and evaluate the solution plan. Be sure to elicit thoughts about the plan and ask these consumers to mark the line on the SCALE Worksheet to indicate their expectations about the likely success or failure of the plan. If success expectations are low, ask why and encourage consumers to test out defeatist expectations by trying the plan and evaluating the outcome. For consumers who did not develop a plan for solving their problem during the group, the at-home practice assignment is to fill out as many steps of a SCALE Worksheet as possible on their own. The first step, Specify, was completed in group during additional training on how to specify problems, so ask consumers to consider possible solutions and write them on the SCALE worksheet for at-home practice. They can complete more of the steps or even execute and evaluate a plan that they develop on their own, but the minimum assignment is to complete the Consider step.

Summarize the Session

The key points to summarize for this session are:

- *Specify:* Breaking problems down into simple steps that can be done in a week makes problems easier to solve. Remember, even the longest journey starts with the first step.
- *Thoughts can get in the way:* If we expect to fail, we are more likely to fail. Test it out by trying a solution to a problem and see what happens.

Ask for Consumer Feedback

Ask whether the SCALE steps are becoming easier to understand and remember with practice. If specific consumers report that they are still struggling, try to spend extra time teaching them the steps when reviewing at-home practice in the next session, and help them begin to fill out their SCALE Worksheet when assigning homework.

Session 4: Consider All Solutions

PROVIDER PLAN FOR THIS SESSION

- Set the Agenda Collaboratively
- Review At-Home Practice: SCALE Worksheet
- Teach Consider All Solutions
  o Brainstorming Exercise: Get the Cat Out of the Tree
- Teach Assess the Best Solution
- In-Session Skill Practice: SCALE Steps
- Assign At-Home Practice: SCALE Worksheet
- Summarize the Session
- Ask for Consumer Feedback

CONDUCTING THE SESSION

Set the Agenda Collaboratively

- Review At-Home Practice: SCALE Worksheet
- Learn to Consider First, Then Assess
- Assign At-Home Practice: SCALE Worksheet
- Additional Agenda Items?

Review At-Home Practice: SCALE Worksheet

The same procedures described in Session 3 for reviewing at-home practice are followed in Session 4. Identify problems during at-home practice review that will be the focus of in-session SCALE practice later in this session.

Teach Consider All Solutions

Teach consumers to brainstorm all possible solutions—at least six—to the specified problem, even those that seem unrealistic or unlikely (See Table 8.4). No solution should be dismissed at this step; *all* must be considered. To do this, consumers are instructed to "Just generate, don't evaluate!" Assessing whether solutions are good or bad is the next step (Assess). One common barrier to successful problem solving is generating one solution, then dismissing it as likely to fail. For example, "I don't have a car, so I can't take a pottery class." Consumers might also generate multiple options sequentially, reject each one based on a limitation, and end up with no options. Generating multiple solutions without initially evaluating them allows one to have multiple options to assess in the next step. "Perseveration," or getting stuck on one solution, is also a common problem in consumers with schizophrenia. Encouraging consumers to generate at least six solutions, even silly ones, without evaluating them, can open up new choices that sometimes are creative solutions

---

TABLE 8.4. Consider

Brainstorm.
- "Just generate, don't evaluate!"
  - Write *all* solutions on the board. Don't censor or evaluate.
  - Encourage unrealistic solutions ("red herrings") to emphasize not to evaluate.
- Be creative; try to get at least six possible solutions.

Pitfalls—defeatist attitudes ("I can't," "It won't work").
- Don't evaluate! The next step is to "Assess."

194

PRACTICAL GUIDE

that otherwise may not have occurred to them. The objective is to get consumers into the habit of "thinking outside the box." The Consider All Solutions step can be explained as follows:

> "Separating the Consider and Assess steps is not easy. When we consider solutions, it is essential that we do not start to assess which solution is best. One of the biggest problems with solving problems is that we come up with one solution, then quickly decide it may not work, so we give up. Try to generate at least six solutions before picking the best one."

In a group setting, it is possible to compensate for perseveration or evaluating solutions by asking all members to call out solutions (brainstorming). If one member is stuck, others can help out. During brainstorming, humor can be used to reduce the tendency to filter or censor certain solutions by offering "red herrings" or humorous alternatives. For example, if the problem is "How do I get to a store to buy a new shirt?," brainstorming might be as follows:

> PROVIDER 1: What are some other possible ways of getting to the store? (Provider 1 writes everything people say on the board, including "red herrings.")
> CONSUMER 1: Ride the bus.
> PROVIDER 2: You could ride a llama.
> CONSUMER 2: You could fly in a helicopter.
> CONSUMER 3: You could ride a bike.
> PROVIDER 2: Ask your roommate to carry you on his back.
> CONSUMER 4: Ask your roommate to give you a ride in his car.

Consumers write the solutions on their SCALE Worksheets. If consumers comment that a solution is silly or bad, remind them that we cannot evaluate solutions or assess whether they are good or bad yet; that is the next step. One of the games in Appendix B (Buzz the Evaluator) is to bring a buzzer to group, and a consumer is assigned the task of buzzing it every time someone makes a comment evaluating a solution during brainstorming. This is a fun way to remind people to "just generate, don't evaluate."

Brainstorming Exercise: Get the Cat Out of the Tree

To practice considering all solutions without assessing, a fun brainstorming exercise is carried out, in which consumers are asked to generate 30 ways to get a cat down from a tree. Providers explain that the problem is "My cat is stuck in a tree," and consumers are instructed as follows:

"Try to think of 30 different ways to get the cat out of the tree. Think up as many ideas as possible without making judgments about them. Don't edit out any ideas because they seem silly or bad. Just let the ideas keep coming. You never know when a 'silly' idea will trigger a good one."

It may seem like a lot of solutions to try to generate, but it is not too difficult to produce many if you allow silly solutions and do not evaluate. The providers can offer solutions, too, and should toss out silly ones, like "Cut down the tree" or "Rescue the cat with a helicopter," to illustrate that the process is to just generate, not evaluate. Once 30 ideas are generated, providers can later refer to this exercise when consumers are struggling to come up with six solutions for a problem on the SCALE Worksheets (e.g., "We came up with 30 solutions to get the cat out of the tree, so we should be able to come up with six for this"). The game How Can I Use This? in Appendix B offers another fun way to practice brainstorming skills.

Teach Assess the Best Solution

After several potential solutions are generated, the pros and cons of each are then assessed to determine the best solution to execute and evaluate (see Table 8.5). Ask the consumer with the problem to review all the solutions generated and select the two "best" solutions to examine in greater detail in the Assess step. The consumer selects only two solutions, because there is not enough time in a session to assess the pros and cons of all possible solutions. In addition, the two solutions selected by the consumer are likely to be solutions he or she is more willing to try out for at-home practice. Silly solutions or those with strong negative reactions can be easily dismissed (cross them out on the board). Occasionally, a consumer may have difficulty narrowing the list to two solutions, so it can be helpful to start by striking through the options that are impractical, humorous, or just unwanted, which reduces the number of choices and makes this step less overwhelming.

Once two possible solutions are selected, consumers generate the pros and cons of each solution. The providers write these on the board (e.g., one column for pros

---

TABLE 8.5. Assess

The consumer with the problem picks two potential solutions.
- Identify the pros and cons of each solution and pick the best one.

Pitfalls—the consumer picks an unrealistic solution to assess.
- Example: The problem is needing rent money, and "playing the lottery" is selected as a potential solution.
- Accept the solution as one of two to evaluate, but solicit (or offer, if necessary) pros and cons to help make it clear that another solution has a higher probability of success.

and the other for cons), and there is a space on the SCALE Worksheet for consumers to write them (see Part III). The process of identifying positive and negative aspects of each of the two solutions is generally easier than the previous two steps for most consumers and can be made even easier in a group format. The unique perspective of different group members can be helpful when identifying the pros and cons of each solution.

To increase the likelihood that consumers will try to execute a solution plan, ask for feedback about possible solutions during the assess process. Ask whether consumers would be willing to try (or have tried) solutions, whether the solutions were helpful, and why or why not. One way of asking for feedback is to ask the consumer to rate solutions on a 10-point scale (see the Provider Tip on this page). The entire group can become involved by asking all group members to come to the board rate each solution. At the end of the session, the group can examine the solutions that people find most helpful and want to try.

In-Session Skill Practice: SCALE Steps

The in-session skill practice follows the same procedures described in Session 2. Select problems to solve for consumers who did not execute and evaluate a solution plan for homework after the last session, and work the first four steps of SCALE together. Unlike Sessions 2 and 3, there is no in-session practice SCALE Worksheet in Session 4 of the Consumer Workbook, because by this session, consumers typically understand how to fill out the SCALE Worksheets, so there is no need to just practice filling out worksheets with information that is not personally relevant. Only the consumers with the problems that are the focus of in-session skills practice fill out SCALE Worksheets (the At-Home Practice: SCALE Worksheet). These consumers then finish the Execute and Evaluate step on this worksheet for at-home practice. Other consumers help brainstorm solutions, identify pros and cons of solutions, and develop a plan for the consumer(s) with the problem, but they do not fill out a worksheet at this point, although they may be asked to help write on the board. If they

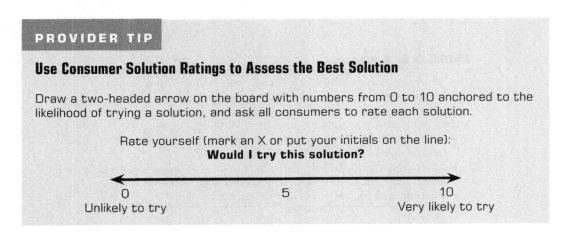

PROVIDER TIP

Use Consumer Solution Ratings to Assess the Best Solution

Draw a two-headed arrow on the board with numbers from 0 to 10 anchored to the likelihood of trying a solution, and ask all consumers to rate each solution.

Rate yourself (mark an X or put your initials on the line):
Would I try this solution?

0   5   10
Unlikely to try   Very likely to try

do not work on a problem in session, they start filling out a worksheet for at-home practice. Consumers are typically able to work through the steps at a faster pace by this point in the module, so providers should try to work the SCALE steps for as many problems as possible during the session.

Assign At-Home Practice: SCALE Worksheet

At-home practice for consumers who worked the SCALE steps during in-session practice is to execute and evaluate the solution plan that was generated. Be sure to elicit thoughts and success expectations about the plan, and address barriers to plan execution. If consumers expect the plan to fail, remind them that this is the "fortune telling" mistake in thinking and that the only way to find out is to try out the plan and see what happens. Even when there has been extensive discussion of the plan, some consumers may bring up other resource barriers at this time (e.g., money, transportation, support person availability, other materials needed to execute the plan), so providers may need to problem-solve and plan further after asking about thoughts about the plan. At-home practice for consumers who have not developed a plan is to work the SCALE steps and fill out as much of the SCALE Worksheet as possible, at a minimum specifying a problem by the next session, but given that this session focused on considering solutions, encourage consumers to try to list some solutions as well.

Summarize the Session

The key point to summarize for this session is:

- When considering all possible solutions, be careful not to skip ahead and start assessing which one is the best. This is when self-defeating thoughts can get in the way (e.g., "That won't work"). You never know until you try.

Ask for Consumer Feedback

Ask about the brainstorming exercises: "Is it easier to generate solutions without evaluating them, now that we practiced? Were they fun?" Emphasize that it can be fun to learn, and it can also be fun to solve problems, if we brainstorm silly solutions and do not get negative and expect our solutions to fail. Also, ask whether the lessons are moving too fast or too slow. At this point in the module, some consumers may find the pace too slow or even express concerns about being bored or annoyed by the redundancy of repeatedly working the SCALE Worksheets in this module. Providers have several options to keep pace with fast learners who understand the skill well. These consumers can be encouraged to try to solve two problems (e.g., complete two goal steps) per week, rather than one. Expert consumers can also be enlisted to help others complete worksheets during group or even meet outside of sessions to help others with at-home practice (this has worked particularly well with consumers who live in the same setting). If the vast majority of consumers in a group find the pace too slow, it may be possible to teach all the content in this module in fewer than 6 sessions and use the additional session time to review content from other modules, add short-term goals or goal steps to the 7–7–7 Goal Jackpot! Worksheet, or move on to the next module after fewer sessions.

Session 5: Lay Out a Plan

PROVIDER PLAN FOR THIS SESSION

- Set the Agenda Collaboratively
- Review At-Home Practice: SCALE Worksheet
- Teach Lay Out a Plan
- In-Session Skill Practice: SCALE Steps
- Assign At-Home Practice: SCALE Worksheet
- Summarize the Session
- Ask for Consumer Feedback

CONDUCTING THE SESSION

Set the Agenda Collaboratively

- Review At-Home Practice: SCALE Worksheet
- Teach Lay Out a Detailed Plan
- Assign At-Home Practice: SCALE Worksheet
- Additional Agenda Items?

Review At-Home Practice: SCALE Worksheet

Follow the same procedures described in Sessions 3 and 4 for reviewing at-home practice. It is not uncommon for obstacles to arise when consumers attempt a solution plan (e.g., someone they needed to talk to was not available; a needed resource such as money, transportation, or even a piece of paper or a pencil was not available). Point out how these obstacles are just problems that can be solved using SCALE and illustrate this by specifying the problem (e.g., "Who else could I talk to?" or "How else can I get there?") and working the steps of scale for this problem during at-home practice review. This will help consumers adapt and solve problems when things do not work out exactly as planned. Chapter 3 offers additional suggestions for increasing adherence with homework assignments.

Teach Lay Out a Plan

The rationale for this problem-solving step can be explained as follows:

> "Sometimes our efforts to solve problems don't work, because we haven't laid out a plan, or our plan isn't detailed enough. No step is too small. We need to think about every little detail; every person, place, and thing we need for the plan."

Consumers need to establish a very detailed plan to carry out the solution (see Table 8.6). For example, ask the consumer, "What will you do first? Second? And then?" Consider all the resources that will be required. Will the consumer need a bus pass, a ride somewhere, specific help from a support person, money, or even a pen and paper? It can be helpful to ask the person to visualize the steps he or she will go through to execute their plan—almost like a test-run in session. The crucial point to remember for this step is that no detail is too small. By identifying all of the necessary steps and resources, consumers reduce the number of unexpected obstacles and increase the likelihood of execution and success. The planning process can be explained as follows:

> "If your plans have not been working, they may need more details. When laying out a plan, think through all the steps necessary, even the ones that seem obvious. Write down each step and how you are going to accomplish it. Think about any resources that may be helpful to you when accomplishing each step. Resources are things that are needed to execute the plan, including people (e.g., your case manager, staff member, friend, or a family member), objects (e.g., pencils, paper, telephone), or even transportation (e.g., a ride or a bus pass)."

Once the initial plan has been laid out, ask about any obstacles the consumer can anticipate getting in the way of his or her plan. Consider whether backup

---

TABLE 8.6. Lay Out a Plan

Write down the steps of the solution plan.
- What will you do first, second, third?
- What resources (people, places and things) are needed?
- NO STEP IS TOO SMALL!
- Set up a time and place to execute the plan (this is the homework for this week).
- Ask consumers to estimate the likelihood of success–failure (on a scale from 0–100% sure of success).

Pitfalls—the consumer expectation is below 90% that the plan will succeed.
- Ask about and address obstacles that are lowering success expectations.

resources might be needed (e.g., if Mary is not home or says "no" to my request to borrow her phone, then I'll ask Jane). For example, after Carol (a case example described in Chapter 5) selected "go to the library to search for animal shelters online" as the solution she would like to plan, she began to lay out the steps of the plan as follows:

1. Go to the library.
2. Search for animal shelters on the computer.
3. Write down a list of shelters near my house.

The provider then began to ask Carol a series of questions to help her consider some additional details that might make the plan more effective and decrease the likelihood of encountering barriers to success.

PROVIDER: On which day and what time will you go to the library? Do you know what times the library is open so you don't arrive when it is closed?

CAROL: I have a doctor's appointment this Monday, so I will go on Tuesday. I know the library opens at 10:00 A.M. I will leave my house at that time so I get there after it opens.

PROVIDER: That sounds like a good day and time to go. You mentioned that the library has a computer lab. Have you used the computers in that lab before?

CAROL: No, but I saw someone working there. Maybe that person can help me.

PROVIDER: Great. Add that step to your plan. The attendant can also help you open an Internet browser to a page where you can search for shelters. Have you done that before?

CAROL: Yes.

PROVIDER: Let's discuss some words you can type on the search page to get a list of local animal shelters.

Carol and the provider continued to examine additional details of Carol's plan. They also discovered that Carol would need to bring money to print the list of the shelters, or a pen and paper to write down the list. This is a small detail, but it would have potentially led to failure of the plan. Carol's plan was much more specific after working through each step with the provider:

1. On Tuesday at 10:00 A.M., walk four blocks from my house to the library on Monroe Avenue.
2. Go to the computer lab on the second floor of the library.
3. Ask the lab attendant for assistance turning on the computer and opening an Internet browser to the search website.
4. Type in the search term "San Diego animal shelters."

5. Using the map on the search results page, locate four shelters that are within walking distance from my house or near a bus route.
6. Write down a list of the shelters, with names, addresses, and phone numbers in my notebook.

In-Session Skill Practice: SCALE Steps

The in-session skill practice is the same as in Session 4. Select problems to solve and work through the first four steps of SCALE together. Consumers have practiced the SCALE steps in three prior sessions, so it is typically possible to solve more than two problems during the session. It is also not necessary for all consumers to write on the worksheet during in-session practice; only the consumer(s) with the problem that is being solved fill out the At-Home Practice: SCALE Worksheet in the Consumer Workbook. Ask consumers to volunteer problems or select from their 7–7–7 Goal Jackpot! Worksheet goal steps or issues they added to the agenda at the start of the session.

Assign At-Home Practice: SCALE Worksheet

As in the prior sessions, the at-home practice for consumers who worked the SCALE steps during in-session practice is to execute and evaluate the solution plan that was generated, and all other consumers fill out as much of the SCALE Worksheet as possible. By this session in the module, consumers should have had enough practice with the SCALE steps to complete more than the first step of the worksheets. Ask them to complete as many as possible; suggest the first three steps (Specify, Consider, and Assess). Be sure to elicit thoughts about their ability to accomplish this. Help them through the first step, if they have serious concerns or still do not know how to convert goal steps from the 7–7–7 Goal Jackpot! Worksheet into problems to solve. By the end of the module (next session), consumers should be able to work all five SCALE steps on their own to execute a plan to solve a problem.

Summarize the Session

The key point to summarize for this session is:

• Sometimes plans do not work out because we missed some details. No problem. Use SCALE to solve problems with the steps and make a new plan.

Ask for Consumer Feedback

Ask about planning: "Is it hard to think of all the details in a plan? Do you think it helps to make detailed plans?" Note that some people like lots of details in their plans, while others like the big picture and do not want to write down many detailed steps. Providers can normalize this by noting that thinking about the details and resources needed for a plan will help the plan succeed, but there is no required amount of detail. Ask whether the SCALE steps and SCALE Worksheets are getting easier to use. If consumers say they find the worksheets to be too much work or that they slow them down, suggest that they try to use the steps to solve a problem "in their head" and report back next session about how the Execute and Evaluate step went, without writing anything down. If the process is already becoming intuitive for some consumers and they can complete goal steps between sessions without writing anything down, then there is no need to fill out the worksheets if problems are getting solved and action plans are executed.

Session 6: Solving Problems Related to Goals

PROVIDER PLAN FOR THIS SESSION

- Set the Agenda Collaboratively
- Review At-Home Practice: SCALE Worksheet
- Solve Problems Related to Consumer Goals
- In-Session Skill Practice: SCALE Steps
- Assign At-Home Practice: SCALE Worksheet
- Summarize the Session
- Ask for Consumer Feedback

CONDUCTING THE SESSION

Set the Agenda Collaboratively

- Review At-Home Practice: SCALE Worksheet
- Solve the Problems Related to Consumer Goals
- Assign At-Home Practice: SCALE Worksheet
- Additional Agenda Items?

Review At-Home Practice: SCALE Worksheet

Always encourage and reinforce consumers for trying solution plans, regardless of their success. We cannot control the outcome, but we can control how hard we try. It is important to discuss solution plans that do not achieve the desired outcome. Normalize failure so that consumers do not catastrophize and assume that problems are impossible to solve because one plan was not successful. Listen for and label mistakes in thinking such as all-or-none thinking and fortune telling mistakes (i.e., "One plan didn't work so no plan will work"). Review the plan and revise it as necessary to address problems the consumer encountered, or pick another solution and make a new plan. Teach consumers to not give up, but to adapt to the situation and environment (see Table 8.7).

Solve Problems Related to Consumer Goals

By this session, consumers may have solved many of the problems related to completing the goal steps on their 7–7–7 Goal Jackpot! Worksheet. Session 6 of this module in the Consumer Workbook provides a number of problems that may be directly related to consumers' long-term goals or may stimulate the identification of additional goal-related problems. Ask consumers to read through the list and mark any that might relate to their goals, or remind them of a problem they need to solve. For example, for the item "You think a coworker wants to get you fired" from the workbook, a consumer might say, "I'm not worried about a coworker, but I think my boss wants to fire me." This can be specified as "How can I find out if my boss wants to fire me?"

In-Session Skill Practice: SCALE Steps

The in-session skill practice is the same as that in Session 5. Consumers developed new problems to solve in the first part of this session, and these problems are solved by working the first four steps of SCALE together for as many problems as possible during the session.

TABLE 8.7. Execute and Evaluate

Evaluate the outcome.
- Did your plan work? How well?
- What went wrong? Can it be fixed or improved?
- Rate success (0–100% successful) and compare pre- and postsuccess ratings, linking thoughts (expectations) to the likelihood of trying to do things ("You were more successful than you thought; maybe next time you don't need to worry so much about failing").

Pitfalls—the plan was not executed.
- Identify and use SCALE to problem-solve about obstacles that got in the way.
- Linking the plan to long-term motivating goals can overcome failure expectations ("Are you willing to do an experiment to test out whether the plan will fail? The only way to know for sure is to try it and see. If you don't try, you will never know if the plan could get you one step closer to your goal").

Assign At-Home Practice: SCALE Worksheet

As in the prior sessions, at-home practice for consumers who worked the SCALE steps during in-session practice is to execute and evaluate the solution plan that was generated, and all other consumers fill out as much of the SCALE Worksheet as possible, even the full worksheet. By this session in the module, consumers should be able to work all five SCALE steps on their own to execute a plan to solve a problem.

Summarize the Session

The key point to summarize for this session is:

- SCALE gives us the tools to solve problems, face challenges, and remove obstacles in the way of our goals. We can use SCALE to solve problems and take steps toward achieving our goals.

Ask for Consumer Feedback

Ask whether consumers feel comfortable working through the SCALE steps on their own: "Is it starting to come naturally, or are you having trouble remembering the steps? Do you think you will use SCALE to solve problems after you graduate from the CBSST program?" If consumers find the skill helpful, celebrate with them and encourage them to use it to solve problems related to goals. If they do not think it will be helpful, ask why. Maybe they have had successes solving problems without marching through steps systematically, so celebrate their strengths in this area. Maybe they find the six steps too much of a burden, or do not think they will remember to do it. Giving out laminated wallet cards with the SCALE steps on them can help remind consumers to use SCALE. Ask whether consumers found any of the specific work on learning to break down problems, brainstorming, or planning helpful to strengthen their problem-solving skills, and suggest that they try to remember the step that was most helpful.

PROVIDER TIP

Module Reminders

- At the beginning of each session, give consumers the skill handout or give them the entire Problem-Solving Skills Module Consumer Workbook, as well as a small laminated card that contains the steps of SCALE for reference in and out of sessions.

- Use a whiteboard or notepad to teach and write down the SCALE steps and/or a poster board displaying the SCALE steps.

- Relate current problems to personalized recovery goals and guide consumers to select problems and solutions that are steps toward achieving their long-term goal.

- Encourage consumers to take action and give lots of praise, especially for completing at-home practice.

- Use the 3C's, mistakes in thinking, and social communication skills with consumers who have learned these skills to facilitate problem solving.

- Use games and experiential learning activities from Appendix B to maintain engagement and make learning fun.

- Get feedback about the exercises:
  - What did they like? Dislike?
  - What was the most difficult part?
  - Was it helpful?

CHAPTER 9

Special Populations

In the Practical Guide (Part II) Chapters 5–8, we have described how the basic CBSST skills can be personalized to help consumers achieve their individual recovery goals. The modules are designed to train general basic skills sets that can be adapted to address a variety of different recovery goals and the unique needs of different individuals. As such, the basic skills in the CBSST program can also be adapted for use with a variety of special populations, which is the focus of this chapter.

YOUNGER CONSUMERS

We recommend several modifications for younger consumers (ages 18–25). First, sessions can usually be shorter and move at a faster pace, and it is usually not necessary to repeat the modules. There is less need for redundancy and repeated skills practice to compensate for severe cognitive impairment or disorganization, and younger consumers can be put off by repeating the content. To provide additional skills practice and promote practical use of the skills in the community without completely repeating the modules, two extra skills practice sessions can be added to the end of each module (e.g., increasing each module to eight sessions). In these sessions, the core skills of the module (e.g., the 3C's, basic communication skills, or SCALE) can be applied to working on goal steps, as described in Chapters 5–8.

Second, our recommendation in Chapter 3 to call groups "classes" to help engage older consumers may not be appropriate for younger consumers, who typically are still in school and attending classes most of the week. Younger consumers may prefer to participate in a "group" or be part of a "social group" or a "meeting."

Avoid stigmatizing labels that can deter engagement (e.g., consumers once told us they did not want to go to the Psychosocial Rehabilitation Center, because they did not like going to a "psycho center"). We have empowered some groups to name programs and meetings themselves. Labels are important, because they can either facilitate or deter engagement.

Third, and related to this, younger consumers are sometimes put off by being asked to set "goals." At their stage in life, asking about "goals" can seem like added pressure to commit to a career path, and to a clear plan and goal for their life. Try setting goals without using the word "goal" (e.g., "What do you really want in your life? What would make your life more enjoyable?"). The 7–7–7 Goal Jackpot! Worksheet can be modified by switching the word "goal" to "want" and "goal steps" to "what I can do to get what I want."

Fourth, we advocate greater use of games and playing music and videos in session to facilitate engagement (see Appendix B and the Provider Tip on this page). Fifth, emphasis on normalization and destigmatization of psychotic symptoms is highly relevant to individuals experiencing these symptoms for the first time. Identifying shared or "me, too" experiences is highly beneficial to younger consumers and can facilitate group cohesion. Sixth, given that younger consumers are often living with their families or typically have much greater contact with their family members than older consumers, involving the family in psychoeducation and other family interventions is important both to support the family and improve outcomes in consumers. Seventh, outings to arcades, parks, or just the cafeteria can promote

PROVIDER TIP

Making It Fun for Younger Consumers

While it is important to make sessions fun for all consumers to promote engagement, younger consumers respond favorably to stimulating and active sessions. There are many ways to do this. Here are some suggestions:

- Include games and activities in every session when possible. Appendix B includes numerous engaging activities that illustrate concepts and provide practice opportunities for the various CBSST skills.
- Make use of technology to connect with younger consumers. If the room has an Internet connection, play funny videos on a video streaming website. Stream music for the start and end of the session through a computer or smartphone. Text-message reminders to complete homework or appointment times. Discuss communication skills as they might apply to communication in social media.
- Group facilitators may need to be more energetic, make the discussions lively, and use humor to keep consumers engaged throughout the session.
- Use presentation software to create multimedia content, such as colorful slides illustrating a skill or a worksheet with or without animation.

engagement, because they are not only fun but they also provide opportunities for skills practice in the community. Finally, include role-play topics and examples of problems relevant to younger adults (e.g., peer interactions at school, academic performance, negotiating with parents), and discuss communication skills in the context of communication on social media websites.

OLDER CONSUMERS

CBSST was originally developed for middle-aged and older consumers (over age 55) and has been found to be effective in this population (see Chapter 2). Important considerations arise in CBSST for older consumers, but not fundamental differences in the CBSST program. First, the educational, collaborative approach of CBSST itself tends to be more acceptable to older people than other forms of psychotherapy. This is one of the reasons we refer to CBSST sessions as "classes" rather than groups with older consumers. Older consumers may be more likely to attend a class on coping or socializing than attend yet another "group" or therapy experience. Second, interventions in the Cognitive Skills Module can be used to modifying ageist beliefs that interfere with treatment. Cohort-related beliefs can devalue therapy (e.g., "Don't air your dirty laundry"), and ageist beliefs held both by therapists and patients (e.g., "I'm too old to learn or change") may interfere with participation in therapy. Thought-challenging interventions such as the 3C's can be used to address these beliefs. Third, a focus on age-relevant content is also necessary, such as age-relevant role-play situations (e.g., talking to a doctor about health concerns or eyeglasses) and age-specific problem solving (e.g., finding transportation, coping with hearing or vision problems, dealing will role changes and loss of friends and family). Some of these can be directly relevant to the group (e.g., a consumer with hearing loss asking other group members to speak up). Issues of loss and isolation, and improving social support, leisure activities, and interpersonal communication skills, can be even more important for older clients. Fourth, transportation and ambulation problems are more common among older clients, so it may be necessary to provide transportation to therapy sessions or conduct therapy at convenient locations in the community. Providing treatment in the community can also reduce stigma associated with going to a mental health clinic, which can especially deter older clients.

Medical problems and cognitive impairments (see the Provider Tip on page 209) also increase as people age, and physical suffering can directly influence mood, anxiety, psychotic symptoms, engagement in rewarding activities, financial resources, daily activities, and interpersonal interactions. All of these problems can also interfere with participation in CBSST, which emphasizes the active practice of new skills. Therefore, CBSST interventions need to focus on increasing consumer activities within the constraints of medical conditions. In addition, Cognitive Skills Module

PROVIDER TIP

Compensating for Cognitive Impairments in Older Consumers

Normal aging and a lifetime of comorbid factors (e.g., poor education, lack of work, physical illness, poor nutrition, poverty) can lead to greater severity of cognitive impairment in older consumers. There are several strategies to compensate for cognitive impairment:

- Simplify and slow the pace of discussions.
- Repeat content, such as a repeating the three modules, and allow for repeated practice of skills during the session.
- Use compensatory aids (e.g., reminder notes, treatment workbooks, wallet cards describing skills, writing down information in session, and acronyms to help with skills recall) to help mitigate the effects of neurocognitive impairments.
- Fine motor, vision, and hearing difficulties are common in older consumers. Materials should use large fonts and ample writing spaces, and providers should frequently check on whether auditory volume is adequate for consumers.

interventions can be beneficial if they help clients to shift perspective from the negative aspects of illness and focus on thinking that can improve their experience in the moment, even in the context of medical problems.

Finally, older consumers who have been ill for thirty years or more can present unique challenges to goal setting (see the following Provider Tip). Older consumers may have experienced a lifetime of failures due to their illness, which can lead to low expectations for success. Information-processing biases also often lead older people to focus on failures and ignore past achievements. By acknowledging a goal, older consumers must accept the risk of yet another failure. Consumers sometimes extrapolate beyond the failure of the specific goal to a risk of symptom exacerbation and rehospitalization as well. In particular, by this stage of illness, older people with psychosis have also been informed that they have a severe, chronic brain disease with little hope of recovery. Older consumers have had much less exposure to modern recovery and psychosocial rehabilitation models that have only recently begun to transform health care systems to focus more on strengths and hope for functional achievement. Hopelessness in providers can be passed on as hopelessness in older, persistently ill consumers.

Suggestions to address these goal-setting challenges were discussed in Chapter 5. In addition, it is critical for success with older consumers that providers first examine their own beliefs, and any unintentional messages that reinforce pessimism about goals. Having open and direct discussion about the experience of living with severe mental illness (SMI) and the influence on expectations about goals can be a very important component of success for older consumers.

PROVIDER TIP

Setting Recovery Goals with Older Consumers

Living, learning, working, and socializing goals evolve with aging. For example:

- Independent living may be defined differently and may be altered to accommodate physical health issues that interfere with independent living. "Independence" may be defined as taking greater control and additional responsibilities at an assisted living facility rather than moving out.
- Work and educational goals may be less focused on long-term vocational development and directed toward increased community involvement by volunteering or taking adult classes.
- Socialization goals may be a higher priority for an older consumer who isolates at home due to lack of interest in socializing, physical limitations, or decreasing social connections with friends or family, or whose close friends have passed away.

While it is important to take these issues into consideration, providers are cautioned to avoid predicting what a consumer can or cannot do. The only way for a consumer to determine if it is an achievable goal is to try.

SUBSTANCE USE

Substance use disorders are common in people with serious mental illness, with 40–60% of consumers experiencing a substance use disorder during their lifetime. The CBSST program can be adapted to target substance use. Substance use relapse prevention interventions can be incorporated by helping individuals identify triggers (e.g., unpleasant feelings, interpersonal pressures, high-risk places) that increase cravings, then teach CBSST skills to cope with these triggers to prevent relapse. The skills in the three CBSST modules can be trained with a focus on substance use. Thought-challenging skills such as the 3C's can be applied to relapse prevention by identifying and challenging thoughts that can trigger cravings or use (e.g., "I can't deal with this without drinking," "Things are going well, so one drink won't hurt," "My friends won't like me if I don't drink with them," "I can't have fun without drinking"). Examples of role plays relevant to substance use include making a positive request that someone stop offering drinks or drugs, making excuses to leave a high-risk situation, and the "Broken Record Technique" (saying "I just don't drink/ use anymore" repeatedly when someone offers or asks about drinking repeatedly). Problem-solving skills (SCALE) can be applied to problems such as finding alternative, fun leisure activities to replace drinking; identifying places to find new friends who are clean and sober; finding an Alcoholics Anonymous/Narcotics Anonymous meeting, or identifying new ways of coping with negative affect. In groups targeting substance use, we recommend that a check-in procedure be incorporated at the beginning of class, whereby consumers report whether they have remained clean and sober since the last session, or whether a relapse (or near miss) has occurred. By discussing use episodes, reviewing triggers, and improving coping attempts, consumers can learn how to prevent future use.

Incorporating substance use into group structure can be done in a number of ways. If possible, it is optimal to have a group in which substance use is a primary focus for every consumer who attends the group. This allows the materials, examples, and role plays to be focused on substance use. However, if not all group members have substance use-related goals, it is still possible to incorporate substance use as an individual goal for those to whom it is relevant, just as consumers do with any other goal.

DISORGANIZED SPEECH

Disorganized speech can be a significant barrier to forming interpersonal relationships, and tangential consumers can derail CBSST sessions with time-consuming attempts to clarify and understand speech. Communication skills training can be an effective intervention to improve disorganized speech. Perseveration, tangentiality, and loose associations can be framed as a communication skills problem. If a consumer is difficult to understand, providers can say, "I'm sorry, I'm having a little trouble understanding," and ask whether others have seemed confused in conversations outside group (or ask consumers in the group for additional feedback). Point out that lengthy, confusing communication can interfere with goals (e.g., job interviews, conversations with friends or dates). This can be hard for some providers to do because of the fear that they will hurt the consumer's feelings by saying they do not understand him or her. As providers, we may also think that we should be able to understand, so we keep waiting while a consumer delivers a long, unclear monologue. It is more helpful (to the consumer and the group) to note ineffective communication quickly and use this as an opportunity to practice the skills. It is typically more harmful to allow ineffective communication to interfere with interpersonal functioning than to gently intervene to improve communication.

The Social Skills Module can be used to teach more concise, "short and sweet" verbal and nonverbal expression, and more focused attention on the cues in others that signal confusion (e.g., looking away). After linking confusing communication to recovery goals, we have found it helpful to make an agreement to work on "short and sweet" communication to achieve goals. For example, ask for permission to interrupt by raising your hand, gesturing with your hands by waving, or using another nonverbal signal when the consumer needs to be "short and sweet" during a role play or at other times during sessions. Some of our favorites are using a "T" sign (like a time-out sign in sports) as a "Tangent" sign, letting the consumer know that he or she is on a tangent, or just moving one's hands together in a gesture to indicate "shorter." After consumers learn to shorten and focus speech when they see these agreed-upon signals, teach other naturally occurring social cues that can

Focusing on Group Process, Not Disorganized Speech Content

Address process when needed and appropriate. Becoming mired in the detailed content of an event or delusion, or becoming sidetracked by a lengthy tangential topic, can quickly disrupt a session. Arguing in group can also disrupt a session. Rather than focusing on the content, take a step back and make a process comment about what you may be observing in the session. For example:

- "I notice that the group and I keep offering evidence against this belief and you offer evidence for it. Maybe we should agree to disagree about whether it is accurate and talk about whether it is helping you reach your goal."
- "I noticed that you became upset after John interrupted you. How did it feel when he did that?"
- "I'm noticing a lot of cross-talk right now. Please remember the group rule about being respectful of other group members and not having side conversations while another group member is talking."
- "I notice that you are talking about a new topic now and people seem confused about what you are saying. Does that happen often to you? Do you want to set a goal to work on clear communication?"

signal confusion in listeners (e.g., facial expressions, loss of eye contact, body language, or questioning). In this way, consumers can learn to be "short and sweet" in response to confusion cues in the listener.

ANXIETY

Anxiety can also interfere with skills performance. Behavioral interventions to reduce anxiety include "graduated exposure," which involves engaging in feared activities according to agreed-upon manageable steps in an organized fashion. Consumers break down a feared activity (e.g., asking for a date, shopping in a store) into specific steps that are arranged from least anxiety provoking to most anxiety provoking (e.g., going to the store but not entering; going to the store and browsing but not buying; shopping in a large grocery store early, when no one else is there; building up to the most anxiety-provoking situations, such as shopping in a small, crowded shop at the busiest time of the day). Consumers practice doing less anxiety-provoking tasks first, until their anxiety level is reduced, then move on to the next task.

For anxiety about doing role plays in groups, consumers can practice talking in group by reading aloud from sections of the Consumer Workbooks, reading the steps of the role play, or giving a specific type of feedback to others about their role plays (e.g., checking for eye contact), then reading a scripted role play before participating in one. As consumers practice a task, asking them to rate their anxiety on a scale from 0 to 10 before, during, and after the task helps them become aware of their anxiety and how it decreases over time when practicing a task.

This progression through the anxiety hierarchy is accompanied by teaching a variety of relaxation techniques, such as progressive muscle relaxation or breathing retraining, to facilitate their management of their anxiety symptoms. To ensure that sufficient time is devoted to learning relaxation training skills, supplemental individual sessions may be needed for anxious consumers. However, this is a skill that other group members could use in anxiety-provoking situations, so adding a group session to teach the entire group relaxation skills may be warranted. Providers can also use the 3C's to dispute anxiety-provoking thoughts, such as "I will say something embarrassing," "I will mess up," or "People will laugh."

A related exercise that has been incorporated into both anxiety and depression treatment, and, to some extent, acceptance interventions for psychosis is mindfulness meditation. "Mindfulness" is defined as paying attention in a purposeful way, in the moment, nonjudgmentally. Consumers are taught to allocate their attention to a particular stimulus (e.g., their breath), and to only attend to this. As distractions arise (e.g., internal thoughts, external sounds), consumers learn to notice these things, as well as their own reaction to them, but not dwell on them. They then return attention to the task at hand (in this case, their breathing). Mindfulness requires practice (likely several supplemental individual or group sessions), but it is a particularly useful skill for helping consumers learn to observe their thoughts. When people notice their thoughts, they can then question the accuracy of them and learn that they do not need to act on those thoughts.

PART III

CBSST Consumer Workbooks

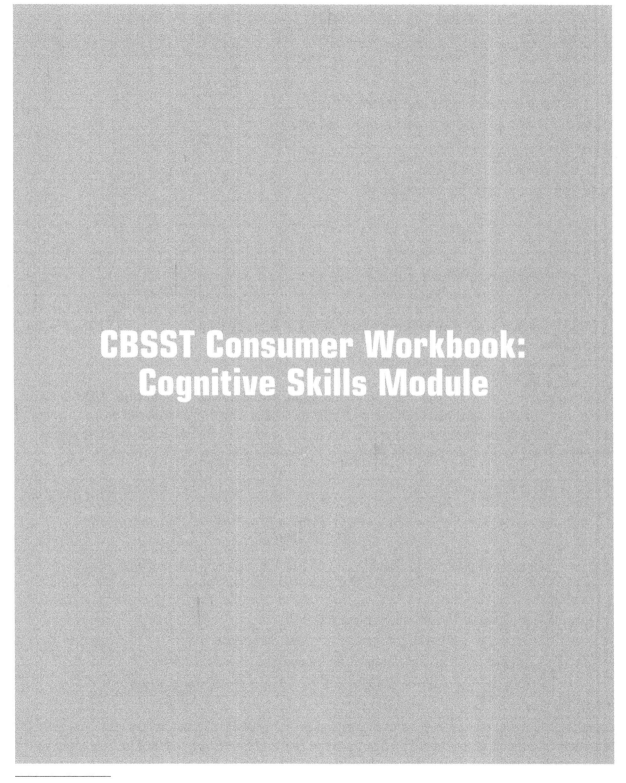

CBSST Consumer Workbook:
Cognitive Skills Module

Session 1: Introduction and Goal Setting

Agenda

- Introductions and Orientation
- CBSST and Changing Unhelpful Thinking
- Review At-Home Practice (previous members only)
- Set Goals
- At-Home Practice: Set Goals
- Do you want to add any agenda items?

    1. _____

    2. _____

What Is Cognitive-Behavioral Social Skills Training (CBSST)?

In CBSST, you will learn how to achieve your personal goals by thinking about your thoughts and learning new skills. You will learn how to change unhelpful thinking, communicate better with others, and solve problems.

Plan to participate actively. **The more you participate, the more you will get from CBSST.** Feel free to ask questions and make comments during discussions and talk about the program with others. Discussing the material with others will help you improve the skills you learn. **It will be very important to practice the skills you learn at home so you can reach your goals.**

What Is Unhelpful Thinking?

DISCUSSION

Scenario: Someone bumps into you on the street and you immediately think the person did it on purpose to hurt you.

1. How would this situation make you feel?
2. Would you shout at the person or shove the person?
3. Would this make you want to be around people more or less?
4. Can you see how the thought influenced your feelings and actions?

Unhelpful thoughts can prevent us from working on our goals and make us feel bad. They can also make it difficult to tell the difference between real and unreal experiences or to interact with other people. Unhelpful thoughts can make it difficult to have relationships, work, or go to school.

Unhelpful thoughts are just mistakes in thinking that can be corrected by testing them out and gathering all the facts. Everyone makes mistakes in thinking. One of the most important skills we will learn in this class is how to change the inaccurate, unhelpful thoughts that are preventing us from achieving our goals.

One of the best ways to improve the quality of our lives is to set goals. In today's class, we are going to set at least one personal goal. The purpose of this program is to help you learn skills that will help you reach your goals.

The best goals are things you really, really want that will improve the quality of your life, such as finding a girlfriend or boyfriend, making a new friend, having more fun with friends, reconnecting with family, living independently, taking a class, getting a job, or volunteering. We can break it down into small steps you can do each week (in 7 days) to accomplish a short-term goal in the next 7 weeks to help you achieve your long-term goal in the next 7 months or more. We call this the 7–7–7 Goal Jackpot! The longest journey starts with the first step, and small steps lead to bigger goals. For example, if you wash the dishes today and pay your own bills tomorrow, then soon you will be taking care of your own apartment.

7–7–7 GOAL JACKPOT! WORKSHEET EXAMPLE

Name: _Jane_   **Date Long-Term Goal Set:** _Oct. 1_

Long-Term (Meaningful) Goal (7 months): _Have a boyfriend_

Short-Term Goals Related to the Long-Term Goal (7 weeks):
(check off steps when you complete them)

1. _Improve hygiene_   **2.** _Improve conversations_

Steps (7 days):   *Steps (7 days):*

1. _Separate clean/dirty laundry_ ✓   1. _Draft list of possible topics_ ✓

2. _Do laundry 2X per week_ ✓   2. _Practice starting conversations_ ✓

3. _Brush teeth_ A.M./P.M. ✓   3. _Practice ending conversations_

4. _Shower daily_ ✓   4. _Practice asking someone for a date_

Let's start filling out your own goal-setting worksheet in class and you can work on it more at home.

7–7–7 GOAL JACKPOT! WORKSHEET

Name: _____   Date Long-Term Goal Set: _____

Long-Term (Meaningful) Goal (7 months): _____

Short-Term Goals Related to the Long-Term Goal (7 weeks):
(check off steps when you complete them)

1. _____	2. _____

Steps (7 days):	*Steps (7 days):*
1. _____	1. _____
2. _____	2. _____
3. _____	3. _____
4. _____	4. _____

Start Date: _____	**Start Date:** _____
Date Reviewed: _____	**Date Reviewed:** _____

Modified/Next Steps:

1. _____	1. _____
2. _____	2. _____
3. _____	3. _____
4. _____	4. _____

Date Reviewed: _____	**Date Reviewed:** _____

Modified/Next Steps:

1. _____	1. _____
2. _____	2. _____
3. _____	3. _____
4. _____	4. _____

Session 2: The Thoughts–Feelings–Behaviors Link

▦ Review At-Home Practice: Setting Goals

▦ What Is the Thoughts–Feelings–Behaviors Link?

▦ Thoughts versus Feelings

▦ At-Home Practice: Identifying Thoughts

▦ Do you want to add any agenda items?

1. _____

2. _____

What Is The Thoughts–Feelings–Behaviors Link?

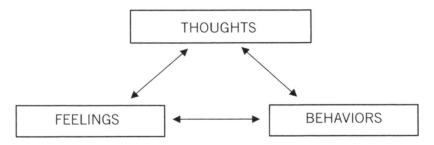

DEFINITIONS

- **Thoughts** are all of the things we tell ourselves. For example, "I think I can achieve my goals."

- **Behaviors** are actions. They are what we do. For example, watching TV, talking to someone, or taking a walk.

- **Feelings** are the many emotions and moods we experience. They can be summed up in one word, such as "happy," "sad," "afraid."

It's important to be sure our thoughts are accurate and helpful. We all make mistakes in thinking. The good news is that we can learn to change our thinking, and that can change what we do and how we feel. Our thoughts can either help us achieve our goals or prevent us from achieving our goals.

⊃ REMEMBER THIS ⊂

Our **thoughts, feelings, and behaviors** affect each other.

221

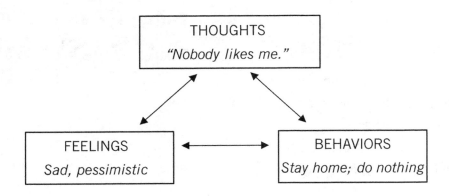

Now, change the inaccurate thought:

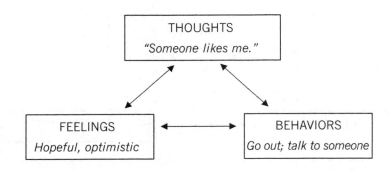

SOME PLEASANT FEELINGS

Happy	Respected	Productive	Worthy
Loved	Caring	Understood	Optimistic
Liked	Empowered	Relieved	Rested
Calm	Satisfied	Needed	Joyful
Useful	Content	Hopeful	Excited
Proud	Relaxed	Encouraged	Helpful

SOME UNPLEASANT FEELINGS

Sad	Rejected	Bored	Anxious
Afraid	Frustrated	Guilty	Lonely
Tired	Disappointed	Angry	Defeated
Hurt	Worried	Betrayed	Overwhelmed
Stressed	Nervous	Annoyed	Embarrassed
Doubtful	Helpless	Hopeless	Irritated

Notice how all the feelings in both lists are only one word. Thoughts, in contrast, are almost always more than one word. Thoughts include all the things you tell yourself. Thoughts can include statements (e.g., "No one likes me"), questions (e.g., "Why is that person staring at me?"), images (e.g., pictures in our minds), and memories.

⊃ **REMEMBER THIS** ⊂

Feelings are one word. **Thoughts** are more than one word.

DISCUSSION

What Were You Feeling This Week?

*Which positive feelings did you have in the past week? Where were you?
Do you remember what you were doing? What were you thinking?*

*Which unpleasant feelings did you have in the past week? Where were you?
Do you remember what you were doing? What were you thinking?*

Summary

- **The Thoughts–Feelings–Behaviors Link:** Our thoughts influence how we feel and what we do.
- **Thoughts can be accurate or inaccurate, helpful or unhelpful.** If you correct inaccurate, unhelpful thoughts, you can feel better and do the things you want to do.
- **Thoughts versus Feelings:** Feelings are one word, and thoughts are more than one word.

Try to do one of the goal steps on your 7–7–7 Goal Jackpot! Worksheet. Try to notice what you are thinking while you try to do the goal step. Write down this **thought** and whether you think it was helpful or unhelpful.

	Goal Step	Thought	Circle one:
Example:	*Say "hi" to someone at the clubhouse.*	*"Nobody would want to be my friend."*	Helpful (Unhelpful)
1. Practice right now			Helpful Unhelpful
2. At-Home Practice			Helpful Unhelpful
3. (optional)			Helpful Unhelpful

Agenda

- Review At-Home Practice: Identifying Thoughts
- The 3C's: Catch It, Check It, Change It
- Catch It: Recognizing Unhelpful Thoughts
- At-Home Practice: Catch the Thought
- Do you want to add any agenda items?

1. _____

2. _____

The 3C's: Catch It, Check It, Change It

The primary skill we will be using to help change our thinking is the 3C's:

1. **Catch It**
2. **Check It**
3. **Change It**

What's "it"? "**It**" is a thought that might be accurate or a mistake. Changing mistakes in thinking is a skill that takes practice, like learning to ride a bike.

Catch It: Catch your thoughts.
 The first *C* is learning how to recognize and write down your thoughts.

Check It: Is the thought accurate or inaccurate? Helpful or unhelpful?
 The second *C* is deciding whether the thought is inaccurate or unhelpful.

Change It: Change mistakes in thinking into accurate, helpful thoughts.
 If a thought is inaccurate or unhelpful, the third *C* is changing it to a more accurate, helpful thought that can help you feel better and do things to achieve your goals.

⊃ REMEMBER THIS ⊂

The **3C's** help you change your unhelpful thoughts and correct common mistakes in thinking that prevent you from achieving your goals and feeling better. The **3C's:**
1. **Catch It**
2. **Check It**
3. **Change It**

225

Catch It: Recognizing Unhelpful Thoughts

Here are some unhelpful thoughts:

- *There's no point in trying. Things will never get better.*
- *I can't trust anyone.*
- *People won't like me because I have a mental illness.*
- *I can't change the way I am. I was born this way.*
- *I'm too sick to do what I need to do or have fun.*

> ### DISCUSSION
>
> *What do you notice about all these thoughts?*
>
> *Would these thoughts help you reach your goals?*

Catch It: Using Feelings as a "Red Flag"

Feelings are important signals that let us know when to catch thoughts. We should look for our thoughts when we have an unpleasant feeling, such as being afraid, angry, or sad, because a thought is linked to the feeling. The bad feeling is a "red flag" to look for thoughts.

> ### ➲ REMEMBER THIS: UNPLEASANT FEELINGS ARE RED FLAGS ➲
>
> **When you have an unpleasant feeling, ask yourself:**
> *"What went through my mind just before I had that feeling?"*

Summary

- The **3C's** is a skill for changing inaccurate or unhelpful thoughts.
- Use feelings as "red flags" to tell you when to catch your thoughts.

Catch a thought when you try to do one of the goal steps on your 7–7–7 Goal Jackpot! Worksheet or when you notice a "red flag" feeling. Note the situation, feeling, and action linked to it.

Situation: What happened? Where was I and when did it happen?	**Feelings:** How was I feeling?
	Actions: What was I doing?

CATCH IT: What was I thinking in this situation? What went through my mind? Which thought best explains how I was feeling or what I was doing?

Situation: What happened? Where was I and when did it happen?	**Feelings:** How was I feeling?
	Actions: What was I doing?

CATCH IT: What was I thinking in this situation? What went through my mind? Which thought best explains how I was feeling or what I was doing?

Session 4: The 3C's—Check It

- Review At-Home Practice: Catch the Thought
- Check It: What's the Evidence for That Thought?
- Mistakes in Thinking
- At-Home Practice: Catch and Check the Thought
- Do you want to add any agenda items?

1. _____

2. _____

Check It

The Check It step is considering all of the evidence to decide if a thought about a situation is accurate.

Our thoughts might be *accurate* or *inaccurate.* Thoughts can also be *helpful* or *unhelpful.* One way to **Check It** is to act like a scientist or a detective. Look at the evidence, the facts for and against a thought.

How do we find *evidence for* a thought? Often this will be the easy step, since we pay more attention to things that confirm the thoughts we have. How do we find *evidence against* a thought? Sometimes this can be very difficult. Try asking yourself:

☐ Are there any alternative explanations?

☐ If someone else had this thought, what would I tell him or her?

☐ Am I missing any facts that contradict my thought?

☐ Is this thought helping me reach my goals or feel better?

Thought: " _____ "	
EVIDENCE FOR	**EVIDENCE AGAINST**

There are several common mistakes we all tend to make in our thinking. These can cause us to have unhelpful or inaccurate thoughts that block us from our goals or make us feel bad.

Common Mistakes in Thinking

☐ All-or-Nothing   ☐ Jumping to Conclusions

☐ Mind Reading   ☐ Catastrophizing

☐ Fortune Telling   ☐ Emotional Reasoning

---

1. **ALL-OR-NOTHING**

   Seeing things as completely good or completely bad. Everything is black or white, with no shades of gray.
   - For example, "I always fail." All-or-nothing thoughts use words like ALWAYS, NEVER, NOBODY, and EVERYBODY. This assumes the thought is true 100% of the time. It only takes ONE instance to prove the thought is false. For example, if you succeed once, it proves you are not ALWAYS a failure.

2. **MIND READING**

   Believing that you know what other people are thinking.
   - For example, someone stares at you or bumps into you and you think, *"He is mad at me or wants to hurt me."* What else could this mean?

3. **FORTUNE TELLING**

   Believing that things in the future will turn out badly.
   - For example, *"I won't learn anything new"* or *"I'll never be able to get a job."* The only way to know whether you can succeed is to try.

4. **JUMPING TO CONCLUSIONS**

   Not gathering enough evidence before making a decision.
   - For example, a voice says it will hurt you if you don't do what it says. You believe the voice, so you do what is says. But what the voice says is not enough evidence that it can hurt you. If it never hurt you before and medications make the voice go away, maybe it can't hurt you.

5. **CATASTROPHIZING**

   Believing that one unfortunate experience is the worst possible thing that could happen. When we jump to conclusions, we are often also catastrophizing.
   - For example, one person turns you down for a date, so you think you will never get a date and you will be alone forever.

6. **EMOTIONAL REASONING**

   Using *feelings* rather than objective evidence as the only basis for what you think or decide.
   - For example, I am feeling afraid, so I think, "Something terrible must be about to happen to me." This may not be true. You may have it backwards. Your fear might be triggered by an inaccurate thought that something bad will happen.

ACTIVITY

What is the common mistake in thinking in the following thoughts?

1. I'll never make any friends.
2. My voices are going to make me do something bad.
3. I'm scared, so something bad is going to happen to me.
4. No one likes me.
5. My doctor doesn't like me.
6. If I leave my room, the voices will get worse.
7. I can never get a job.
8. I know she was talking about me, because she stopped talking when I came in.

DISCUSSION

Was there a time this week when you were feeling bad? Can you remember what you were thinking? Was it a mistake in thinking?

We each have thinking mistakes that have become habits. Is there a particular mistake in thinking that you make most often? Write your favorite mistake here:

Summary

- **Check It** means to examine all the evidence for and against the thought, then decide whether the thought is accurate or not.
- We all make **mistakes in thinking** and have a favorite mistake we make most often.
- If we **check and correct mistakes in thinking** that lead to negative feelings and interfere with our goals, we can improve our lives.

Catch and Check a thought when you are having an unpleasant feeling or when you try to do one of the goal steps on your 7–7–7 Goal Jackpot! Worksheet.

Situation: What was happening? Where and when?	**Feelings:** How was I feeling at the time?
	Actions: What was I doing?

CATCH IT: What was I thinking in this situation? What went through my mind? Which thought best explains how I was feeling or what I was doing?

CHECK IT: Check to see if the thought is accurate by listing the evidence for and against it. Also, check to see if the thought is a mistake in thinking.

EVIDENCE FOR	EVIDENCE AGAINST	MISTAKES IN THINKING (Check any that apply)
		☐ All-or-Nothing ☐ Mind Reading ☐ Fortune Telling ☐ Jumping to Conclusions ☐ Catastrophizing ☐ Emotional Reasoning ☐ Other: _____

Session 5: The 3C's—Change It

Agenda

▦ Review At-Home Practice: Catch and Check the Thought
▦ Change It
▦ Practice Generating Alternatives
▦ At-Home Practice: 3C's
▦ Do you want to add any agenda items?

1. _____

2. _____

Change It

The final step of the 3C's is **Change It**. In the Change It step, you develop a more helpful, more accurate thought that is a better match with the evidence you found in the Check It step. It is important that the *new thought* you develop is realistic, helpful and makes sense to you.

It is helpful to ask yourself:

- What alternative thought is a better match with the evidence?
- What alternative thought might help me achieve my goals?

For any unhelpful, inaccurate thoughts you might have, there are many other thoughts that may be more accurate and helpful. Let's look at an example of how to do this and then we'll practice changing thoughts.

Generating Alternatives

┌───┐
│   ⊃ REMEMBER THIS ⊂   │
│   │
│   Don't jump to conclusions!   │
│ Consider all alternatives before you decide the best explanation. │
└───┘

232

ACTIVITY
GENERATING ALTERNATIVE THOUGHTS

Situation: Why would people look at me at the mall?

Thought: "They think I am strange and will laugh at me."

Alternative Explanations:

1. They may think I look like someone they know and want to say 'hi.'
2. They may not be looking at me but at the store behind me.
3. They may think I look attractive.
4. _____
5. _____

Situation: My SSI check didn't come in the mail on the day I expected it.

Thought: "Someone is stealing my mail."

Alternative Explanations:

1. It was a holiday so the mail was delayed.
2. _____
3. _____

Situation: Why would someone say "no" when I ask for a date?

Thought: "Nobody would want to date me."

Alternative Explanations:

1. _____
2. _____
3. _____

Situation: Why would someone bump into me walking down a sidewalk?

Thought: "He or she wants to hurt me."

Alternative Explanations:

1. _____
2. _____
3. _____

The 3C's Example:

Situation: What was happening? Where and when?	**Feelings:** How was I feeling at the time?
Going to community college to sign up for a class	Pessimistic; hopeless
	Actions: What was I doing?
	Didn't sign up for the class; went back home

CATCH IT: What was I thinking in this situation? What went through my mind? Which thought best explains how I was feeling or what I was doing?

"I will fail the class."

CHECK IT: Check to see if the thought is accurate by listing the evidence for and against it. Also, check to see if the thought is a mistake in thinking.

EVIDENCE FOR	EVIDENCE AGAINST	MISTAKES IN THINKING (Check any that apply)
1. I got a bad grade in the last class I took. 2. People tell me school will be too hard for me.	1. I have had good grades before. 2. Some classes are easier than others.	☐ All-or-Nothing ☐ Mind Reading ☑ Fortune Telling ☑ Jumping to Conclusions ☐ Catastrophizing ☐ Emotional Reasoning ☐ Other: _____

CHANGE IT: What would be a more accurate and helpful thought? If there was mistake in thinking or if the thought was inaccurate, develop a more helpful thought based on the evidence you listed.

"It may be hard, but I may learn something if I try."

Summary

- If we change inaccurate thoughts to more accurate helpful thoughts, we can feel better and achieve our goals.
- Practice makes it easier to generate alterative thoughts.

Use the 3C's to examine at least one thought when you are having an unpleasant feeling or when trying to do a goal step on your 7–7–7 Goal Jackpot! Worksheet.

Situation: What was happening? Where and when?	**Feelings:** How was I feeling at the time?
	Actions: What was I doing?

CATCH IT: What was I thinking in this situation? What went through my mind? Which thought best explains how I was feeling and what I was doing?

CHECK IT: Check to see if the thought is accurate by listing the evidence for and against it. Also, check to see if the thought is a mistake in thinking and do an experiment to test it out.

EVIDENCE FOR	EVIDENCE AGAINST	MISTAKES IN THINKING (Check any that apply)
		☐ All-or-Nothing ☐ Mind Reading ☐ Fortune Telling ☐ Jumping to Conclusions ☐ Catastrophizing ☐ Emotional Reasoning ☐ Other: _____

CHANGE IT: What would be a more accurate and helpful thought? If there was mistake in thinking or if the thought was inaccurate, develop a more helpful thought based on the evidence you listed.

Session 6: 3C's Practice

Agenda

■ Review At-Home Practice: 3C's

■ Doing Experiments to Check It

■ Practice the 3C's to Achieve Goals

■ At-Home Practice: 3C's

■ Do you want to add any agenda items?

1. _____

2. _____

Doing Experiments to Check It

One way to gather evidence on whether thoughts are accurate is to design an **experiment**. Just like any experiment, the purpose is to set up a test for a hypothesis which in this case is the thought.

➲ REMEMBER THIS ☾

You can be a scientist and design an experiment to test your beliefs and thoughts. Here are the steps:

1. *Specify the thought to be tested.* Make a prediction about what will happen if you do something. Your prediction comes from your thought or belief.

2. *Experiment:* **DO** something to test it out.

3. *Results and Conclusion:* How did it turn out? Do the results support or dispute your hypothesis?

EXAMPLE: EXPERIMENT ABOUT PARANOIA

1. **Specify the belief and hypothesis being tested.**
   Belief: "Someone is stealing my mail."
   Hypothesis: "No mail should come for me."

2. **Devise an experiment to test the belief.**
   Send myself a letter; if the letter comes, nobody is taking my mail.

3. **Record results and make conclusions about the hypothesis and belief.**
   Letter arrived, so mail was not stolen, so belief is not accurate.

EXAMPLE: AFRAID TO MEET SOMEONE NEW

Catch It!

Unhelpful thought: "I'm not going to act right, so they will laugh at me."

Check It! Is this thought true?
- I act right and speak well in CBSST (talking in class is an experiment).
- Lots of people don't laugh at me.
- What **Mistake in Thinking** is this? (Fortune Telling)

Change It! to a more helpful thought.

"I'll try and test it out even though I'm scared."

EXAMPLE: VOICES

Catch It!

Unhelpful thoughts: "The voices I hear are very powerful."
"I can't control the voices."

Check It! Is this thought true?
- **Experiment:** Can you turn the voices off by humming, listening to music, repeating the voices, taking medications?
- What **Mistake(s) in Thinking** is this? (All-or-None Thinking; Jumping to Conclusions)

Change It! to a more helpful thought.

"If I can turn these voices off and on, then they can't be all powerful."

EXAMPLE: WORKING

Catch It!

Unhelpful thought: "They will never hire me."

Check It! Is this thought true?
- I used to do a similar job. I am a hard worker.
- Experiment: Go to the interview and see if they hire you.
- What **Mistake in Thinking** is this? (Fortune Telling)

Change-It! to a more helpful thought.

"Maybe I can get a job if I fill out an application."

Summary

- One way to Check our thoughts is to design **experiments** to test them out.
- Doing experiments and correcting mistakes in thinking using the 3C's gets easier with practice.

Use the 3C's to examine a thought when you are having an unpleasant feeling or trying to do a goal step on your 7–7–7 Goal Jackpot! Worksheet.

Situation: What was happening? Where and when?	Feelings: How was I feeling at the time?
	Actions: What was I doing?

CATCH IT: What was I thinking in this situation? What went through my mind? Which thought best explains how I was feeling and what I was doing?

CHECK IT: Check to see if the thought is accurate by listing the evidence for and against it. Also, check to see if the thought is a mistake in thinking and do an experiment to test it out.

EVIDENCE FOR	EVIDENCE AGAINST	MISTAKES IN THINKING (Check any that apply)
		☐ All-or-Nothing ☐ Mind Reading ☐ Fortune Telling ☐ Jumping to Conclusions ☐ Catastrophizing ☐ Emotional Reasoning ☐ Other: _____

EXPERIMENT: What can I do to test out this thought?

CHANGE IT: What would be a more accurate and helpful thought? If there was mistake in thinking or if the thought was inaccurate, develop a more helpful thought based on the evidence you listed.

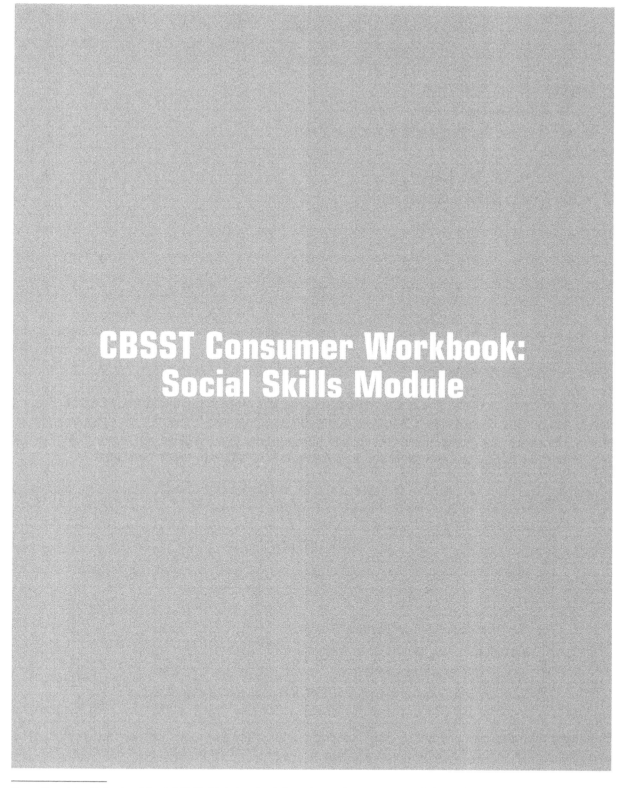

CBSST Consumer Workbook:
Social Skills Module

Session 1: Introduction and Goal Setting

Agenda

- Introductions and Orientation
- CBSST and Changing Unhelpful Thinking
- Review At-Home Practice (previous members only)
- Set Goals
- At-Home Practice: Set Goals
- Do you want to add any agenda items?

1. _____

2. _____

What Is Cognitive-Behavioral Social Skills Training (CBSST)?

In CBSST, you will learn how to achieve your personal goals by thinking about your thoughts and learning new skills. You will learn how to change unhelpful thinking, communicate better with others, and solve problems.

Plan to participate actively. **The more you participate, the more you will get from CBSST.** Feel free to ask questions and make comments during discussions, and talk about the program with others. Discussing the material with others will help you improve the skills you learn. **It will be very important to practice the skills you learn at home, so you can reach your goals.**

What Is Unhelpful Thinking?

DISCUSSION

Scenario: Someone bumps into you on the street and you immediately think the person did it on purpose to hurt you.

1. How would this situation make you feel?
2. Would you shout at the person or shove the person?
3. Would this make you want to be around people more or less?
4. Can you see how the thought influenced your feelings and actions?

Unhelpful thoughts can prevent us from working on our goals and make us feel bad. They can also make it difficult to tell the difference between real and unreal experiences or to cope and interact with other people. Unhelpful thoughts can make it difficult to have relationships, work or go to school.

Unhelpful thoughts are just mistakes in thinking that can be corrected by testing them out and gathering all the facts. Everyone makes mistakes in thinking. One of the most important skills we will learn in this class is how to change the inaccurate, unhelpful thoughts that are preventing us from achieving our goals.

Setting Goals

One of the best ways to improve the quality of our lives is to set goals. In today's class, we are going to set at least one personal goal. The purpose of this program is to help you learn skills that will help you reach your goals.

The best goals are things you really, really want that will improve the quality of your life, such as finding a girlfriend or boyfriend, making a new friend, having more fun with friends, reconnecting with family, living independently, taking a class, getting a job, or volunteering. We can break it down into small steps you can do each week (in 7 days) to accomplish a short-term goal in the next 7 weeks to help you achieve your long-term goal in the next 7 months or more. We call this the 7–7–7 Goal Jackpot! The longest journey starts with the first step, and small steps lead to bigger goals. For example, if you wash the dishes today and pay your own bills tomorrow, then soon you will be taking care of your own apartment.

7–7–7 GOAL JACKPOT! WORKSHEET EXAMPLE

Name: _Jane_ **Date Long-Term Goal Set:** _Oct. 1_

Long-Term (Meaningful) Goal (7 months): _Have a boyfriend_

Short-Term Goals Related to the Long-Term Goal (7 weeks):
(check off steps when you complete them)

1. _Improve hygiene_

Steps (7 days):

1. _Separate clean/dirty laundry ✓_
2. _Do laundry 2X per week ✓_
3. _Brush teeth A.M./P.M. ✓_
4. _Shower daily ✓_

2. _Improve conversations_

Steps (7 days):

1. _Draft list of possible topics ✓_
2. _Practice starting conversations ✓_
3. _Practice ending conversations_
4. _Practice asking someone for a date_

Let's start filling out your own goal-setting worksheet in class, and you can work on it more at home.

7–7–7 GOAL JACKPOT! WORKSHEET

Name: _____   Date Long-Term Goal Set: _____

Long-Term (Meaningful) Goal (7 months): _____

Short-Term Goals Related to the Long-Term Goal (7 weeks):
(check off steps when you complete them)

1. _____   **2.** _____

Steps (7 days):   *Steps (7 days):*

1. _____   1. _____

2. _____   2. _____

3. _____   3. _____

4. _____   4. _____

Start Date: _____   **Start Date:** _____

Date Reviewed: _____   **Date Reviewed:** _____

Modified/Next Steps: **Modified/Next Steps:**

1. _____   1. _____

2. _____   2. _____

3. _____   3. _____

4. _____   4. _____

Date Reviewed: _____   **Date Reviewed:** _____

Modified/Next Steps: **Modified/Next Steps:**

1. _____   1. _____

2. _____   2. _____

3. _____   3. _____

4. _____   4. _____

Session 2: Communicate Effectively to Achieve Our Goals

Agenda

- Review At-Home Practice: Goal Setting
- Why Learn to Communicate?
- Learn Nonverbal Communication Skills
- Practice Active Listening Skills
- At-Home Practice: Active Listening
- Do you want to add any agenda items?

1. _____

2. _____

Why Communicate Well with Others?

DISCUSSION

- *How can communication skills help you achieve your goals?*
- *What communication skills would you like to improve in yourself?*
- *Do you feel better when people understand you or do what you ask them to do?*

It is important to communicate our thoughts and feelings well to others, because that is how we get our needs met. If we communicate well, people are more likely to understand us and help us. We will learn how best to express feelings and ask others to do things for us, so we can get what we need to achieve our goals. For example, if we practice asking someone to go on a date, then we are more likely to get dates successfully and may eventually get a girlfriend or boyfriend.

Also, if you are feeling upset, it usually helps to talk to someone. When you are feeling down, what kind of thoughts are you having?

"I'm no good," "I'll never get over this," "Here we go again."

Checking out these thoughts with others (friends, family, case manager, doctor, therapist) can make you feel better, because they may not be accurate.

Nonverbal Communication Skills

To communicate well, we need to learn the best words to say, as well has how act when we say them. Nonverbal communication skills are the things we do when we are talking with others. These skills include the following:

Eye Contact   Look people in the eyes; don't stare.

Posture   Stand or sit up straight facing the other person, relaxed, but upright.

Gestures	Use appropriate body movements and gestures when talking. Gestures are movements of the hands or body that emphasize what is being said.
Facial Expressions	*Facial expression*s tell others what you are feeling and should match the discussion. Smiles and head nods tell people you are listening.
Voice Volume and Tone	Voice volume should be pleasant, not too loud or soft, and the pitch of your voice should go up and down naturally with emotions and emphasis. Avoid speaking in a monotone.
Speech Pace and Duration	Maintain a smooth *pace*; don't talk too fast or slow and pause to let others speak. **Be short and sweet.**

My best nonverbal skill is: _____

My priority nonverbal skill to practice is: _____

Active Listening

When you hold conversations with others, pay attention to the discussion to understand what others mean and how they are feeling. This is called "active listening." It is the best way to show another person that you are paying attention to what they are saying.

Active Listening Skills:
1. MAINTAIN EYE CONTACT.
2. NOD YOUR HEAD.
3. SAY "UH-HUH," "OK," OR "I SEE."
4. REPEAT WHAT THE PERSON SAID IN YOUR OWN WORDS.

Let the other person finish speaking and let the person know what you heard him or her say before offering your own comment.

Practice Active Listening Skills

> ### ROLE PLAY: ACTIVE LISTENING
>
> Practice **Active Listening** and **Nonverbal Communication Skills** in a role play in which one person talks and the other listens.
>
> **Goals of the Role Play:**
> - Do all four steps of the **Active Listening Skill.**
> - Practice your **Priority Nonverbal Communication Skill.**

Summary

- Much communication is nonverbal. It involves our facial expressions, eye contact, posture, gestures, voice volume, pace, and tone.
- Active listening can help people in our lives feel understood, which improves our relationships.

At least once during the week, use the **Active Listening Skills** when someone is talking to you. Fill out the first three boxes of the form now with your provider, then fill out the last two boxes when you practice at home.

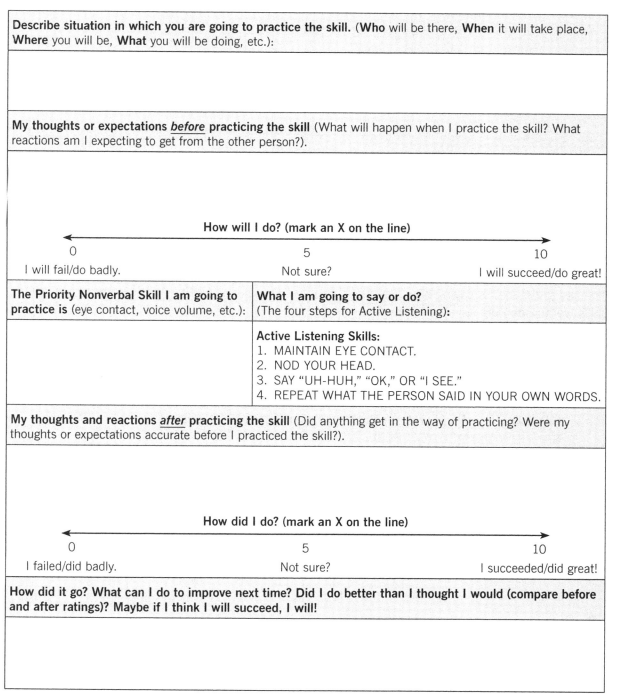

Describe situation in which you are going to practice the skill. (**Who** will be there, **When** it will take place, **Where** you will be, **What** you will be doing, etc.):

My thoughts or expectations *before* practicing the skill (What will happen when I practice the skill? What reactions am I expecting to get from the other person?).

How will I do? (mark an X on the line)

0	5	10
I will fail/do badly.	Not sure?	I will succeed/do great!

The Priority Nonverbal Skill I am going to practice is (eye contact, voice volume, etc.):	**What I am going to say or do?** (The four steps for Active Listening):
	Active Listening Skills: 1. MAINTAIN EYE CONTACT. 2. NOD YOUR HEAD. 3. SAY "UH-HUH," "OK," OR "I SEE." 4. REPEAT WHAT THE PERSON SAID IN YOUR OWN WORDS.

My thoughts and reactions *after* practicing the skill (Did anything get in the way of practicing? Were my thoughts or expectations accurate before I practiced the skill?).

How did I do? (mark an X on the line)

0	5	10
I failed/did badly.	Not sure?	I succeeded/did great!

How did it go? What can I do to improve next time? Did I do better than I thought I would (compare before and after ratings)? Maybe if I think I will succeed, I will!

Session 3: Expressing Pleasant Feelings

■ Review At-Home Practice: Active Listening
■ Learn Expressing Pleasant Feelings Skill
■ At-Home Practice: Expressing Pleasant Feelings
■ Do you want to add any agenda items?

1. _____

2. _____

Expressing Pleasant Feelings

Expressing pleasant feelings means telling someone that something he or she **did** made you **feel** good! This communication skill helps us start and maintain friendships and relationships. If we want to keep our friends, we need to tell them how important they are to us and how they make us happy. If we tell people that we appreciate them and feel happy because of what they do, they are more likely to keep doing what makes us happy again and again!

The key to the skill is saying how the things people **DO** make us **FEEL**. All the communication skills we are learning follow similar steps:

"When you **DO** _____, I **FEEL** _____."

Expressing Pleasant Feelings Skill:
1. MAINTAIN EYE CONTACT.
2. SAY EXACTLY WHAT THE PERSON **DID** THAT PLEASED YOU.
3. SAY HOW IT MADE YOU **FEEL.**

It can sometimes feel uncomfortable to express how we really feel to someone else. We may not know how to say it, or we may be concerned about how someone will react. We may have thoughts such as "The person doesn't want to know how I'm feeling" or "The person might get mad." The only way to find out if these thoughts are correct is to express pleasant feelings and test it out. We will learn how to express pleasant feelings and how to correct unhelpful thoughts that get in the way expressing them.

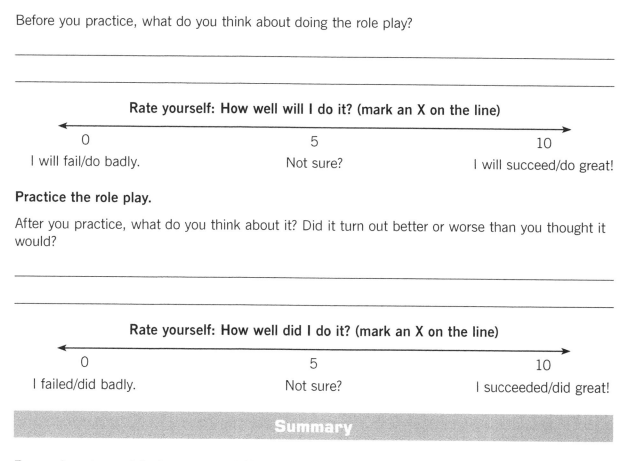

ROLE PLAY: EXPRESSING PLEASANT FEELINGS

Practice **Expressing Pleasant Feelings** and **Nonverbal Communication Skills** in a role play. Tell another person about something he or she did (e.g., driving you somewhere) that made you feel happy (or another pleasant feeling). The other person practices **Active Listening Skills.**

Goals of Role play:
- Practice **Nonverbal Communication Skills.**
- Do all three steps of the **Expressing Pleasant Feelings Skills.**
- Remember to say what the person **DID** (his or her actions).
- Use the list of **Pleasant Feelings** to label your feelings.

Before you practice, what do you think about doing the role play?

_____

_____

Rate yourself: How well will I do it? (mark an X on the line)

0   5   10

I will fail/do badly.   Not sure?   I will succeed/do great!

Practice the role play.

After you practice, what do you think about it? Did it turn out better or worse than you thought it would?

_____

_____

Rate yourself: How well did I do it? (mark an X on the line)

0   5   10

I failed/did badly.   Not sure?   I succeeded/did great!

Summary

Expressing pleasant feelings means telling people about the things they **do** that make us **feel good**, which will make them keep doing what makes us feel good!!

At least once during the week, use the **Expressing Pleasant Feelings Skill.** Fill out the first three boxes of the form now with your provider, then fill out the last two boxes when you practice at home.

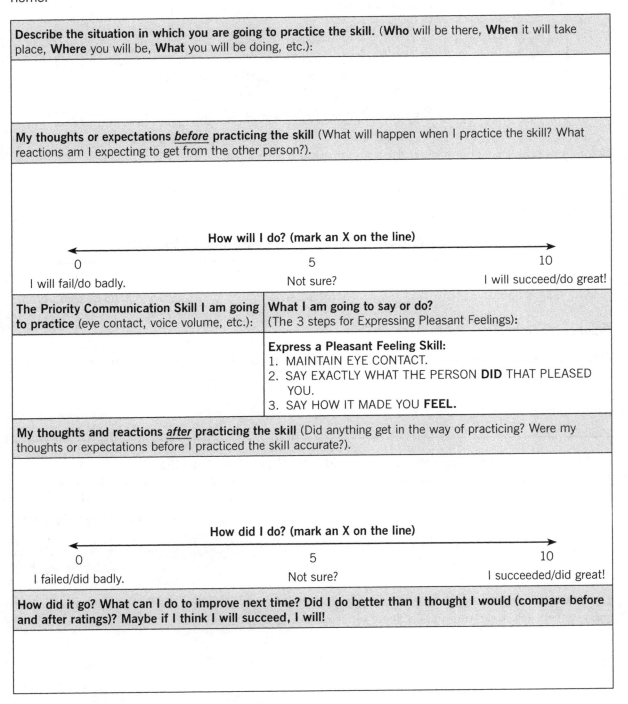

Describe the situation in which you are going to practice the skill. (Who will be there, **When** it will take place, **Where** you will be, **What** you will be doing, etc.):
My thoughts or expectations _before_ practicing the skill (What will happen when I practice the skill? What reactions am I expecting to get from the other person?).

How will I do? (mark an X on the line)

0 — 5 — 10

I will fail/do badly.　　　Not sure?　　　I will succeed/do great!

The Priority Communication Skill I am going to practice (eye contact, voice volume, etc.):	**What I am going to say or do?** (The 3 steps for Expressing Pleasant Feelings):
	Express a Pleasant Feeling Skill: 1. MAINTAIN EYE CONTACT. 2. SAY EXACTLY WHAT THE PERSON **DID** THAT PLEASED YOU. 3. SAY HOW IT MADE YOU **FEEL.**

My thoughts and reactions _after_ practicing the skill (Did anything get in the way of practicing? Were my thoughts or expectations before I practiced the skill accurate?).

How did I do? (mark an X on the line)

0 — 5 — 10

I failed/did badly.　　　Not sure?　　　I succeeded/did great!

How did it go? What can I do to improve next time? Did I do better than I thought I would (compare before and after ratings)? Maybe if I think I will succeed, I will!

From *Cognitive-Behavioral Social Skills Training for Schizophrenia* by Eric L. Granholm, John R. McQuaid, and Jason L. Holden. Copyright © 2016 by The Guilford Press.

- Review At-Home Practice: Expressing Pleasant Feelings
- Learn Making a Positive Request Skill
- At-Home Practice: Making a Positive Request
- Do you want to add any agenda items?

1. _____

2. _____

Making a Positive Request

Making a positive request is asking someone to do something that would help you achieve your goals and feel good! Everyone needs to ask others for help. Sometimes we want to ask someone to do something fun with us to make us feel good. If we learn how to make positive requests well, we are more likely to get others to help us and do fun activities with us.

The key to the skill is saying how the things people might **DO** would make us **FEEL**. All the skills we are learning follow similar "WHEN YOU **DO** _____, I **FEEL** _____" steps:

Making a Positive Request skill:
1. MAINTAIN EYE CONTACT.
2. SAY EXACTLY WHAT YOU WOULD LIKE THE PERSON TO **DO**.
3. SAY HOW IT WOULD MAKE YOU **FEEL**.

It can sometimes feel uncomfortable to ask others to do things for us. We may not know how to say it or we may be concerned about how someone will react. We may have thoughts such as "The person will just say no," "The person doesn't care about me or like me," or "The person might get mad." The only way to find out whether these thoughts are correct is to make the positive request and test it out. We will learn how to make positive requests and how to correct the unhelpful thoughts that get in the way of making them.

ROLE PLAY: MAKING A POSITIVE REQUEST

Describe a situation in your life in which you want to make a positive request:

_____

Practice **Making a Positive Request** and **Nonverbal Communication Skills** in a role play of this situation, while the other person practices **Active Listening Skills.** It will be much easier to do this if you practice it.

Goals of Role Play:
- *Practice **Nonverbal Communication Skills.***
- *Do all three steps of the **Making a Positive Request Skill.***
- *Remember to SAY WHAT YOU WANT THE PERSON TO **DO** (his or her actions).*
- *Use the **List of Pleasant Feelings** to label your feelings.*

Before you practice, what do you think about doing the role play?

_____

_____

Rate yourself: How well will I do it? (mark an X on the line)

0	5	10
I will fail/do badly.	Not sure?	I will succeed/do great!

Practice the role play.

After you practice, what do you think about it? Did it turn out better or worse than you thought it would?

_____

_____

Rate yourself: How well did I do it? (mark an X on the line)

0	5	10
I failed/did badly.	Not sure?	I succeeded/did great!

Summary

- People may not do what you ask them, but by using the Making a Positive Request Skill, you will have the best chance of getting people to do things to help you reach your goals.

At least once during the week, use the **Making a Positive Request Skill.** Fill out the first three boxes of the form now with your provider, then fill out the last two boxes when you practice at home.

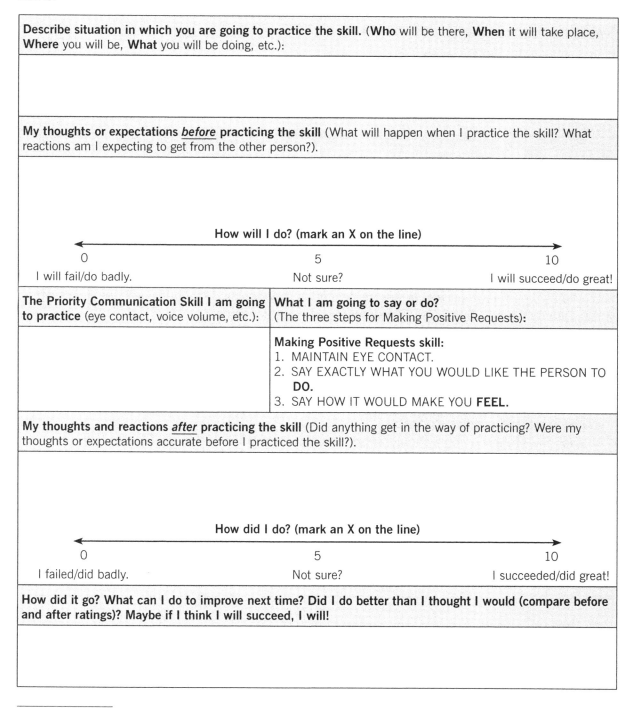

Describe situation in which you are going to practice the skill. (Who will be there, **When** it will take place, **Where** you will be, **What** you will be doing, etc.):

My thoughts or expectations _before_ **practicing the skill** (What will happen when I practice the skill? What reactions am I expecting to get from the other person?).

How will I do? (mark an X on the line)

0 — 5 — 10

I will fail/do badly.   Not sure?   I will succeed/do great!

The Priority Communication Skill I am going to practice (eye contact, voice volume, etc.):	**What I am going to say or do?** (The three steps for Making Positive Requests):
	Making Positive Requests skill: 1. MAINTAIN EYE CONTACT. 2. SAY EXACTLY WHAT YOU WOULD LIKE THE PERSON TO **DO.** 3. SAY HOW IT WOULD MAKE YOU **FEEL.**

My thoughts and reactions _after_ **practicing the skill** (Did anything get in the way of practicing? Were my thoughts or expectations accurate before I practiced the skill?).

How did I do? (mark an X on the line)

0 — 5 — 10

I failed/did badly.   Not sure?   I succeeded/did great!

How did it go? What can I do to improve next time? Did I do better than I thought I would (compare before and after ratings)? Maybe if I think I will succeed, I will!

Session 5: Asking for Help with Your Goals

- Review At-Home Practice: Making a Positive Request
- Talking to Others about Goals
- At-Home Practice: Making a Positive Request
- Do you want to add any agenda items?

1. _____

2. _____

Getting Help to Achieve Our Goals

There are many people who might be able to help us achieve our goals. Some support persons are professionals (doctors, case managers, work counselors, teachers, bosses). Other support persons are family members and friends who are close to us. Still other support persons can help with professional matters, such as getting a job, taking a class, or moving to a new place to live. Some of them may know us well enough to be able to notice changes in our moods, behaviors, and thinking (sometimes even before we notice it ourselves). These support persons can be very helpful to us when we don't realize we are becoming overwhelmed by stress or if our illness gets worse. Different support persons are helpful for different concerns.

How do you choose a support person to help you?

- Think of people who know you well, whom you can trust, and who are willing to help you without being critical.
- Think of people who are open-minded and understanding about your illness and able to give you accurate and positive feedback.
- At least one of these people should be someone you see often and is available to help you.
- They can be friends, spouses, other relatives, health-team members, or other professionals in the community—anyone you can think of whom you can ask for help with your goals.

MY SUPPORT PERSONS		
NAME	RELATIONSHIP	PHONE NUMBER
_____	_____	_____
_____	_____	_____
_____	_____	_____
_____	_____	_____
_____	_____	_____
_____	_____	_____

252

Now that you have identified the support people in your life, here is a list of the types of help you can possibly get from them:

- Help with finding better housing
- Help with transportation to appointments (e.g., taking bus rides, getting directions)
- Help with sobriety
- Writing letters or making phone calls to keep communication open
- Making time for weekly outings (e.g., going to the beach or to dinner)
- Filling your time with fun activities (working, volunteering, school, leisure activities)
- Finding a job
- Help with finances or problems with benefits
- Registering for a class
- Helping you notice illness warning signs

What else would you like to do or discuss with a support person?

1. _____

2. _____

3. _____

4. _____

5. _____

ROLE PLAY: MAKING A POSITIVE REQUEST

What do you want to ask a support person to do to help you with your goal?

_____

Practice **Making a Positive Request** and **Nonverbal Communication Skills** in a role play of this situation, while the other person practices **Active Listening Skills.**

Goals of the Role Play:
- Practice basic **Nonverbal Communication Skills.**
- Do all three steps of the **Making a Positive Request Skill.**
- Remember to SAY WHAT YOU WANT THE PERSON TO **DO** (the person's actions).
- Use the list of **Pleasant Feelings** to label your feelings.

Before you practice, what do you think about doing the role play?

_____

_____

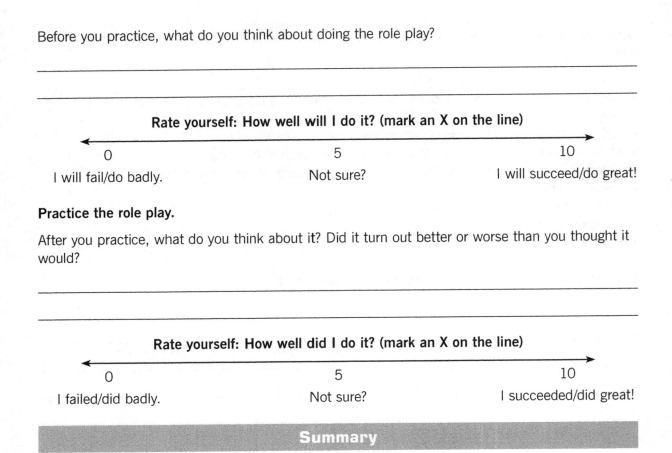

Rate yourself: How well will I do it? (mark an X on the line)

0   5   10

I will fail/do badly.   Not sure?   I will succeed/do great!

Practice the role play.

After you practice, what do you think about it? Did it turn out better or worse than you thought it would?

_____

_____

Rate yourself: How well did I do it? (mark an X on the line)

0   5   10

I failed/did badly.   Not sure?   I succeeded/did great!

Summary

- If we make positive requests of the support persons in our lives, we will make progress toward our goals.

At least once during the week, use the **Making a Positive Request Skill.** Fill out the first three boxes of the form now with your provider, then fill out the last two boxes when you practice at home.

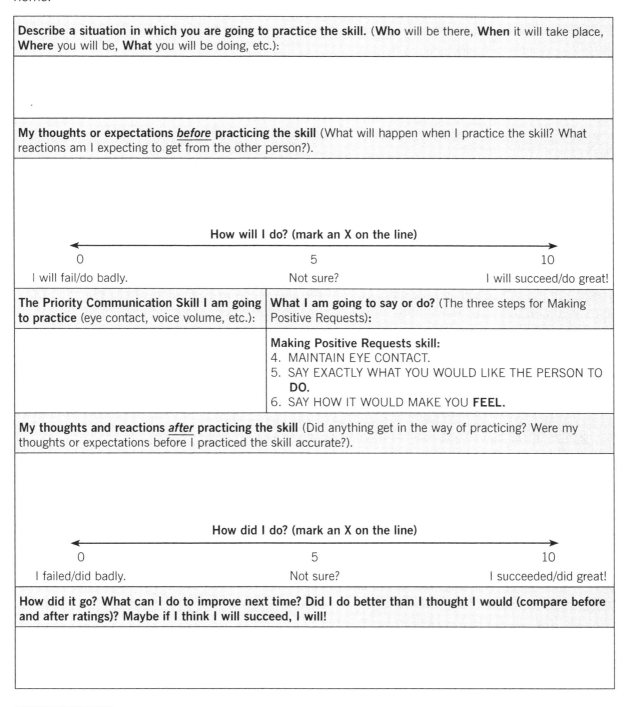

Describe a situation in which you are going to practice the skill. (Who will be there, **When** it will take place, **Where** you will be, **What** you will be doing, etc.):

My thoughts or expectations _before_ practicing the skill (What will happen when I practice the skill? What reactions am I expecting to get from the other person?).

How will I do? (mark an X on the line)

0   5   10
I will fail/do badly.   Not sure?   I will succeed/do great!

The Priority Communication Skill I am going to practice (eye contact, voice volume, etc.):	**What I am going to say or do?** (The three steps for Making Positive Requests):
	Making Positive Requests skill: 4. MAINTAIN EYE CONTACT. 5. SAY EXACTLY WHAT YOU WOULD LIKE THE PERSON TO **DO.** 6. SAY HOW IT WOULD MAKE YOU **FEEL.**

My thoughts and reactions _after_ practicing the skill (Did anything get in the way of practicing? Were my thoughts or expectations before I practiced the skill accurate?).

How did I do? (mark an X on the line)

0   5   10
I failed/did badly.   Not sure?   I succeeded/did great!

How did it go? What can I do to improve next time? Did I do better than I thought I would (compare before and after ratings)? Maybe if I think I will succeed, I will!

Session 6: Expressing Unpleasant Feelings

- Review At-Home Practice: Making a Positive Request
- Learn Expressing Unpleasant Feelings Skill
- At-Home Practice: Expressing Unpleasant Feelings
- Do you want to add any agenda items?

1. _____

2. _____

Expressing Unpleasant Feelings

Expressing Unpleasant Feelings is telling someone that something he or she did made us feel bad (like sad or angry). This is important, because telling others that we feel sad or angry because of what they did may get them to stop doing it. If we never ask people to stop and never suggest that they do something more helpful for us, how do they know that we want them to do something different?

The key to the skill is saying how the things people **DID** made us **FEEL** and what they could **DO** to make us **FEEL** better. Remember, all the communication skills we are learning follow similar steps:

"When you **DO** _____, I **FEEL** _____."

Expressing Unpleasant Feelings Skill:
1. MAINTAIN EYE CONTACT. SPEAK FIRMLY BUT CALMLY.
2. SAY EXACTLY WHAT THE PERSON **DID** THAT UPSET YOU.
3. SAY HOW IT MADE YOU **FEEL.**
4. SUGGEST WHAT THE PERSON SHOULD **DO** TO PREVENT THIS FROM HAPPENING AGAIN.

It can feel uncomfortable to express unpleasant feelings, because you may not know how to say it; you may be concerned about how others will react. You might have thoughts such as "They won't stop, so why bother," "They don't care what I want," or "They might get mad." These are common thoughts. The only way to find out whether these thoughts are correct is to test them by trying the skill. We will learn how to express unpleasant feelings and how to correct the unhelpful thoughts that get in the way of expressing them.

ROLE PLAY: EXPRESSING UNPLEASANT FEELINGS

Describe a situation in your life when you are upset by something someone does:

_____

Practice *Expressing Unpleasant Feelings* and *Nonverbal Communication Skills* in a role play of this situation, while the other person practices *Active Listening Skills*.

Goals of Role play:
- Practice basic **Nonverbal Communication Skills.**
- Do all four steps of the **Expressing Unpleasant Feelings Skill.**
- Remember to SAY WHAT THE PERSON **DID** AND WHAT YOU WANT THE PERSON TO **DO** DIFFERENTLY (the person's actions).
- Use the **List of Unpleasant Feelings** to label your feelings.

Before you practice, what do you think about doing the role play?

_____

_____

Rate yourself: How well will I do it? (mark an X on the line)

```
←————————————————————————————————————————————→
0                        5                       10
I will fail/do badly.    Not sure?    I will succeed/do great!
```

Practice the role play.

After you practice, what do you think about it? Did it turn out better or worse than you thought it would?

_____

_____

Rate yourself: How well did I do it? (mark an X on the line)

```
←————————————————————————————————————————————→
0                        5                       10
I failed/did badly.      Not sure?    I succeeded/did great!
```

Summary

People may not do what you ask them, but by using the Expressing Unpleasant Feelings Skill, you will have the best chance of getting people to stop doing the things that make you feel bad.

At least once during the week, use the **Expressing Unpleasant Feelings Skill.** Fill out the first three boxes of the form now with your provider, then fill out the last two boxes when you practice at home.

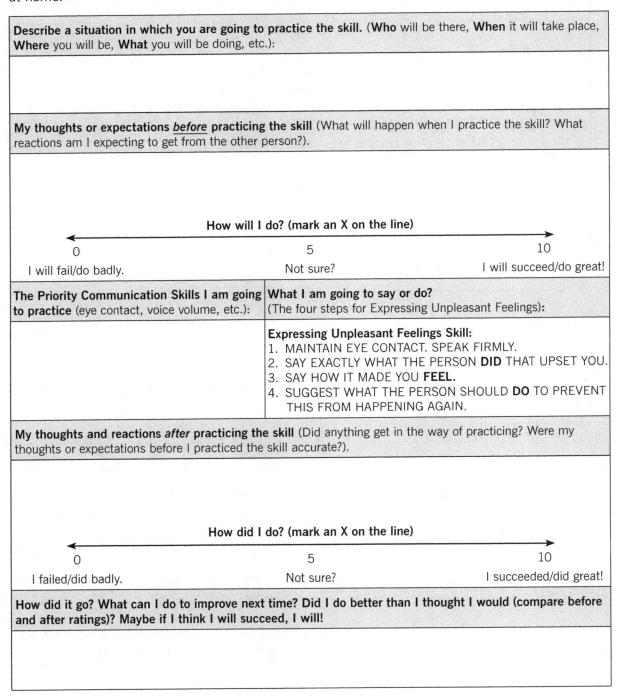

Describe a situation in which you are going to practice the skill. (**Who** will be there, **When** it will take place, **Where** you will be, **What** you will be doing, etc.):

My thoughts or expectations *before* practicing the skill (What will happen when I practice the skill? What reactions am I expecting to get from the other person?).

How will I do? (mark an X on the line)

0	5	10
I will fail/do badly.	Not sure?	I will succeed/do great!

The Priority Communication Skills I am going to practice (eye contact, voice volume, etc.):	What I am going to say or do? (The four steps for Expressing Unpleasant Feelings):
	Expressing Unpleasant Feelings Skill: 1. MAINTAIN EYE CONTACT. SPEAK FIRMLY. 2. SAY EXACTLY WHAT THE PERSON **DID** THAT UPSET YOU. 3. SAY HOW IT MADE YOU **FEEL**. 4. SUGGEST WHAT THE PERSON SHOULD **DO** TO PREVENT THIS FROM HAPPENING AGAIN.

My thoughts and reactions *after* practicing the skill (Did anything get in the way of practicing? Were my thoughts or expectations before I practiced the skill accurate?).

How did I do? (mark an X on the line)

0	5	10
I failed/did badly.	Not sure?	I succeeded/did great!

How did it go? What can I do to improve next time? Did I do better than I thought I would (compare before and after ratings)? Maybe if I think I will succeed, I will!

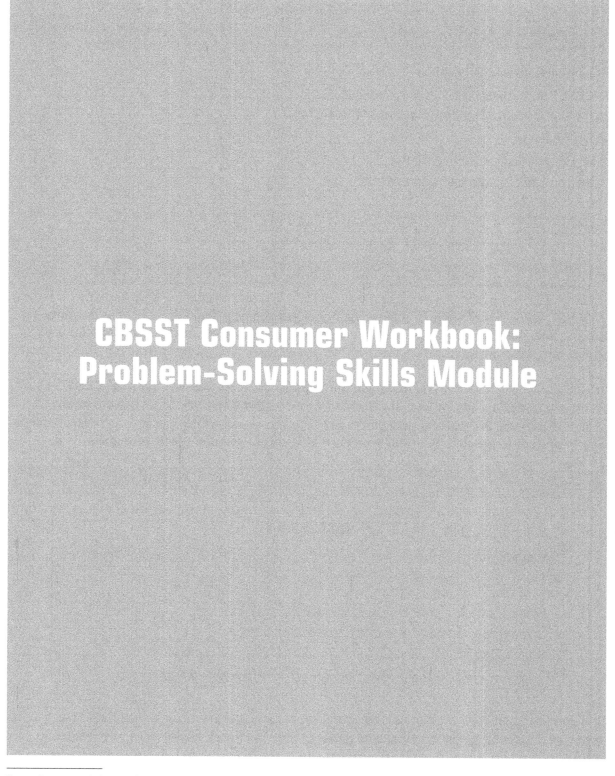

CBSST Consumer Workbook:
Problem-Solving Skills Module

Session 1: Introduction and Goal Setting

Agenda

- Introductions and Orientation
- CBSST and Changing Unhelpful Thinking
- Review At-Home Practice (previous members only)
- Set Goals
- At-Home Practice: Setting Goals
- Do you want to add any agenda items?

   1. _____

   2. _____

What is Cognitive-Behavioral Social Skills Training (CBSST)?

In CBSST, you will learn how to achieve your personal goals by thinking about your thoughts and learning new skills. You will learn how to change unhelpful thinking, communicate better with others, and solve problems.

Plan to participate actively. **The more you participate, the more you will get from CBSST.** Feel free to ask questions and make comments during discussions and talk about the program with others. Discussing the material with others will help you improve the skills you learn. **It will be very important to practice the skills you learn at home so you can reach your goals.**

What Is Unhelpful Thinking?

DISCUSSION

Scenario: *Someone bumps into you on the street and you immediately think the person did it on purpose to hurt you.*

1. *How would this situation make you feel?*
2. *Would you shout at the person or shove the person?*
3. *Would this make you want to be around people more or less?*
4. *Can you see how the thought influenced your feelings and actions?*

Unhelpful thoughts can prevent us from working on our goals and make us feel bad. They can also make it difficult to tell the difference between real and unreal experiences or to cope and interact with other people. Unhelpful thoughts can make it difficult to have relationships, work or go to school.

Unhelpful thoughts are just mistakes in thinking that can be corrected by testing them out and gathering all the facts. Everyone makes mistakes in thinking. One of the most important skills we will learn in this class is how to change the inaccurate, unhelpful thoughts that are preventing us from achieving our goals.

Setting Goals

One of the best ways to improve the quality of our lives is to set goals. In today's class, we are going to set at least one personal goal. The purpose of this program is to help you learn skills that will help you reach your goals.

The best goals are things that you really, really want, that will improve the quality of your life, such as finding a girlfriend or boyfriend, making a new friend, having more fun with friends, reconnecting with family, living independently, taking a class, getting a job or volunteering. We can break it down into small steps you can do each week (in 7 days) to accomplish a short-term goal in the next 7 weeks that will help you achieve your long-term goal in the next 7 months or more. We call that the 7–7–7 Goal Jackpot! The longest journey starts with the first step, and small steps lead to bigger goals. For example, if you wash the dishes today and pay your own bills tomorrow, then soon you will be taking care of your own apartment.

7–7–7 GOAL JACKPOT! WORKSHEET EXAMPLE

Name: _Jane_   **Date Long-Term Goal Set:** _Oct. 1_

Long-Term (Meaningful) Goal (7 months): _Have a boyfriend_

Short-Term Goals Related to the Long-Term Goal (7 weeks):
(check off steps when you complete them)

1. _Improve hygiene_   **2.** _Improve conversations_

Steps (7 days):   *Steps (7 days):*

1. _Separate clean/dirty laundry ✓_   1. _Draft list of possible topics ✓_
2. _Do laundry 2X per week ✓_   2. _Practice starting conversations ✓_
3. _Brush teeth A.M./P.M. ✓_   3. _Practice ending conversations_
4. _Shower daily ✓_   4. _Practice asking someone for a date_

Let's start filling out your own goal-setting worksheet in class and you can work on it more at home.

7–7–7 GOAL JACKPOT! WORKSHEET

Name: _____   Date Long-Term Goal Set: _____

Long-Term (Meaningful) Goal (7 months): _____

Short-Term Goals Related to the Long-Term Goal (7 weeks):
(check off steps when you complete them)

1. _____   **2.** _____

Steps (7 days):   *Steps (7 days):*

1. _____   1. _____
2. _____   2. _____
3. _____   3. _____
4. _____   4. _____

Start Date: _____   Start Date: _____

Date Reviewed: _____ Date Reviewed: _____

Modified/Next Steps: **Modified/Next Steps:**

1. _____   1. _____
2. _____   2. _____
3. _____   3. _____
4. _____   4. _____

Date Reviewed: _____ Date Reviewed: _____

Modified/Next Steps: **Modified/Next Steps:**

1. _____   1. _____
2. _____   2. _____
3. _____   3. _____
4. _____   4. _____

Session 2: Introduction to SCALE

- Review At-Home Practice: Goal Setting
- Learn Problem-Solving Skills: SCALE
- In-Session Practice: SCALE Worksheet
- Check Your Thoughts about the Plan
- At-Home Practice: SCALE Worksheet
- Do you want to add any agenda items?

1. _____

2. _____

Steps to Follow to Solve Problems: SCALE

The problem-solving steps spell out **SCALE**, like your efforts to **SCALE** the mountain (i.e., your problem, challenge or goal step).

Specify: What's the problem? Frame it as a question. Don't make it too big. Make it a specific but important step toward achieving your goals that you can accomplish by next week.

Consider all possible solutions: Brainstorm all possible solutions; just generate, don't evaluate. We will evaluate on the next step.

Assess the best solution: Identify positives and negatives of each possible solution and pick the best one.

Lay out a plan: What will you do first, second, third? Who will do what, how, and when? What will you need (e.g., time, support persons, things, transportation, money)?

Execute and **E**valuate: Did your plan work? How well did it work? Can it be improved? Do you need to try another solution? Use SCALE to solve problems and challenges that come up.

SCALE EXAMPLE: *Find Transportation*

Specify: Define the problem; be specific.
- How can I get to the store to buy a new shirt for my interview?

Consider all possible solutions; Brainstorm alternatives; just generate, don't evaluate.
- Take the bus
- Walk
- Ask my roommate for a ride
- Ask my case manager to take me
- Borrow a bicycle

---

*A*ssess *the best solution*: Pick two solutions that you like the most and identify positives and negatives of each.

1. Take the bus.

   Positive: I don't need to rely on anyone else.
   I can go there on my schedule.

   Negative: I don't have a bus pass, so it will cost me money.
   It is a long ride.

2. Ask my roommate for a ride.

   Positive: It will be the fastest way to get to the store.

   Negative: I may have to give my roommate gas money.
   He may not be able to go when I want to go.

   Assessment: Solution 1 seems best.

*L*ay *out a plan*: What will you do first, second, third?

1. Ask my roommate how much the bus fare will be.
2. Set aside enough money from my check for the fare.
3. Identify the correct bus and route to get to the store. How do I do that? May need to use SCALE again for this problem.
4. Choose a time to go that doesn't conflict with my appointments.

*E*xecute *and E*valuate: Did your plan work? How well did it work? Can it be improved? What went wrong? How can you fix it? Do you need to try another solution?

After we lay out a plan, we check out our thoughts about the plan. On the SCALE Worksheet, mark the arrow line to indicate how successful you think the plan will be. If you think a plan will fail, you might not try it out. The only way to know for sure whether a plan will work is to execute it and evaluate whether it was successful or not. For SCALE to work well, we must check out our thoughts about each plan to make sure unhelpful thoughts do not stop us from trying out the plan.

Summary

SCALE: Specify the problem, **C**onsider all possible solutions, **A**ssess the best solution, **L**ay out a plan, and **E**xecute and **E**valuate the outcome. These are the five steps to simplify and solve problems to achieve goals.

Specify the problem: What's the problem? Frame it as a question. Be specific.

Consider *all* possible solutions: Brainstorm alternatives. Just generate, don't evaluate!

1.	4.
2.	5.
3.	6.

Assess the best solution: Pick two you like and identify positives and negatives of each.

1:	2:
Pros:	Pros:
1.	1.
2.	2.
3.	3.
Cons:	Cons:
1.	1.
2.	2.
3.	3.

Lay out a plan: Select one of the two solutions and plan how you will try it out. What will you do first, second, third, and so forth? List everything and everyone you will need. No detail is too small!

Rate yourself (mark an X on the line):
Will I succeed?

0	5	10
I will fail/do poorly.	Not sure?	I will succeed/do great!

Execute and **E**valuate: Did your plan work? What went well/not well? Need another solution?

Rate yourself (mark an X on the line):
Did I succeed?

0	5	10
I failed/did poorly.	Not sure?	I succeeded/did great!

Specify the problem: What's the problem? Frame it as a question. Be specific.

Consider *all* possible solutions: Brainstorm alternatives. Just generate, don't evaluate!

1.	4.
2.	5.
3.	6.

Assess the best solution: Pick two you like and identify positives and negatives of each.

1:	**2:**
Pros:	**Pros:**
1.	1.
2.	2.
3.	3.
Cons:	**Cons:**
1.	1.
2.	2.
3.	3.

Lay out a plan: Select one of the two solutions and plan how you will try it out. What will you do first, second, third, etc.? List everything and everyone you will need. No detail is too small!

Rate yourself (mark an X on the line):
Will I succeed?

0   5   10
I will fail/do poorly.   Not sure?   I will succeed/do great!

Execute and **E**valuate: Did your plan work? What went well/not well? Need another solution?

Rate yourself (mark an X on the line):
Did I succeed?

0   5   10
I failed/did poorly.   Not sure?   I succeeded/did great!

Session 3: Specify the Problem

Agenda

▓ Review At-Home Practice: SCALE Worksheet

▓ Learn to Specify Problems

▓ How Do Thoughts Relate to Problems?

▓ In-Session Practice: SCALE Worksheet

▓ At-Home Practice: SCALE Worksheet

▓ Do you want to add any agenda items?

1. _____

2. _____

How to Specify the Problem

Problems that are not specific are very difficult to solve:

- Not specific: "I'm bored."
- Specific: "Where can I meet new people?"
- Not specific: "I need to keep my apartment clean."
- Specific: "How can I make sure I wash the dishes every day?"

Sometimes, it helps to specify problems as questions that need to be answered. To specify problems, consider your goals, the steps you have identified to achieve goals, and what obstacles stand in the way of your goals.

EXERCISE: SPECIFY PROBLEMS

Review your 7–7–7 Goal Jackpot! Worksheet to help you identify your goal steps. Write a step as specific problem here:

_____

How we think about our problems will influence how hard we work on solving them. Changing inaccurate, self-defeating thoughts about problems can help us try harder to solve problems, face challenges, and work toward our goals.

DISCUSSION: THOUGHTS THAT INTERFERE WITH GOALS

Thought (A):
"Even though I take my medications regularly, I still hear these voices sometimes. I'm never going to get better."

Thought (B):
"Even though I sometimes still hear these voices, overall I am feeling much better since I started taking my medication regularly."

Which thought is more accurate? More helpful? Why?

Thought (A):
"Why bother, I'm just going to fail. I have too many problems."

Thought (B):
"I might do really well. I'll never know if I don't try."

Which thought is more accurate? More helpful? Why?

Thought (A)
"I'm going to sound weird, stupid, or strange."

Thought (B)
"I'm going to be able to express some things and someone may like me."

Which thought is more accurate? More helpful? Why?
Which thoughts would make us try harder to solve problems?

Summary

- **Specify:** Breaking problems down into simple steps that can be done in a week makes problems easier to solve. Remember, even the longest journey starts with the first step.
- **Thoughts can get in the way:** If we expect to fail we are more likely to fail. Test it out by trying a solution to a problem and see what happens.

Specify the problem: What's the problem? Frame it as a question. Be specific.

Consider *all* possible solutions: Brainstorm alternatives. Just generate, don't evaluate!

1.	4.
2.	5.
3.	6.

Assess the best solution: Pick two you like and identify positives and negatives of each.

1:	**2:**
Pros:	**Pros:**
1.	1.
2.	2.
3.	3.
Cons:	**Cons:**
1.	1.
2.	2.
3.	3.

Lay out a plan: Select one of the two solutions and plan how you will try it out. What will you do first, second, third, etc.? List everything and everyone you will need. No detail is too small!

Rate yourself (mark an X on the line):
Will I succeed?

0   5   10
I will fail/do poorly.   Not sure?   I will succeed/do great!

Execute and **E**valuate: Did your plan work? What went well/not well? Need another solution?

Rate yourself (mark an X on the line):
Did I succeed?

0   5   10
I failed/did poorly.   Not sure?   I succeeded/did great!

At-Home Practice: SCALE Problem-Solving Worksheet

Specify the problem: What's the problem? Frame it as a question. Be specific.

Consider *all* possible solutions: Brainstorm alternatives. Just generate, don't evaluate!

1.	4.
2.	5.
3.	6.

Assess the best solution: Pick two you like and identify positives and negatives of each.

1:	**2:**
Pros:	**Pros:**
1.	1.
2.	2.
3.	3.
Cons:	**Cons:**
1.	1.
2.	2.
3.	3.

Lay out a plan: Select one of the two solutions and plan how you will try it out. What will you do first, second, third, etc.? List everything and everyone you will need. No detail is too small!

Rate yourself (mark an X on the line):
Will I succeed?

0 — I will fail/do poorly.   5 — Not sure?   10 — I will succeed/do great!

Execute and **E**valuate: Did your plan work? What went well/not well? Need another solution?

Rate yourself (mark an X on the line):
Did I succeed?

0 — I failed/did poorly.   5 — Not sure?   10 — I succeeded/did great!

Session 4: Consider All Solutions

- Review At-Home Practice: SCALE Worksheet
- Learn to Consider First, then Assess
- At-Home Practice: SCALE Worksheet
- Do you want to add any agenda items?

1. _____

2. _____

Consider All Solutions, Then Assess

Separating the Consider and Assess steps is not easy. When we consider solutions, it is essential that we do not at the same time start to assess which solution is best. One big difficulty with solving problems is when we come up with one solution, we quickly decide it may not work, and then give up.

⟳ REMEMBER THIS: ⟲

JUST GENERATE, DON'T EVALUATE!

After you have a long list of solutions, then—and only then—pick two that you like the most and are most likely to try out, and identify the positive and negatives of these two solutions.

EXERCISE: PRACTICE CONSIDERING ALL SOLUTIONS

Problem: My cat is stuck in a tree.

Try to think of 30 different ways to get the cat out of the tree.

Think of as many ideas as possible without making judgments about them. Don't edit out any ideas because they seem silly or bad. Just let the ideas keep coming. You never know when a silly idea will trigger a good one.

Summary

When you consider all solutions, be careful not to skip ahead and start assessing which is the best one. This is when self-defeating thoughts can get in the way, such as "That won't work." You never know until you try.

Specify the problem: What's the problem? Frame it as a question. Be specific.

Consider *all* possible solutions: Brainstorm alternatives. Just generate, don't evaluate!

1.	4.
2.	5.
3.	6.

Assess the best solution: Pick two you like and identify positives and negatives of each.

1:	**2:**
Pros:	**Pros:**
1.	1.
2.	2.
3.	3.
Cons:	**Cons:**
1.	1.
2.	2.
3.	3.

Lay out a plan: Select one of the two solutions and plan how you will try it out. What will you do first, second, third, etc.? List everything and everyone you will need. No detail is too small!

Rate yourself (mark an X on the line): **Will I succeed?**	0 ⟵——————————— 5 ——————————⟶ 10
	I will fail/do poorly. Not sure? I will succeed/do great!

Execute and **E**valuate: Did your plan work? What went well/not well? Need another solution?

Rate yourself (mark an X on the line): **Did I succeed?**	0 ⟵——————————— 5 ——————————⟶ 10
	I failed/did poorly. Not sure? I succeeded/did great!

Session 5: Lay Out a Plan

Agenda

- Review At-Home Practice: SCALE Worksheet
- Learn to Lay Out a Detailed Plan
- At-Home Practice: SCALE Worksheet
- Do you want to add any agenda items?

1. _____

2. _____

Lay Out a Detailed Plan

If your plans have not been working, they may need more details. When laying out a plan, think through all the steps necessary, even the ones that seem obvious. Write down each step and how you are going to accomplish it. Also think about any resources that may be helpful to you when accomplishing each step. Resources are things that are needed to execute the plan, including people (e.g., your case manager, staff member, friend, or a family member), objects (e.g., pencils, paper, telephone), or even transportation (e.g., a ride or a bus pass).

Did one of your plans not work out? Review the plan and lay out more detailed steps. You may need to use SCALE to solve problems related to the steps in the plan.

Summary

Sometimes plans don't work out because we missed some details. No problem, use SCALE to solve problems with the steps and make a new plan.

At-Home Practice: SCALE Problem-Solving Worksheet

Specify the problem: What's the problem? Frame it as a question. Be specific.

Consider *all* possible solutions: Brainstorm alternatives. Just generate, don't evaluate!

1.	4.
2.	5.
3.	6.

Assess the best solution: Pick two you like and identify positives and negatives of each.

1:	**2:**
Pros:	**Pros:**
1.	1.
2.	2.
3.	3.
Cons:	**Cons:**
1.	1.
2.	2.
3.	3.

Lay out a plan: Select one of the two solutions and plan how you will try it out. What will you do first, second, third, etc.? List everything and everyone you will need. No detail is too small!

Rate yourself (mark an X on the line): **Will I succeed?**

0	5	10
I will fail/do poorly.	Not sure?	I will succeed/do great!

Execute and **E**valuate: Did your plan work? What went well/not well? Need another solution?

Rate yourself (mark an X on the line): **Did I succeed?**

0	5	10
I failed/did poorly.	Not sure?	I succeeded/did great!

Session 6: Solving Problems Related to Goals

- Review At-Home Practice: SCALE Worksheet
- Solving Problems Related to Your Goals
- At-Home Practice: SCALE Worksheet
- Do you want to add any agenda items?

1. _____

2. _____

Solving Problems Related to Your Goals

The following is a list of common problems that may get in the way of your goals. Go through and put a ✓ in the boxes next to the problems that are related to your goals. If you don't see one that relates to your goals, use your 7–7–7 Goal Jackpot! Worksheet to identify a goal step or obstacle related to a step.

☐ You would like to go on a picnic in the park with some family and friends and have a barbecue. You are not quite sure how to prepare for this. What are the steps you need to take to go on a picnic?

☐ You have a pain in your side, and you want to find out if you have a medical problem.

☐ You have been sober for a few months, but a good friend has continued to use alcohol. You want to hang out with your friend, but whenever you go out, this person drinks in front of you and sometimes pressures you to drink.

☐ You don't have a ride to your appointment, so you need to find another way to get there.

☐ You've been taking your medication regularly, but your problems become worse anyway. You're very concerned and make an appointment with your doctor, but it is not for 3 weeks.

☐ Your roommate or someone you live with won't do any household chores or bothers you in some way.

☐ Your phone has no dial tone, and you need to call a friend.

☐ You want to take a class on using computers.

☐ You think a coworker wants to get you fired.

☐ You've just moved into a new place. Your neighbors are really noisy and keep you awake at night.

☐ You have been sober for 6 months, but recently, your voices have gotten worse. In the past, you used street drugs and alcohol to quiet the voices, and you are tempted to use them now.

☐ You spend most of your days alone and want to find a way to socialize more with others.

☐ A friend invites you to go out with another person with whom you don't get along. How do you handle this situation?

☐ You are having difficulty managing your money but feel embarrassed to ask for help.

☐ You want to live on your own but do not know how to find an apartment.

☐ A friend borrowed money from you and promised to return it immediately. You need the money, but your friend has not mentioned paying you back.

☐ You got a job interview but do not have the right clothes to wear and cannot afford to buy some.

☐ You want to talk with a family member about something, but the family member doesn't want to talk with you.

Summary

- SCALE gives us the tools to solve problems, face challenges, and remove obstacles in the way of our goals. We can use SCALE to solve problems and take steps toward achieving our goals.

Specify the problem: What's the problem? Frame it as a question. Be specific.

Consider *all* possible solutions: Brainstorm alternatives. Just generate, don't evaluate!

1.	4.
2.	5.
3.	6.

Assess the best solution: Pick two you like and identify positives and negatives of each.

1:	**2:**
Pros:	**Pros:**
1.	1.
2.	2.
3.	3.
Cons:	**Cons:**
1.	1.
2.	2.
3.	3.

Lay out a plan: Select one of the two solutions and plan how you will try it out. What will you do first, second, third, etc.? List everything and everyone you will need. No detail is too small!

Rate yourself (mark an X on the line):
Will I succeed?

0	5	10
I will fail/do poorly.	Not sure?	I will succeed/do great!

Execute and **E**valuate: Did your plan work? What went well/not well? Need another solution?

Rate yourself (mark an X on the line):
Did I succeed?

0	5	10
I failed/did poorly.	Not sure?	I succeeded/did great!

APPENDIX A

Assessment Measures

COMPREHENSIVE MODULES TEST (CMT)   281

Scoring: Instructions for scoring the CMT are included on the interview for the total score and individual module scores. Higher scores indicate greater skills knowledge; range is 0–11 per module and 0–33 total.

DEFEATIST PERFORMANCE ATTITUDES SCALE (DPAS)   287

The full name of this measure does not appear on the assessment form to reduce possible response bias. **Scoring:** First, reverse-score item 9 (i.e., 7 = 1, 6 = 2, 5 = 3, 4 = 4), then add ratings for all items. Higher scores indicate greater severity of defeatist performance attitudes; range 15–105.

ASOCIAL BELIEFS SCALE (ABS)   289

The full name of this measure does not appear on the assessment form to reduce possible response bias. **Scoring:** Add 1 point for each True response, after reverse-scoring items 5, 11, and 13 (i.e., add 1 point for a False response to these three items). Higher scores indicate greater severity of asocial beliefs; range 0–15.

COMPREHENSIVE MODULES TEST (CMT)

Name/ID#: _____   **Date of Rating:** _____

NOTES:

_____

_____

_____

Instructions: Some of the questions I will be asking are about CBSST. You may or may not have learned the answers to these questions in CBSST, so I don't expect you to know all the answers. Do your best to answer as many questions as you can. Take a guess if you need to.

SOCIAL SKILLS MODULE TEST

1. Name five nonverbal communication behaviors. *If consumer asks for a definition of* nonverbal: *"communicating without using words."*

_____

_____

_____

Acceptable answers: A verbal/nonverbal answer that includes gestures, eye contact, body posture, body orientation, facial expression, speech pace, voice volume OR that describes or demonstrates a behavior such as "turn your body toward someone," "smile at another person," "nod your head," "hold your hand out." Demonstration of hand gesture(s) = 1 acceptable; demonstration of facial expression(s) = 1 acceptable.

Scoring: 1 point for 2–3 acceptable; 2 points for 4–5 .... ☐

2. Why is it important to make eye contact when talking to someone?

_____

_____

_____

Acceptable answers: It gets (or keeps) the other person's attention OR lets the other person know you are talking to them or listening to them.

Scoring: 1 point total for either acceptable answer .... ☐

3. What can you tell from a person's body posture and the direction he or she is facing?

_____

_____

_____

Acceptable answers: Whether the person wants to talk to you, is listening, is interested; no other responses (e.g., mood) acceptable.

Scoring: 1 point total for any acceptable answer .... ☐

(continued)

4. Explain what "speech pace and duration" means and why it is important.

_____

_____

_____

Acceptable answers: How fast or slow you talk, how long you talk, or any answer using the phrase "short and sweet"—so people can understand you better.

Scoring: 1 point total for capturing one aspect of pace or duration AND saying why. .... ☐

5. What are the important things to do and say to express unpleasant feelings to someone?

_____

_____

_____

Acceptable answers: *Look* at person or make eye contact, *say* exactly what he or she *did* that bothered you, *say* how it made you *feel*, and *say* what you want them to *do* differently.

Scoring: 1 point for 1–2 acceptable; 2 points for all 4 elements .... ☐

6. What are the important things to do and say when you make a positive request or ask someone to do something for you?

_____

_____

_____

Acceptable answers: *Look* at person or make eye contact, *say* exactly what you would like him or her to do, tell how it would make you *feel*.

Scoring: 1 point for 1–2 acceptable; 2 points for all 3 elements .... ☐

7. What are the important things to do and say when you need to listen actively to what someone is saying?

_____

_____

_____

Acceptable answers: *Look* at person or make eye contact, *nod and say*, "uh-huh," *ask* clarifying questions, *summarize*/check out what you heard.

Scoring: 1 point for 1–2 acceptable; 2 points for 3–4 elements .... ☐

SOCIAL SKILLS MODULE TOTAL (max. of 11) .... ☐

PROBLEM-SOLVING SKILLS MODULE TEST

1. What are the steps to follow when solving a problem?

_____

_____

_____

(continued)

Acceptable answers: (SCALE) **S**pecify (a concise problem), **C**onsider (compile/brainstorm alternatives without evaluating), **A**ssess (evaluate/choose the best one; pros and cons), **L**ay out a plan (specific resources, details, etc.), **E**xecute and **E**valuate (do it and see if it worked).

Scoring: 1 point for 2–3 steps; 2 points for 4–5 steps .... ☐

2. What is the best way to be specific or "specify" a problem you want to solve?

_____

_____

_____

Acceptable answers: Essential is the notion of breaking the problem down into something the consumer can DO with a high probability of success within a week.

Scoring: 1 point for breaking down a problem into a simple step; 2 points if consumer also says he or she can accomplish it in a week .... ☐

3. How do you come up with different solutions? *If consumer gives a vague answer (e.g., "think about it"), ask what he or she means*

_____

_____

_____

Acceptable answers: It is essential is to generate or brainstorm SEVERAL solutions without evaluating them.

Scoring: 1 point for generating or brainstorming; 2 points if add without evaluating. .... ☐

4. How do you decide the best solution to solve a problem?

_____

_____

_____

Acceptable answers: List or examine the pros and cons of solutions and pick the one with more pros than cons.

Scoring: 1 point for listing pros and cons of solutions .... ☐

5. After you decide on a solution, what do you do next?

_____

_____

_____

Acceptable answers: Plan/decide what resources (people, things) you need to carry out the solution and decide on a plan to do it.

Scoring: 1 point for resources or plan; 2 points for both .... ☐

6. What should you do after you try your solution to a problem?

_____

_____

_____

(continued)

Acceptable answers: Evaluate if it worked/was effective.

Scoring: 1 point for evaluate outcome .... □

7. What things can you do to help yourself solve problems?

_____

_____

Acceptable answers: ONLY fill out a problem-solving or SCALE Worksheet, a description of a SCALE step, "use SCALE" or ask someone to help me use SCALE/problem-solving steps; use of 3C's not acceptable.

Scoring: 1 point for any acceptable answer .... □

PROBLEM-SOLVING SKILLS MODULE TOTAL (max. of 11) .... □

COGNITIVE SKILLS MODULE TEST

1. What is the main focus of the cognitive skills in cognitive behavioral social skills training (CBSST)?

_____

_____

Acceptable answers: *Thoughts/beliefs/attitudes;* or how thoughts relate to actions and/or feelings (anything related to examining thoughts to get better or achieve goals).

Scoring: 1 point for any acceptable answer .... □

2. What are the 3C's?

_____

_____

Acceptable answer: "Catch It, Check It, Change It"

Scoring: 0 points for 0 or 1 answer, 1 point for 2 answers; 2 points for all three .... □

3. What is a mistake in thinking? *If consumer gives an example, ask for the name of the example or for a definition.*

_____

_____

Acceptable answers: A thought that is not accurate/no evidence for it; all-or-nothing thinking, jumping to conclusions, mind reading, fortune telling, emotional reasoning.

Scoring: 1 point for any acceptable answer .... □

(continued)

284

4. What should you do when you have an unhelpful thought? *Query (Tell me what you mean?):* "Stop and think about it." Or "Use the 3C's."

_____

_____

_____

Acceptable answers: *Examine evidence* for and against it, use the 3C's to check the accuracy; *examine/ check it* alone is acceptable, but NOT just catch or change it.

Scoring: 1 point for any acceptable answer .... ☐

5. What is a helpful way to deal with paranoid thoughts or suspiciousness?

_____

_____

_____

Acceptable answers: Do reality checking to see if the thought is really true, check the evidence, use the 3C's to check the accuracy.

Scoring: 1 point for any acceptable answer .... ☐

6. Give an example of an unhelpful thought.

_____

_____

_____

Acceptable answer: Any dysfunctional thought; a thought that would lead to an unpleasant feeling or unhelpful behavior (e.g., withdrawal or avoidance of goal-directed activity).

Scoring: 1 point for any acceptable dysfunctional thought .... ☐

7. Give an example of a feeling.

_____

_____

_____

Acceptable answer: Any emotion (emotions are one word).

Scoring: 1 point for any acceptable answer .... ☐

8. How would you deal with this problem: You want to ask someone to do something fun with you, but you think they will say no or laugh at you?

_____

_____

_____

Acceptable answer: Use the 3C's to check the thought; any answer involving checking the accuracy of the thought to change defeatist thinking. NOT just ask doctor, friend, etc. (don't query either).

Scoring: 1 point for any acceptable answer .... ☐

(continued)

9. Role play: I'd like to do a role play with you in which you will support a friend who needs help.

   Q1. I'll act as the friend. "Hi [*consumer's name*], I really need to talk with you. I saw this guy with a bulge in his jacket on the bus. I think he had a gun and wanted to hurt me. I think I should stay off the bus, don't you?"

   _____

   _____

   _____

   Acceptable answers: Identifying jumping to conclusions as a mistake in thinking; any attempt to evaluate evidence for or against the thought about the gun or avoiding the bus (e.g., "you should use the 3C's to check that out"); if participant also offers an alternative answer, do not ask the next question and give 1 point for the answer in Q2.

   Scoring: 1 point for any acceptable answer .... ☐

   Q2. What do you think could have been in his jacket?

   _____

   _____

   _____

   Acceptable answers: Any alternative nonthreatening answer (e.g., wallet, glasses, handkerchief, gloves).

   Scoring: 1 point for any acceptable answer, even if "gun" is also offered .... ☐

COGNITIVE SKILLS MODULE TOTAL (max. of 11) .... ☐

COMPREHENSIVE MODULES TEST TOTAL (sum of all three modules; max of 33). .... ☐

DPAS

Name/ID#: _____ Date of Rating: _____

NOTES:

_____

_____

_____

Instructions: This questionnaire lists different attitudes or beliefs that people sometimes hold. Read **EACH** statement carefully and decide how much you agree or disagree with the statement. For each of the attitudes, circle the number that **BEST DESCRIBES HOW YOU THINK**. Be sure to choose only one answer for each attitude. Because people are different, there is no right answer or wrong answer to these statements. To decide whether a given attitude is typical of your way of looking at things, simply keep in mind what you are like **MOST OF THE TIME**.

---

1. It is difficult to be happy unless one is good looking, intelligent, rich, and creative.

1	2	3	4	5	6	7
disagree totally	disagree very much	disagree slightly	neutral	agree slightly	agree very much	agree totally

---

2. People will probably think less of me if I make a mistake.

1	2	3	4	5	6	7
disagree totally	disagree very much	disagree slightly	neutral	agree slightly	agree very much	agree totally

---

3. If I do not do well all the time, people will not respect me.

1	2	3	4	5	6	7
disagree totally	disagree very much	disagree slightly	neutral	agree slightly	agree very much	agree totally

---

4. Taking even a small risk is foolish, because the loss is likely to be a disaster.

1	2	3	4	5	6	7
disagree totally	disagree very much	disagree slightly	neutral	agree slightly	agree very much	agree totally

---

5. If a person asks for help, it is a sign of weakness.

1	2	3	4	5	6	7
disagree totally	disagree very much	disagree slightly	neutral	agree slightly	agree very much	agree totally

---

6. If I do not do as well as other people, it means I am an inferior human being.

1	2	3	4	5	6	7
disagree totally	disagree very much	disagree slightly	neutral	agree slightly	agree very much	agree totally

(continued)

Based on Grant and Beck (2009). Original items from Weissman and Beck (1978). Reprinted with permission from the authors.

7. **If I fail at my work, then I am a failure as a person.**

1	2	3	4	5	6	7
disagree totally	disagree very much	disagree slightly	neutral	agree slightly	agree very much	agree totally

8. **If you cannot do something well, there is little point in doing it at all.**

1	2	3	4	5	6	7
disagree totally	disagree very much	disagree slightly	neutral	agree slightly	agree very much	agree totally

9. **Making mistakes is fine, because I can learn from them.**

1	2	3	4	5	6	7
disagree totally	disagree very much	disagree slightly	neutral	agree slightly	agree very much	agree totally

10. **If I fail partly, it is as bad as being a complete failure.**

1	2	3	4	5	6	7
disagree totally	disagree very much	disagree slightly	neutral	agree slightly	agree very much	agree totally

11. **People should have a reasonable likelihood of success before undertaking anything.**

1	2	3	4	5	6	7
disagree totally	disagree very much	disagree slightly	neutral	agree slightly	agree very much	agree totally

12. **If I don't set the highest standards for myself, I am likely to end up a second-rate person.**

1	2	3	4	5	6	7
disagree totally	disagree very much	disagree slightly	neutral	agree slightly	agree very much	agree totally

13. **If I am to be a worthwhile person, I must be truly outstanding in one major respect.**

1	2	3	4	5	6	7
disagree totally	disagree very much	disagree slightly	neutral	agree slightly	agree very much	agree totally

14. **People who have good ideas are more worthy than those who do not.**

1	2	3	4	5	6	7
disagree totally	disagree very much	disagree slightly	neutral	agree slightly	agree very much	agree totally

15. **If I ask a question, it makes me look inferior.**

1	2	3	4	5	6	7
disagree totally	disagree very much	disagree slightly	neutral	agree slightly	agree very much	agree totally

ABS

Name/ID#: _____ Date of Rating: _____

NOTES:

_____

_____

_____

Instructions: For each of the following statements, please indicate whether the statement is true or false of you. Circle the answer (True or False) that comes closest to how the item describes you.

1. I prefer hobbies and leisure activities that do not involve other people.	True	False
2. There are few things more important to me than privacy.	True	False
3. Making new friends isn't worth the energy it takes.	True	False
4. I prefer watching television to going out with other people.	True	False
5. I like to make long-distance phone calls to friends and relatives.	True	False
6. In many ways, I prefer the company of pets to the company of other people.	True	False
7. Having close friends is not as important as most people say.	True	False
8. People are usually better off if they stay aloof from emotional involvements with most others.	True	False
9. People sometimes think I'm shy, when I really just want to be left alone.	True	False
10. I could be happy living all alone in a cabin in the woods or mountains.	True	False
11. When things are bothering me, I like to talk to other people about it.	True	False
12. There are a few things more tiring than to have a long, personal discussion with someone.	True	False
13. If given the choice, I would much rather be with others than be alone.	True	False
14. I find that people too often assume that their daily activities and opinions will be interesting to me.	True	False
15. I attach very little importance to having close friends.	True	False

Based on Grant and Beck (2010). Original items from Eckblad, Chapman, Chapman, and Mishlove (1982). Reprinted with permission from the authors.

Games to Engage and Teach

These experiential learning games and activities help engage consumers by making learning more fun than a lecture, and they facilitate learning by transforming abstract constructs into concrete activities that illustrate important principles. They are particularly helpful for engaging consumers with negative symptoms and compensating for cognitive impairments. People are more likely to attend sessions if they are fun and engaging.

GOAL SETTING

Goal-Setting Collage

Purpose: To identify personal values and goals.

Materials: Plain paper or construction paper, magazines or newspapers, glue sticks.

Procedure: Consumers select pictures or words from magazines that represent personal values, things they would like to change in their lives, or things they would like to have in their lives. Cut or tear them out, and glue them onto paper. Consumers then take turns sharing their collages with the group. Providers look for themes and help the consumer identify possible recovery goals based on his or her collage. The long-term goal that can develop through this process may then be added to the consumer's 7–7–7 Goal Jackpot! Worksheet.

Thumbs-Up versus Thumbs-Down Game

Purpose: To identify aspects of life in which change is desired and translate this into recovery goals.

Materials: Pen and paper or whiteboard and markers.

Procedure: Start a discussion about aspects of life that people often want to change to improve their quality of life, including relationships, work, school, living situation, recreation activities, and so forth. Consumers "rate" how satisfied they are with each aspect of life by giving it a thumbs-up or thumbs-down (or ratings on a scale from 1 to 10). Engage each consumer in a discussion about why he or she is satisfied or not satisfied with each aspect and whether/how he or she would like to change it. Ask each consumer to rank all aspects that were given a thumbs-down rating (e.g., "Which area do you want to change the most?") and guide the formulation of a long-term recovery goal for that area.

Music/Video to Accompany Goal-Setting Activities

Purpose: To increase fun, promote engagement, emphasize themes, and facilitate recall of session content (compensate for memory problems).

Materials: Computer with audio tracks or Internet access (e.g., for YouTube videos).

Procedure: Choose a song or video related to session content and play it in session, for example:

- Listen to the "Wannabe" (Spice Girls) lyric, "Tell me what you want; what you really, really want," and emphasize how long-term goals should be something you really want.
- Listen to "Ain't No Mountain High Enough" (Marvin Gaye and Tammi Terrell) and emphasize that the only way to find out whether you can achieve your long-term goal is to try to achieve it by completing goal steps each week and find out if you succeed (e.g., "If you believe in yourself, you are more likely to succeed"). This song is applicable to all goals but works particularly well with the goal to find a partner (e.g., "Ain't no mountain high enough to keep me from you").
- View the video of the scene from the movie *Rocky,* in which Rocky climbs the steps while the inspirational movie theme music is playing, and emphasize how hard he trained each day to achieve his goal.
- Be creative and ask consumers to volunteer options for music or videos.

Variation: Use videos and music when teaching skills in other modules. For example, the scene from *Rocky* is also applicable to teaching SCALE (e.g., "Like Rocky, who trained hard by scaling the steps to achieve his goal of winning the fight, you can train to use the SCALE steps to achieve your goal").

COGNITIVE SKILLS MODULE

Ball Toss Game (one of our favorite games)

Purpose: To teach how failure expectations (defeatist thoughts) impact goal-directed actions and how behavioral experiments can be used to correct defeatist thoughts.

Materials: Two bowls, one large, the other small; some ping pong balls; and a napkin.

Procedure: Before the session, place the napkin in the bottom of the smaller bowl, so the balls are less likely to bounce out of that bowl (consumers are not aware of this before the game). Try out the game first to confirm that balls are more likely to stay in the small bowl. Place the empty bowls on a table. Say to consumers, "Toss balls into the bowls and try to get as many balls in either of the bowls as possible." Most people initially try to toss more balls into the larger bowl, because it appears easier than the smaller bowl. However, after tossing a few, people often try the smaller bowl, and experience teaches them that it is actually easier to get them to stay in the smaller bowl, so they toss more at the smaller bowl. After everyone who wants a turn is done, make this observation, then ask, "Why do you think people tossed the balls at the big bowl first and then switched to the little one?" Guide the discussion to point out that people tossed the balls at the larger bowl because they *thought* it would be *easier,* and avoided tossing at the smaller bowl because they *thought* it was more *difficult* and they would *fail.* That is, defeatist attitudes or failure expectations guided behavior. This is normal; nobody wants to fail. Point out the link (draw this on a whiteboard or piece of paper) between the failure expectations and goal choice. Also, guide the discussion to point out that people did an experiment to test out their failure expectations. Once they tossed at the smaller bowl and tried it out, the data (more balls stayed in the smaller bowl) indicated that failure expectations were incorrect, so they changed their behavior and tried things they initially thought were too difficult for them.

Variation: Start far away from the bowls, toss, then take a "baby step" closer; toss, then a step closer; toss, and so forth. Point out how long-term goals far away in time seem impossible, but taking easy baby steps toward long-term goals makes them easier to achieve. Use this game to demonstrate the importance of breaking goals down into attainable goal steps.

Funny Videos Activity

Purpose: To demonstrate how thoughts impact actions and feelings, and make sessions fun to promote engagement.

Materials: Computer or tablet and humorous videos on DVD or streamed on the Internet (e.g., *America's Funniest Home Videos* clips).

Procedure: Before watching a video, ask how enjoyable consumers expect it will be, and after watching the video, ask how enjoyable it was. Note any differences between expectations about how enjoyable an activity might be (pleasure predicting) and how enjoyable it actually was. Emphasize that people are less likely to try an activity if they don't think it will be fun, and note that people usually think things will be less fun than they actually are. This is why we should try things to find out how fun they might be.

Variations: This game can be used to promote engagement in the Introduction and Goal-Setting Session and all three modules (e.g., for humorous examples of poor communication skills in the Social Skills Module or funny failed solutions in the Problem-Solving Skills Module, such as Wile E. Coyote's solutions).

Jumping to Conclusions Game

Purpose: To illustrate the jumping to conclusions mistake in thinking and stimulate discussion about the hazards of making hasty decisions based on limited information.

Materials: Large paper grocery bag containing a set of colored pieces of paper (thick paper or card stock) cut into two different shapes with two different colors (e.g., 8 orange circles, 8 green circles, 8 orange squares, 8 green squares).

Procedure: Draw an orange circle and a green square from the bag, and explain, "The bag contains 32 pieces of paper in two different shapes and two different colors." Place the pieces back in the bag. Invite a volunteer to close his or her eyes, reach into the bag, "draw seven orange pieces," and hand them to the provider one at a time. People typically jump to the conclusion that all circles are orange and pull circles from the bag, some of which will be green. In a group format, show the items to the group, but ask group members to remain quiet while the items are drawn. When the seven pieces have been drawn, ask the consumer to open his or her eyes, show the consumer the pieces selected (which will likely be a mixture of all four pieces), then, in a humorous way, ask, "Where did all the green pieces come from?" Discuss observations about the exercise and mention that it is common for someone to jump to the conclusion that all squares are green after seeing the first green square displayed by the group leader. Ask consumers when they jump to conclusions in their own lives. Do they make quick and stereotyped conclusions about other people? Do others make the same mistakes about them? Emphasize the point that we are often misled into making quick decisions or conclusions based upon little information, such as a person's appearance.

Headbands Game

Purpose: To learn to identify mistakes in thinking.

Materials: Headband for each consumer, blank index cards.

Procedure: Write one mistake in thinking on each card and attach one card to each consumer's headband facing forward, without the consumer seeing what is written on the card. The consumer then asks "yes" or "no" questions of other consumers to try to get clues about which mistake is on their headband. It is helpful to put the definitions of each mistake on the whiteboard or a poster board in the front of the room.

Spinner Game

Purpose: To illustrate connections among thoughts, feelings, and behaviors, and how they influence each other.

Materials: A repurposed board game spinner or a piece of cardboard with a drawing of a dial, several feelings written on it, and a spinner.

Procedure: A provider takes the first turn to demonstrate the game, spinning the dial to select a feeling and saying aloud a thought that could lead to the feeling. Consumers take turns spinning the dial and generating thoughts that might lead to the feeling. The same type of game can be played with mistakes in thinking or behaviors in place of feelings. One can also draw a dial on a whiteboard and ask volunteers cover or close their eyes when selecting a feeling (on a pretend spinner) or roll dice to randomly select a number that corresponds to numbered feelings listed on the board, or reach in a hat or bowl to select feelings written on pieces of paper.

Catch a Thought Game

Purpose: To teach the Catch It step of the 3C's and learn how to identify moment-to-moment or automatic thoughts.

Materials: A very soft ball.

Procedure: The provider tosses the ball to a consumer and asks what the person is thinking right at the moment he or she catches the ball—Catch It. The provider asks, "What just went through your mind?" He or she tosses the ball just short of the consumer, to the side, or a little too hard or too short, then asks about the consumer's thoughts. Did a different type of toss (situation) result in a different thought? Emphasize how different thoughts (interpretations) about situations can lead to different feelings or behaviors.

Variation: Write an example of a thought on a piece of paper, crumble it up, and toss it to a consumer, who literally catches a thought. The consumer reads the example thought out loud. Include some silly or humorous examples as well. Consumers can also write thoughts on papers and toss them to each other. After catching the thought, consumers discuss the feelings or behaviors that might follow if a person has that thought.

Thoughts versus Feelings Flash Card Game

Purpose: To learn how to differentiate thoughts and feelings.

Materials: Numerous cards with examples of thoughts and feelings written on each one.

Procedure: Someone reads the thought or feeling on the card to the group. Everyone then votes on whether it is a thought or a feeling. Feeling cards can also be linked to the thoughts that might produce them.

Jenga Game (Thoughts)

Purpose: To learn the link between thoughts and feelings.

Materials: Jenga blocks or other stackable blocks on which one can write.

Procedure: Write an emotion or a thought on each block, and stack the blocks into a tower. Consumers take turns pulling out pieces one at a time and have to generate a thought that would lead to a feeling or a feeling that would stem from the thought. They continue until the tower topples.

Catch It Red-Flag Ball Game

Purpose: To learn the link between thoughts and feelings.

Materials: A medium-sized red ball (e.g., a standard playground kick ball) with all the feelings from the pleasant and unpleasant feelings list (Appendix C) written on it with a permanent marker (alternatively, write common thoughts from Appendix C on it instead).

Procedure: People toss the ball around, and when they "Catch It," they look at the feeling under their hand and have to generate a thought that might lead to the feeling (or feeling that might arise from the thought).

Thinking Error Dice

Purpose: To learn how to differentiate thoughts and feelings.

Materials: One or more small, square boxes with examples of mistakes in thinking written on each side (e.g., "I'll never be happy," "They shouldn't have done that").

Procedure: Consumers take turns rolling the dice. They then say the mistake in thinking that is represented by the example.

Change It Optical Illusion

Purpose: Develop understanding that there are multiple ways of seeing or perceiving things.

Materials: Collections of optical illusions can be found on several websites (e.g., *http://kids. niehs.nih.gov/games/illusions/index.htm*).

Procedure: Present the images and ask consumers to describe what they see. When more than one description is reported, use Socratic questioning to discuss what this tells us about perceptions, and how this might relate to other topics (e.g., things people say, ambiguous situations).

Mistaken Monologue

Purpose: To learn to identify unhelpful thoughts and behaviors, and to identify healthier responses.

Materials: YouTube sitcom dialogue (e.g., "Modern Family" can be good for both unhelpful beliefs and ineffective communication skills).

Procedure: Watch a brief clip. Ask consumers to identify:

- Mistakes in thinking
- Poor communication
- Poor listening
- Poor positive requests
- Backhanded compliments
- Aggressive behavior
- Passive communication
- Any healthy communication

Make the Triangle Game

Purpose: Review the cognitive model of thoughts–feelings–actions links.

Materials: Post-it notes or cards with tacks. On each card, list a common thought (from Appendix C), a pleasant or unpleasant feeling (from Appendix C) or an action (e.g., stay at home; go out, avoid people, go to school). Three big cardstock bidirectional arrows. Bulletin board or whiteboard on which to put them.

Procedure: Put the three arrows on the board in the shape of a triangle. Ask consumers to sort the cards into thoughts, feelings, and actions, then place them on the board at each corner of the triangle, by linking thoughts to feelings and behaviors.

SOCIAL SKILLS MODULE

Facial Emotion Drawing Game

Purpose: To learn how to create and recognize facial expressions associated with specific emotions.

Materials: Large whiteboard; plain paper (several sheets for each player).

Procedure: Explain that the game focuses on drawing different facial emotion expressions. Discuss how facial expressions and emotions are linked and how facial expressions help us communicate by signaling to each other how we feel. Ask consumers to draw a large oval shape on their papers, while you draw an oval on a piece of paper or the whiteboard to illustrate the scale and ask everyone to draw a nose in the middle. Then, using the List of Pleasant and Unpleasant Feelings (Appendix C), model an emotion (make the face) and ask everyone to start drawing the eyes, mouth, and eyebrow shapes that are the key facial features for that emotion (drawings can be cartoon-like). Tell members there will be cues (e.g., a clap or bell) at certain times when they will be asked to pass their drawing to the person on their right, so different parts of the faces will be drawn by different people. Each completed face is examined (which can be surprising and funny), and consumers try to express the emotion in the drawings. It can be helpful to bring in hand-held mirrors for people to see the emotion features in their own faces.

You + Me = Us Activity

Purpose: To identify commonalities among group members.

Materials: Paper and pens.

Procedure: Ask people to sit in pairs. Show the following Venn diagram below:

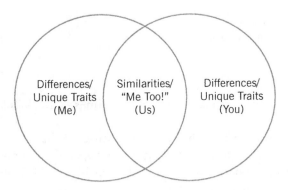

Ask one person in each pair to list things he or she likes that are important to him or her and discuss this list with the other partner in the dyad to discover their similarities and differences. Encourage partners to develop their own Venn diagrams to share with the larger group.

One-Minute Interview Activity

Purpose: To develop listening and communication skills.

Materials: None.

Procedure: Everyone is instructed to find a partner whom he or she does not know very well. One is the speaker and the other is the listener. The listener gets 1 minute to find out all he or she can about the speaker. After the minute, the listener shares with the group all the information he or she discovered. Listener and speaker then switch roles.

Emotional Charades

Purpose: To practice emotional speech prosody and facial affect expression.

Materials: Index cards with one of the six basic emotions (happy, sad, afraid, angry, surprised, and disgusted) on top and a neutral descriptive sentence on the bottom (e.g., "We are going shopping," "You bought a new car today?").

Procedure: A player secretly picks a card with one of the six basic emotions and a sentence. The player then reads the sentence, displaying the emotion indicated. The group discusses and guesses which emotion the player displayed, and why. The group provides positive and corrective feedback to the player about how he or she sounded. The provider lists the six emotions on the whiteboard to help the group guess the emotion.

Variation 1: Players try reading the same sentence, displaying each of the six emotions (e.g., "You bought a new car today?").

Variation 2: Instead of reading a sentence with emotional prosody, the player makes a face to express the emotion, while the group guesses the emotion.

Send a Message Game

Purpose: To teach active listening skills.

Materials: None.

Procedure: Ask the group members to form a circle. The group leader then whispers a message into the ear of the person to his or her left. The message should be whispered only once. That person then passes what he or she heard along to the person to the left, and so on, until the phrase comes around to the person on the group leader's right. The message that made it around the circle is repeated out loud. The group members see how the message has changed. They try again.

A What? Game

Purpose: To teach active listening skills, problem solving, and cooperation.

Materials: Several objects to pass around (pencil, ball, stuffed animal, toy, etc.).

Procedure: This game demonstrates that even simple messages can get confused and muddled during a conversation, especially when there are distractions. Group members are seated in a close circle. An object such as a pencil is passed around the circle. The provider starts by showing it to the first consumer while saying, "This is a banana," or any other object the provider chooses to say, as long as it is not "a pencil." The consumer asks, "A what?" "A banana," says the provider. The first consumer takes the pencil (or other object), turns to the second consumer, and shows him or her the pencil, repeating, "This is a banana." When the second consumer replies, "A what?" the first consumer turns back to the provider and asks again, "A what?" The provider once more informs the first consumer that it is "a banana," which the first consumer repeats to the second and passes the pencil. The second consumer shows the pencil to the third person; the same "This is a banana" statement, with the "A what?" response is repeated and travels back to the provider, who gives the "a banana" response, which, along with the pencil, travels back to the last person to hold the pencil. The banana proceeds around the circle in this back-and-forth fashion. After a few consumers receive the first object, the provider sends another object, such as a ball, in the opposite direction in the same way, announcing, "This is an apple." The challenge and fun begins when the two objects meet and cross as they move around the circle and everyone tries to keep track of which item is which. For a real challenge, try it with more than two objects.

Jenga Game (Conversation Starter)

Purpose: Practice initiating a conversation.

Materials: Jenga or other stacking blocks with conversation starters written on them (e.g., "Hi, I'm [insert name]"; "I like that jacket. Where did you get it?"; "Do you mind if I sit here?").

Procedure: Stack the blocks into a tower and consumers take turns pulling pieces out of the tower until it topples. Each consumer uses the line on the block they pulled out to start a conversation with someone in the group. The two consumers try to keep the conversation going for 30 seconds.

PROBLEM-SOLVING MODULE

How Can I Use This?

Purpose: To teach brainstorming skills and group cooperation.

Materials: Paper and pens or whiteboard and markers.

Procedure: Divide the group in half and ask the two teams to list as many possible uses as they can think of for specific object (e.g., a paper clip, a wood block, an umbrella, a loaf of bread). Allow 5 minutes to generate uses for the object. Describe the rules for brainstorming:

- Share any ideas that come to mind.
- Don't filter or censor any ideas that come to mind.
- Be creative, spontaneous, and even silly.
- Don't evaluate the ideas. That is, don't judge, critique, or discuss the ideas.
- Use ideas that other group members have offered to build on and generate additional ideas.
- Generate as many ideas as possible during the allotted time period.

After the teams share their lists, stimulate discussion about how we often have more options available to solve problems than we first realize, and how much more effectively we find solutions when we don't evaluate ideas or dismiss the first idea that comes to mind because we think it won't work.

Buzz the Evaluator

Purpose: To practice generating solutions without evaluating them.

Materials: A loud buzzer or loud voice to make a buzzer sound.

Procedure: When brainstorming solutions, assign someone to listen for people evaluating potential solutions (e.g., "I tried that and it didn't work" or "That is too expensive"), and playfully sound a buzzer (like what happens when someone gets the wrong answer in a game show) to remind people not to assess the best solution until the next step. Just generate, don't evaluate.

Video/Music for Fun Problem Solving

See variations of the Music/Video to Accompany Goal-Setting Activities and Funny Videos Activity above.

LAST SESSION OF ANY MODULE

Jeopardy Review Game

Purpose: To review CBSST skills knowledge.

Materials: On a whiteboard/chalkboard, make column headings of module skills topics (e.g., mistakes in thinking, steps of SCALE, nonverbal communication skills, making positive requests) and write 100, 200, and 300 in columns under each topic. Generate and write items and answers on cards for each point value in the columns (e.g., for mistakes in thinking, use thoughts as items: item—"Nobody likes me"; answer—"What is all-or-nothing thinking?"; for SCALE Steps: item—"Generate but don't evaluate ways to solve it"; answer—"What is Consider?"; for nonverbal communication skills, item—"Moving your hands"; answer—"What are gestures?").

Procedure: Providers have cards with items and answers corresponding to all items in the columns on the board and call on consumers or teams of consumers to select an item (e.g., "SCALE for 200 points"). Providers erase each selected item on the board and read the item for consumers to answer in the form of a question. Give hints as needed and keep a tally of points.

APPENDIX C

Additional Handouts and Materials

COMMON THOUGHTS CHECKLIST

In the list below there are many common automatic thoughts about different situations. Please put a ✓ by the thoughts you have experienced in each situation. You may add others in the extra space provided at the end of the checklist.

Situation: Learning a new skill	
What thoughts do you have?	
☐ What do you expect?—I have too many problems.	☐ I can still learn some new things, despite my problems.
☐ It doesn't matter what I do; it's not going to change the fact that I'm just not good enough.	☐ OK, so I'm not perfect, but everyone has imperfections.
☐ Why bother?—I'm going fail.	☐ I might do really well.
☐ It's more trouble than it's worth.	☐ Yes, it's hard, but it could be worth it.
☐ It takes too much effort to try.	☐ Most things take some effort.
☐ It's too hard.	☐ It's tough, but I'm tougher.

Situation: Introducing yourself to others	
What thoughts do you have?	
☐ I'm not going to be good enough.	☐ I'll do my best.
☐ I'm not going to sound right, I'll have nothing to say.	☐ I'll try even though I feel scared.
☐ I can't do it.	☐ I can do some of it.
☐ Interacting with other people will lead to unhappiness.	☐ It might be fun to mingle with others.
☐ It's best not to get involved.	☐ I could learn more about others.

Situation: Taking a class in school	
What thoughts do you have?	
☐ If I fail, I am a failure as a person.	☐ It might be hard, but at least I can try.
☐ If I cannot do something well, there is little point to doing it at all.	☐ I know I'm not good at this sort of thing, but I can still try to learn something.
☐ If I fail partly, it is as bad as being a complete failure.	☐ No one knows all the answers.
☐ If a person asks for help, it is a sign of weakness.	☐ I can learn more about things I don't know if I ask for help.
☐ If I do not do as well as other people, it means I am an inferior human being.	☐ Everyone has strengths and weaknesses.
☐ Taking even a small risk is foolish, because the loss is likely to be a disaster.	☐ Sometimes, I may need to take a risk to experience new things.
☐ People will probably think less of me if I make a mistake.	☐ Everyone makes mistakes.
☐ Asking questions makes you look foolish.	☐ Asking questions is a good way for me to learn.
☐ I should be upset if I make a mistake.	☐ I could learn from making mistakes.

(continued)

Some items from Weissman and Beck (1978). Reprinted with permission from the authors.

Situation: Going to the grocery store
What thoughts do you have?

☐ It's too much work.	☐ I can handle it.
☐ It's not worth the effort.	☐ I'll give it my best shot.
☐ Why bother?—it's just a hassle.	☐ It might be fun.
☐ If I can't find something, I'll look like a fool.	☐ Asking for help is a good way to find things.
☐ I'll mess up and be embarrassed.	☐ Nobody does it perfectly every time.

Situation: Expressing your feelings to someone who has upset you
What thoughts do you have?

☐ If I show my feelings, others will see my inadequacy.	☐ It sometimes feels good to express my feelings.
☐ I'm not going to find the right words to express myself.	☐ I'll do my best to express myself.
☐ I take so long to get my point across that it's boring.	☐ Others may be interested in what I have to say.
☐ My face will appear stiff and contorted to others.	☐ I'll try to relax when I talk with others.
☐ I'm going to sound weird, stupid, strange.	☐ I'm going to be able to express some of my thoughts.
☐ I don't have the ability to express my feelings.	☐ I can talk with some people about how I feel.
☐ It takes too much effort to talk.	☐ Talking with others can be hard, but I'm willing to give it my best shot.

Situation: Going to a party
What thoughts do you have?

☐ What's the point?	☐ It could be fun.
☐ Why should I bother?	☐ It might be worth it.
☐ It's too much work.	☐ It's not that hard.
☐ I won't enjoy it around all those people.	☐ I may make new friends and have fun.
☐ I'll mess up and be embarrassed.	☐ Nobody's perfect, I'll keep trying.

SOME PLEASANT FEELINGS

Happy	Respected	Productive	Worthy
Loved	Caring	Understood	Optimistic
Liked	Empowered	Relieved	Rested
Calm	Satisfied	Needed	Joyful
Useful	Content	Hopeful	Excited
Proud	Relaxed	Encouraged	Helpful

SOME UNPLEASANT FEELINGS

Sad	Rejected	Bored	Anxious
Afraid	Frustrated	Guilty	Lonely
Tired	Disappointed	Angry	Defeated
Hurt	Worried	Betrayed	Overwhelmed
Stressed	Nervous	Annoyed	Embarrassed
Doubtful	Helpless	Hopeless	Irritated

References

Aarons, G. A. (2004). Mental health provider attitudes toward adoption of evidence-based practice: The Evidence-Based Practice Attitude Scale (EBPAS). *Mental Health Services Research, 6,* 61–74.

Aarons, G. A., Fettes, D. L., Flores, L. E., Jr., & Sommerfeld, D. H. (2009). Evidence-based practice implementation and staff emotional exhaustion in children's services. *Behaviour Research and Therapy, 47,* 954–960.

Addington, J., Marshall, C., & French, P. (2012). Cognitive behavioral therapy in prodromal psychosis. *Current Pharmaceutical Design, 18,* 558–565.

Andreasen, N. C. (1982). Negative symptoms in schizophrenia: Definition and reliability. *Archives of General Psychiatry, 39,* 784–788.

Andreasen, N. C., Carpenter, W. T., Jr., Kane, J. M., Lasser, R. A., Marder, S. R., & Weinberger, D. R. (2005). Remission in schizophrenia: Proposed criteria and rationale for consensus. *American Journal of Psychiatry, 162,* 441–449.

Arns, P., Rogers, E. S., Cook, J., & Mowbray, C. (2001). The IAPSRS toolkit: Development, utility, and relation to other performance measurement systems (Members of the IAPSRS Research Committee, International Association of Psychological Rehabilitation Services). *Psychiatric Rehabilitation Journal, 25,* 43–52.

Avery, R., Startup, M., & Calabria, K. (2009). The role of effort, cognitive expectancy appraisals and coping style in the maintenance of the negative symptoms of schizophrenia. *Psychiatry Research, 167,* 36–46.

Bandura, A. (1969). Social-learning theory of identificatory processes. In D. A. Goslin (Ed.), *Handbook of socialization theory and research* (pp. 213–262). Chicago: Rand McNally.

Bandura, A. (1986). *Social foundations of thought and action: A social cognitive theory.* Englewood Cliffs, NJ: Prentice-Hall.

Bandura, A. (1997). *Self-efficacy: The exercise of control.* New York: Freeman.

Beck, A. T., Baruch, E., Balter, J. M., Steer, R. A., & Warman, D. M. (2004). A new instrument for measuring insight: The Beck Cognitive Insight Scale. *Schizophrenia Research, 68,* 319–329.

Beck, A. T., & Rector, N. A. (2000). Cognitive therapy of schizophrenia: A new therapy for the new millennium. *American Journal of Psychotherapy, 54,* 291–300.

Beck, A. T., Rector, N. A., Stolar, N. M., & Grant, P. M. (2009). *Schizophrenia: Cognitive theory, research, and therapy.* New York: Guilford Press.

Beck, A. T., & Steer, R. A. (1990). *Manual for the Beck Anxiety Inventory.* San Antonio, TX: Psychological Corporation.

Beck, A. T., Steer, R. A., & Brown, G. K. (1996). *Beck Depression Inventory—Second Edition Manual*. San Antonio, TX: Psychological Corporation.

Bellack, A. S. (2002). Skills training for people with severe mental illness. *Psychiatric Rehabilitation, 7,* 375–391.

Bellack, A. S., & Mueser, K. T. (1993). Psychosocial treatment for schizophrenia. *Schizophrenia Bulletin, 19,* 317–336.

Bellack, A. S., Mueser, K. T., Gingerich, S., & Agresta, J. (2004). *Social skills training for schizophrenia: A step-by-step guide* (2nd ed.). New York: Guilford Press.

Bellack, A. S., Mueser, K. T., Morrison, R. L., Tierney, A., & Podell, K. (1990). Remediation of cognitive deficits in schizophrenia. *American Journal of Psychiatry, 147,* 1650–1655.

Bellack, A. S., Sayers, M., Mueser, K. T., & Bennett, M. (1994). Evaluation of social problem solving in schizophrenia. *Journal of Abnormal Psychology, 103,* 371–378.

Benton, M. K., & Schroeder, H. E. (1990). Social skills training with schizophrenics: A meta-analytic evaluation. *Journal of Consulting and Clinical Psychology, 58,* 741–747.

Bilker, W. B., Brensinger, C., Kurtz, M. M., Kohler, C., Gur, R. C., Siegel, S. J., et al. (2003). Development of an abbreviated schizophrenia quality of life scale using a new method. *Neuropsychopharmacology, 28,* 773–777.

Birchwood, M., Smith, J., Cochrane, R., Wetton, S., & Copestake, S. (1990). The Social Functioning Scale: The development and validation of a new scale of social adjustment for use in family intervention programmes with schizophrenic patients. *British Journal of Psychiatry, 157,* 853–859.

Birchwood, M., Smith, J., Drury, V., Healy, J., Macmillan, F., & Slade, M. (1994). A self-report Insight Scale for psychosis: Reliability, validity and sensitivity to change. *Acta Psychiatrica Scandinavica, 89,* 62–67.

Birchwood, M., Todd, P., & Jackson, C. (1998). Early intervention in psychosis: The critical period hypothesis. *British Journal of Psychiatry, 172*(Suppl. 33), 53–59.

Bleuler, M. (1968). A 23-year long longitudinal study of 208 schizophrenics and impressions in regard to the nature of schizophrenia. *Journal of Psychiatric Research, 6,* 3–12.

Bowie, C. R., Reichenberg, A., Patterson, T. L., Heaton, R. K., & Harvey, P. D. (2006). Determinants of real-world functional performance in schizophrenia subjects: Correlations with cognition, functional capacity, and symptoms. *American Journal of Psychiatry, 163,* 418–425.

Brabban, A., Tai, S., & Turkington, D. (2009). Predictors of outcome in brief cognitive behavior therapy for schizophrenia. *Schizophrenia Bulletin, 35,* 859–864.

Bradshaw, W. H. (1993). Coping-skills training versus a problem-solving approach with schizophrenic patients. *Hospital and Community Psychiatry, 44,* 1102–1104.

Burns, A. M., Erickson, D. H., & Brenner, C. A. (2014). Cognitive-behavioral therapy for medication-resistant psychosis: A meta-analytic review. *Psychiatric Services, 65,* 874–880.

Cane, D. B., Olinger, L. J., Gotlib, I. H., & Kuiper, N. A. (2006). Factor structure of the dysfunctional attitude scale in a student population. *Journal of Clinical Psychology, 42,* 307–309.

Carrion, R. E., McLaughlin, D., Goldberg, T. E., Auther, A. M., Olsen, R. H., Olvet, D. M., et al. (2013). Prediction of functional outcome in individuals at clinical high risk for psychosis. *JAMA Psychiatry, 70,* 1133–1142.

Ciompi, L. (1980). Catamnestic long-term study on the course of life and aging of schizophrenics. *Schizophrenia Bulletin, 6,* 606–618.

Couture, S. M., Blanchard, J. J., & Bennett, M. E. (2011). Negative expectancy appraisals and defeatist performance beliefs and negative symptoms of schizophrenia. *Psychiatry Research, 189,* 43–48.

Dilk, M. N., & Bond, G. R. (1996). Meta-analytic evaluation of skills training research for individuals with severe mental illness. *Journal of Consulting and Clinical Psychology, 64,* 1337–1346.

Dixon, L. B., Dickerson, F., Bellack, A. S., Bennett, M., Dickinson, D., Goldberg, R. W., et al. (2010). The 2009 schizophrenia PORT psychosocial treatment recommendations and summary statements. *Schizophrenia Bulletin, 36,* 48–70.

Drake, R. E., Bond, G. R., & Essock, S. M. (2009). Implementing evidence-based practices for people with schizophrenia. *Schizophrenia Bulletin, 35,* 704–713.

Drury, V., Birchwood, M., Cochrane, R., & Macmillan, F. (1996). Cognitive therapy and recovery from acute psychosis: A controlled trial: II. Impact on recovery time. *British Journal of Psychiatry, 169,* 602–607.

D'Zurilla, T. J., & Nezu, A. M. (2010). Problem-solving therapy. In K. S. Dobson (Ed.), *Handbook of cognitive-behavioral therapies* (3rd ed., pp. 197–225). New York: Guilford Press.

Eckblad, M. L., Chapman, L. J., Chapman, J. P., & Mishlove, M. (1982). *The Revised Social Anhedonia Scale.* Unpublished test (copies available from T. R. Kwapil, Department of Psychology, UNCG, P.O. Box 26170, Greensboro, NC 27402-6170).

Edwards, J., Maude, D., McGorry, P. D., Harrigan, S. M., & Cocks, J. T. (1998). Prolonged recovery in first-episode psychosis. *British Journal of Psychiatry, 172*(Suppl. 33), 107–116.

Ekman, P. (1999). Basic emotions. In T. Dalgleish & M. Powers (Eds.), *Handbook of cognition and emotion* (pp. 45–60). Sussex, UK: Wiley.

Faerden, A., Nesvåg, R., & Marder, S. R. (2008). Definitions of the term "recovered" in schizophrenia and other disorders. *Psychopathology, 41,* 271–278.

Forbes, C., Blanchard, J. J., Bennett, M., Horan, W. P., Kring, A., & Gur, R. (2010). Initial development and preliminary validation of a new negative symptom measure: The Clinical Assessment Interview for Negative Symptoms (CAINS). *Schizophrenia Research, 124,* 36–42.

Fowler, D., Hodgekins, J., Painter, M., Reilly, T., Crane, C., Macmillan, I., et al. (2009). Cognitive behaviour therapy for improving social recovery in psychosis: A report from the ISREP MRC Trial Platform Study (Improving Social Recovery in Early Psychosis). *Psychological Medicine, 39,* 1627–1636.

Frese, F. J., III, Knight, E. L., & Saks, E. (2009). Recovery from schizophrenia: With views of psychiatrists, psychologists, and others diagnosed with this disorder. *Schizophrenia Bulletin, 35,* 370–380.

Friedman, J. I., Harvey, P. D., Coleman, T., Moriarty, P. J., Bowie, C., Parrella, M., et al. (2001). Six-year follow-up study of cognitive and functional status across the lifespan in schizophrenia: A comparison with Alzheimer's disease and normal aging. *American Journal of Psychiatry, 158,* 1441–1448.

Gaebel, W., Weinmann, S., Sartorius, N., Rutz, W., & McIntyre, J. S. (2005). Schizophrenia practice guidelines: International survey and comparison. *British Journal of Psychiatry, 187,* 248–255.

Garety, P., Fowler, D., Kuipers, E., Freeman, D., Dunn, G., Bebbington, P., et al. (1997). London–East Anglia randomised controlled trial of cognitive-behavioural therapy for psychosis: II. Predictors of outcome. *British Journal of Psychiatry, 171,* 420–426.

Gingerich, S., & Mueser, K. T. (Eds.). (2011). *Illness management and recovery: Personalized skills and strategies for those with mental Illness* (3rd ed.). Center City, MN: Hazelden.

Glynn, S. M., Marder, S. R., Liberman, R. P., Blair, K., Wirshing, W. C., Wirshing, D. A., et al. (2002). Supplementing clinic-based skills training with manual-based community support sessions: Effects on social adjustment of patients with schizophrenia. *American Journal of Psychiatry, 159,* 829–837.

Gould, R. A., Mueser, K. T., Bolton, E., Mays, V., & Goff, D. (2001). Cognitive therapy for psychosis in schizophrenia: An effect size analysis. *Schizophrenia Research, 48,* 335–342.

Granholm, E., Ben-Zeev, D., Fulford, D., & Swendsen, J. (2013). Ecological momentary assessment of social functioning in schizophrenia: Impact of performance appraisals and affect on social interactions. *Schizophrenia Research, 145,* 120–124.

Granholm, E., Ben-Zeev, D., & Link, P. C. (2009). Social disinterest attitudes and group cognitive-behavioral social skills training for functional disability in schizophrenia. *Schizophrenia Bulletin, 35,* 874–883.

Granholm, E., Holden, J., Link, P. C., & McQuaid, J. R. (2014). Randomized clinical trial of cognitive behavioral social skills training for schizophrenia: Improvement in functioning and experiential negative symptoms. *Journal of Consulting and Clinical Psychology, 82*(6), 1173–1185.

Granholm, E., Holden, J., Link, P. C., McQuaid, J. R., & Jeste, D. V. (2013). Randomized controlled trial of cognitive behavioral social skills training for older consumers with schizophrenia: Defeatist performance attitudes and functional outcome. *American Journal of Geriatric Psychiatry, 21,* 251–262.

Granholm, E., Loh, C., Link, P. C., & Jeste, D. V. (2010). Feasibility of implementing cognitive behavioral therapy for psychosis on assertive community treatment teams: A controlled pilot study. *International Journal of Cognitive Therapy, 3,* 294–302.

Granholm, E., McQuaid, J. R., Link, P. C., Fish, S., Patterson, T., & Jeste, D. V. (2008). Neuropsychological predictors of functional outcome in Cognitive Behavioral Social Skills Training for older people with schizophrenia. *Schizophrenia Research, 100,* 133–143.

Granholm, E., McQuaid, J. R., McClure, F. S., Auslander, L. A., Perivoliotis, D., Pedrelli, P., et al. (2005). A randomized, controlled trial of cognitive behavioral social skills training for middle-aged and older outpatients with chronic schizophrenia. *American Journal of Psychiatry, 162,* 520–529.

Granholm, E., McQuaid, J. R., McClure, F. S., Link, P. C., Perivoliotis, D., Gottlieb, J. D., et al. (2007). Randomized controlled trial of cognitive behavioral social skills training for older people with schizophrenia: 12-month follow-up. *Journal of Clinical Psychiatry, 68,* 730–737.

Granholm, E., McQuaid, J. R., McClure, F. S., Pedrelli, P., & Jeste, D. V. (2002). A randomized controlled pilot study of cognitive behavioral social skills training for older patients with schizophrenia. *Schizophrenia Research, 53,* 167–169.

Grant, C., Addington, J., Addington, D., & Konnert, C. (2001). Social functioning in first- and multiepisode schizophrenia. *Canadian Journal of Psychiatry, 46,* 746–749.

Grant, P. M., & Beck, A. T. (2009). Defeatist beliefs as a mediator of cognitive impairment, negative symptoms, and functioning in schizophrenia. *Schizophrenia Bulletin, 35,* 798–806.

Grant, P. M., & Beck, A. T. (2010). Asocial beliefs as predictors of asocial behavior in schizophrenia. *Psychiatry Research, 177,* 65–70.

Green, M. F. (1996). What are the functional consequences of neurocognitive deficits in schizophrenia? *American Journal of Psychiatry, 153,* 321–330.

Green, M. F., Hellemann, G., Horan, W. P., Lee, J., & Wynn, J. K. (2012). From perception to functional outcome in schizophrenia: Modeling the role of ability and motivation. *Archives of General Psychiatry, 69,* 1216–1224.

Green, M. F., Kern, R. S., Braff, D. L., & Mintz, J. (2000). Neurocognitive deficits and functional outcome in schizophrenia: Are we measuring the "right stuff"? *Schizophrenia Bulletin, 26,* 119–136.

Green, M. F., Kern, R. S., & Heaton, R. K. (2004). Longitudinal studies of cognition and functional outcome in schizophrenia: Implications for MATRICS. *Schizophrenia Research, 72,* 41–51.

Green, M. F., Penn, D. L., Bentall, R., Carpenter, W. T., Gaebel, W., Gur, R. C., et al. (2008). Social cognition in schizophrenia: An NIMH workshop on definitions, assessment, and research opportunities. *Schizophrenia Bulletin, 34,* 1211–1220.

Greenwood, K. E., Sweeney, A., Williams, S., Garety, P., Kuipers, E., Scott, J., et al. (2010). CHoice of Outcome In Cbt for psychosEs (CHOICE): The development of a new service user-led outcome measure of CBT for psychosis. *Schizophrenia Bulletin, 36,* 126–135.

Guo, X., Zhai, J., Liu, Z., Fang, M., Wang, B., Wang, C., et al. (2010). Effect of antipsychotic medication alone vs combined with psychosocial intervention on outcomes of early-stage schizophrenia: A randomized, 1-year study. *Archives of General Psychiatry, 67,* 895–904.

Haddock, G., Devane, S., Bradshaw, T., McGovern, J., Tarrier, N., Kinderman, P., et al. (2001). An investigation into the psychometric properties of the Cognitive Therapy Scale for Psychosis (Cts-Psy). *Behavioural and Cognitive Psychotherapy, 29,* 221–233.

Haddock, G., McCarron, J., Tarrier, N., & Faragher, E. B. (1999). Scales to measure dimensions of hallucinations and delusions: The Psychotic Symptom Rating Scales (PSYRATS). *Psychological Medicine, 29,* 879–889.

Harding, C. M. (1988). Course types in schizophrenia: An analysis of European and American studies. *Schizophrenia Bulletin, 14,* 633–643.

Harding, C. M., Brooks, G. W., Ashikaga, T., Strauss, J., & Breier, A. (1987). The Vermont longitudinal study of persons with severe mental illness: II. Long-term outcome of subjects who retrospectively met DSM-III criteria for schizophrenia. *Journal of Psychiatry, 144,* 727–735.

Harris, R. (2009). *ACT made simple: An easy-to-read primer on acceptance and commitment therapy.* New York: New Harbinger.

Harrison, G., Gunnell, D., Glazebrook, C., Page, K., & Kwiecinski, R. (2001). Association between schizophrenia and social inequality at birth: Case–control study. *British Journal of Psychiatry,* *179,* 346–350.

Harrison, G., Hopper K., Craig, T., Laska, E., Siegel, C., Wanderling, J., et al. (2001). Recovery from psychotic illness: A 15- and 25-year international follow-up study. British *Journal of Psychiatry,* *178,* 501–517.

Harrow, M., Grossman, L. S., Jobe, T. H., & Herbener, E. S. (2005). Do patients with schizophrenia ever show periods of recovery? A 15-year multi-follow-up study. *Schizophrenia Bulletin, 2005,* 723–734.

Harvey, P. D., & Bellack, A. S. (2009). Toward a terminology for functional recovery in schizophrenia: Is functional remission a viable concept? *Schizophrenia Bulletin, 35,* 300–306.

Harvey, P. D., Heaton, R. K., Carpenter, W. T., Jr., Green, M. F., Gold, J. M., & Schoenbaum, M. (2012). Functional impairment in people with schizophrenia: Focus on employability and eligibility for disability compensation. *Schizophrenia Research, 140,* 1–8.

Harvey, P. D., Raykov, T., Twamley, E. W., Vella, L., Heaton, R. K., & Patterson, T. L. (2011). Validating the measurement of real-world functional outcomes: Phase I results of the VALERO study. *American Journal of Psychiatry, 168,* 1195–1201.

Harvey, P. D., & Strassnig, M. (2012). Predicting the severity of everyday functional disability in people with schizophrenia: Cognitive deficits, functional capacity, symptoms, and health status. *World Psychiatry, 11,* 73–79.

Hegarty, J. D., Baldessarini, R. J., Tohen, M., Waternaux, C., & Oepen, G. (1994). One hundred years of schizophrenia: A meta-analysis of the outcome literature. *American Journal of Psychiatry, 151,* 1409–1416.

Heinrichs, D. W., Hanlon, T. E., & Carpenter, W. T., Jr. (1984). The Quality of Life Scale: An instrument for rating the schizophrenic deficit syndrome. *Schizophrenia Bulletin, 10,* 388–398.

Heinssen, R. K., Liberman, R. P., & Kopelowicz, A. (2000). Psychosocial skills training for schizophrenia: Lessons from the laboratory. *Schizophrenia Bulletin, 26,* 21–46.

Horan, W. P., Rassovsky, Y., Kern, R. S., Lee, J., Wynn, J. K., & Green, M. F. (2010). Further support for the role of dysfunctional attitudes in models of real-world functioning in schizophrenia. *Journal of Psychiatric Research, 44,* 499–505.

Huber, G., Gross, G., & Schuttler, R. (1975). A long-term follow-up study of schizophrenia: Psychiatric course of illness and prognosis. *Acta Psychiatrica Scandinavica, 52,* 49–57.

Hutton, P., & Taylor, P. J. (2014). Cognitive behavioural therapy for psychosis prevention: A systematic review and meta-analysis. *Psychological Medicine, 44,* 449–468.

Jääskeläinen, E., Juola, P., Hirvonen, N., McGrath, J. J., Saha, S., Isohanni, M., et al. (2013). A systematic review and meta-analysis of recovery in schizophrenia. *Schizophrenia Bulletin, 39,* 1296–1306.

Jauhar, S., McKenna, P. J., Radua, J., Fung, E., Salvador, R., & Laws, K. R. (2014). Cognitive-behavioural therapy for the symptoms of schizophrenia: Systematic review and meta-analysis with examination of potential bias. *British Journal of Psychiatry, 204,* 20–29.

Jones, C., Hacker, D., Cormac, I., Meaden, A., & Irving, C. B. (2012). Cognitive behavior therapy versus other psychosocial treatments for schizophrenia. *Schizophrenia Bulletin, 38,* 908–910.

Kahn, R. S., Fleischhacker, W. W., Boter, H., Davidson, M., Vergouwe, Y., Keet, I. P., et al. (2008). Effectiveness of antipsychotic drugs in first-episode schizophrenia and schizophreniform disorder: An open randomised clinical trial. *Lancet, 371,* 1085–1097.

Kay, S. R., Fiszbein, A., & Opler, L. A. (1987). The positive and negative syndrome scale (PANSS) for schizophrenia. *Schizophrenia Bulletin, 13,* 261–276.

Kelly, J. A., & Lamparski, D. M. (1985). Outpatient treatment of schizophrenics: Social skills and problem-solving training. In M. Hersen & A. S. Bellack (Eds.), *Handbook of clinical behavior therapy with adults* (pp. 485–506). New York: Plenum Press.

Kern, R. S., Green, M. F., & Satz, P. (1992). Neuropsychological predictors of skills training for chronic psychiatric patients. *Psychiatry Research, 43,* 223–230.

Kirkpatrick, B., Fenton, W. S., Carpenter, W. T., Jr., & Marder, S. R. (2006). The NIMH-MATRICS consensus statement on negative symptoms. *Schizophrenia Bulletin, 32,* 214–219.

Kopelowicz, A., Liberman, R. P., & Zarate, R. (2006). Recent advances in social skills training for schizophrenia. *Schizophrenia Bulletin, 32*(Suppl. 1), S12–S23.

Kopelowicz, A., Zarate, R., Gonzalez Smith, V., Mintz, J., & Liberman, R. P. (2003). Disease management in Latinos with schizophrenia: A family-assisted, skills training approach. *Schizophrenia Bulletin, 29*, 211–227.

Kurtz, M. M. (2011). Neurocognition as a predictor of response to evidence-based psychosocial interventions in schizophrenia: What is the state of the evidence? *Clinical Psychology Review, 31*, 663–672.

Kurtz, M. M., Moberg, P. J., Ragland, J. D., Gur, R. C., & Gur, R. E. (2005). Symptoms versus neurocognitive test performance as predictors of psychosocial status in schizophrenia: A 1- and 4-year prospective study. *Schizophrenia Bulletin, 31*, 167–174.

Kurtz, M. M., & Mueser, K. T. (2008). A meta-analysis of controlled research on social skills training for schizophrenia. *Journal of Consulting and Clinical Psychology, 76*, 491–504.

Laozi. (1963). *The way of Lao Tzu* (W.-t. Chan, Trans.). Indianapolis, IN: Bobbs-Merrill.

Leucht, S., & Lasser, R. (2006). The concepts of remission and recovery in schizophrenia. *Pharmacopsychiatry, 39*, 161–170.

Liberman, R. P. (1991). *Psychiatric Rehabilitation Consultants: Modules in the UCLA social and independent living skill series.* Camarillo, CA: Psychiatric Rehabilitation Consultants.

Liberman, R. P. (1994). Psychosocial treatments for schizophrenia. *Psychiatry—Interpersonal and Biological Processes, 57*, 104–114.

Liberman, R. P. (2008). *Recovery from disability: Manual of psychiatric rehabilitation.* Arlington, VA: American Psychiatric Publishing.

Liberman, R. P., Glynn, S., Blair, K. E., Ross, D., & Marder, S. R. (2002). In vivo amplified skills training: Promoting generalization of independent living skills for clients with schizophrenia. *Psychiatry, 65*, 137–155.

Liberman, R. P., & Kopelowicz, A. (2005). Sustained remission of schizophrenia. *American Journal of Psychiatry, 162*, 1763–1764.

Lieberman, J., Jody, D., Geisler, S., Alvir, J., Loebel, A., Szymanski, S., et al. (1993). Time course and biological correlates of treatment response in first-episode schizophrenia. *Archives of General Psychiatry, 50*, 369–376.

Lincoln, T. M., Ziegler, M., Mehl, S., Kesting, M.-L., Lüllmann, E., Westermann, S., et al. (2012). Moving from efficacy to effectiveness in cognitive behavioral therapy for psychosis: A randomized clinical practice trial. *Journal of Consulting and Clinical Psychology, 80*, 674–686.

Lipsey, M. W., & Wilson, D. B. (1993). The efficacy of psychological, educational, and behavioral treatment: Confirmation from meta-analysis. *American Psychologist, 48*, 1181–1209.

Loebel, A. D., Lieberman, J. A., Alvir, J. M., Mayerhoff, D. I., Geisler, S. H., & Szymanski, S. R. (1992). Duration of psychosis and outcome in first-episode schizophrenia. *American Journal of Psychiatry, 149*, 1183–1188.

Lukoff, D., Nuechterlein, K. H., & Ventura, J. (1986). Manual for the expanded Brief Psychiatric Rating Scale. *Schizophrenia Bulletin, 12*, 594–602.

Lynch, D., Laws, K. R., & McKenna, P. J. (2010). Cognitive behavioural therapy for major psychiatric disorder: Does it really work? A meta-analytical review of well-controlled trials. *Psychological Medicine, 40*, 9–24.

Marshall, M., & Rathbone, J. (2011). Early intervention for psychosis. *Schizophrenia Bulletin, 37*, 1111–1114.

Mausbach, B. T., Harvey, P. D., Goldman, S. R., Jeste, D. V., & Patterson, T. L. (2007). Development of a brief scale of everyday functioning in persons with serious mental illness. *Schizophrenia Bulletin, 33*, 1364–1372.

Mayang, A. (1990). *The effects of problem-solving skills training with chronic schizophrenic patients.* Master's thesis available from ProQuest Dissertations and Theses database (UMI No. 1342752).

McEvoy, J. P. (2008). Functional outcomes in schizophrenia. *Journal of Clinical Psychiatry, 69*(Suppl. 3), 20–24.

McGorry, P. D., Edwards, J., Mihalopoulos, C., Harrigan, S. M., & Jackson, H. J. (1996). EPPIC: An evolving system of early detection and optimal management. *Schizophrenia Bulletin, 22*, 305–326.

McGorry, P. D., & Yung, A. R. (2003). Early intervention in psychosis: An overdue reform. *Australian and New Zealand Journal of Psychiatry, 37*, 393–398.

McGurk, S. R., Twamley, E. W., Sitzer, D. I., McHugo, G. J., & Mueser, K. T. (2007). A meta-analysis of cognitive remediation in schizophrenia. *American Journal of Psychiatry, 164,* 1791–1802.

McKee, M., Hull, J. W., & Smith, T. E. (1997). Cognitive and symptom correlates of participation in social skills training groups. *Schizophrenia Research, 23,* 223–229.

McQuaid, J. R., Granholm, E., McClure, F. S., Roepke, S., Pedrelli, P., Patterson, T. L., et al. (2000). Development of an integrated cognitive-behavioral and social skills training intervention for older patients with schizophrenia. *Journal of Psychotherapy Practice and Research, 9,* 149–156.

Medalia, A., & Bellucci, D. M. (2012). Neuropsychologically informed interventions to treat cognitive impairment in schizophrenia. In B. A. Marcopulos & M. M. Kurtz (Eds.), *Clinical neuropsychological foundations of schizophrenia* (pp. 275–302). New York: Psychology Press.

Medalia, A., & Choi, J. (2009). Cognitive remediation in schizophrenia. *Neuropsychology Review, 19,* 353–364.

Medalia, A., Revheim, N., & Casey, M. (2002). Remediation of problem-solving skills in schizophrenia: Evidence of a persistent effect. *Schizophrenia Research, 57,* 165–171.

Menezes, N. M., Arenovich, T., & Zipursky, R. B. (2006). A systematic review of longitudinal outcome studies of first-episode psychosis. *Psychological Medicine, 36,* 1349–1362.

Meyer, P. S., Gingerich, S., & Mueser, K. T. (2010). A guide to implementation and clinical practice of illness management and recovery for people with schizophrenia. In A. Rubin, D. W. Springer, & K. R. Trawver (Eds.), *Psychosocial treatment of schizophrenia* (pp. 23–87). New York: Wiley.

Mishlove, M., & Chapman, L. J. (1985). Social anhedonia in the prediction of psychosis proneness. *Journal of Abnormal Psychology, 94,* 384–396.

Moore, R. C., Fazeli, P. L., Patterson, T. L., Depp, C. A., Moore, D. J., Granholm, E., et al. (2015). UPSA-M: Development and initial validation of a mobile application of the UCSD Performance-Based Skills Assessment. *Schizophrenia Research, 164*(1–3), 187–192.

Morrison, A. P., & Barratt, S. (2010). What are the components of CBT for psychosis?: A Delphi study. *Schizophrenia Bulletin, 36,* 136–142.

Morrison, A. P., Renton, J. C., Williams, S., Dunn, H., Knight, A., Kreutz, M., et al. (2004). Delivering cognitive therapy to people with psychosis in a community mental health setting: An effectiveness study. *Acta Psychiatrica Scandinavica, 110,* 36–44.

Morrison, A. P., Turkington, D., Pyle, M., Spencer, H., Brabban, A., Dunn, G., et al. (2014). Cognitive therapy for people with schizophrenia spectrum disorders not taking antipsychotic drugs: A single-blind randomised controlled trial. *Lancet, 383,* 1395–1403.

Morrison, A. P., Turkington, D., Wardle, M., Spencer, H., Barratt, S., Dudley, R., et al. (2012). A preliminary exploration of predictors of outcome and cognitive mechanisms of change in cognitive behaviour therapy for psychosis in people not taking antipsychotic medication. *Behaviour Research and Therapy, 50,* 163–167.

Morrison, R. L., Bellack, A. S., Wixted, J. T., & Mueser, K. T. (1990). Positive and negative symptoms in schizophrenia: A cluster-analytic approach. *Journal of Nervous and Mental Disease, 178,* 377–384.

Mueser, K. T., & Bellack, A. S. (1998). Social skills and social functioning. In K. T. Mueser & N. Tarrier (Eds.), *Handbook of social functioning in schizophrenia* (pp. 79–96). Needham Heights, MA: Allyn & Boston.

Mueser, K. T., Bellack, A. S., Douglas, M. S., & Wade, J. H. (1991). Prediction of social skill acquisition in schizophrenic and major affective disorder patients from memory and symptomatology. *Psychiatry Research, 37,* 281–296.

Mueser, K. T., Bond, G. R., Drake, R. E., & Resnick, S. G. (1998). Models of community care for severe mental illness: A review of research on case management. *Schizophrenia Bulletin, 24,* 37–74.

Mueser, K. T., Deavers, F., Penn, D. L., & Cassisi, J. E. (2013). Psychosocial treatments for schizophrenia. *Annual Review of Clinical Psychology, 9,* 465–497.

Mueser, K. T., Meyer, P. S., Penn, D. L., Clancy, R., Clancy, D. M., & Salyers, M. P. (2006). The Illness Management and Recovery program: Rationale, development, and preliminary findings. *Schizophrenia Bulletin, 32*(Suppl. 1), S32–S43.

Muñoz, R. F., Ying, Y., Perez-Stable, E. J., & Miranda, J. (1993). *The prevention of depression: Research and practice.* Baltimore, MD: Johns Hopkins University Press.

Naeem, F., Farooq, S., & Kingdon, D. (2014). Cognitive behavioral therapy (brief vs. standard duration) for schizophrenia. *Schizophrenia Bulletin, 40*, 958–959.

Naeem, F., Kingdon, D., & Turkington, D. (2008). Predictors of response to cognitive behavior therapy in the treatment of schizophrenia: A comparison of brief and standard interventions. *Cognitive Therapy and Research, 32*, 651–656.

Newton-Howes, G., & Wood, R. (2013). Cognitive behavioural therapy and the psychopathology of schizophrenia: Systematic review and meta-analysis. *Psychology and Psychotherapy, 86*, 127–138.

Nuechterlein, K. H., Miklowitz, D. J., Ventura, J., Gitlin, J. G., Stoddard, M., & Lukoff, D. (2006). Classifying episodes in schizophrenia and bipolar disorder: Criteria and remission applied to recent onset samples. *Psychiatry Research, 144*, 153–166.

O'Connell, M., Tondora, J., Croog, G., Evans, A., & Davidson, L. (2005). From rhetoric to routine: Asessing perceptions of recovery-oriented practices in a state mental health and addiction system. *Psychiatric Rehabilitation Journal, 28*, 378–386.

Ogawa, K., Miya, M., Watarai, A., Nakazawa, M., Yuasa, S., & Utena, H. (1987). A long-term follow-up study of schizophrenia in Japan with special reference to the course of social adjustment. *British Journal of Psychiatry, 151*, 758–765.

Ozer, E. M., Adams, S. H., Gardner, L. R., Mailloux, D. E., Wibbelsman, C. J., & Irwin, C. E., Jr. (2004). Provider self-efficacy and the screening of adolescents for risky health behaviors. *Journal of Adolescent Health, 35*, 101–107.

Patterson, T. L., Moscona, S., McKibbin, C. L., Davidson, K., & Jeste, D. V. (2001). Social skills performance assessment among older patients with schizophrenia. *Schizophrenia Research, 48*, 351–360.

Penn, D. L., Corrigan, P. W., Bentall, R. P., Racenstein, J. M., & Newman, L. (1997). Social cognition in schizophrenia. *Psychological Bulletin, 121*, 114–132.

Perivoliotis, D., Grant, P. M., Peters, E. R., Ison, R., Kuipers, E., & Beck, A. T. (2010). Cognitive insight predicts favorable outcome in cognitive behavioral therapy for psychosis. *Psychosis: Psychological, Social and Integrative Approaches, 2*, 23–33.

Perris, C., & Skagerlind, L. (1994). Cognitive therapy with schizophrenic patients. *Acta Psychiatrica Scandinavica Supplementum, 382*, 65–70.

Pfammatter, M., Junghan, U. M., & Brenner, H. D. (2006). Efficacy of psychological therapy in schizophrenia: Conclusions from meta-analyses. *Schizophrenia Bulletin, 32*(Suppl. 1), S64–S80.

Pharoah, F., Mari, J., Rathbone, J., & Wong, W. (2006, October 18). Family intervention for schizophrenia. *Cochrane Database of Systematic Reviews, 12*, CD000088.

Pilling, S., Bebbington, P., Kuipers, E., Garety, P., Geddes, J., Martindale, B., et al. (2002). Psychological treatments in schizophrenia: II. Meta-analyses of randomized controlled trials of social skills training and cognitive remediation. *Psychological Medicine, 32*, 783–791.

Pinkham, A. E., Penn, D. L., Green, M. F., Buck, B., Healey, K., & Harvey, P. D. (2014). The social cognition psychometric evaluation study: Results of the expert survey and RAND Panel. *Schizophrenia Bulletin, 40*, 813–823.

Pinninti, N. R., Fisher, J., Thompson, K., & Steer, R. A. (2010). Feasibility and usefulness of training assertive community treatment team in cognitive behavioral therapy. *Community Mental Health Journal, 46*, 337–341.

Quinlan, T., Roesch, S., & Granholm, E. (2014). The role of dysfunctional attitudes in models of negative symptoms and functioning in schizophrenia. *Schizophrenia Bulletin, 157*, 182–189.

Rathod, S., Kingdon, D., Smith, P., & Turkington, D. (2005). Insight into schizophrenia: The effects of cognitive behavioral therapy on the components of insight and association with sociodemographics—data on a previously published randomised controlled trial. *Schizophrenia Research, 74*, 211–219.

Rector, N. A., & Beck, A. T. (2012). Cognitive behavioral therapy for schizophrenia: An empirical review. *Journal of Nervous and Mental Disease, 200*, 832–839.

Rector, N. A., Beck, A. T., & Stolar, N. (2005). The negative symptoms of schizophrenia: A cognitive perspective. *Canadian Journal of Psychiatry, 50*, 247–257.

Revheim, N., Schechter, I., Kim, D., Silipo, G., Allingham, B., Butler, P., et al. (2006). Neurocognitive and symptom correlates of daily problem-solving skills in schizophrenia. *Schizophrenia Research, 83*, 237–245.

Robinson, D. G., Woerner, M. G., McMeniman, M., Mendelowitz, A., & Bilder, R. M. (2004). Symptomatic and functional recovery from a first episode of schizophrenia or schizoaffective disorder. *American Journal of Psychiatry, 161*, 473–479.

Rodewald, K., Rentrop, M., Holt, D. V., Roesch-Ely, D., Backenstrass, M., Funke, J., et al. (2011). Planning and problem-solving training for patients with schizophrenia: A randomized controlled trial. *BMC Psychiatry, 11*, 73.

Rollinson, R., Haig, C., Warner, R., Garety, P., Kuipers, E., Freeman, D., et al. (2007). The application of cognitive-behavioral therapy for psychosis in clinical and research settings. *Psychiatric Services, 58*, 1297–1302.

Rosenheck, R., Leslie, D., Keefe, R., McEvoy, J., Swartz, M., Perkins, D., et al. (2006). Barriers to employment for people with schizophrenia. *American Journal of Psychiatry, 163*, 411–417.

Saks, E. (2007, August 27). A memoir of schizophrenia. Retrieved from *www.time.com/time/arts/article/0,8599,1656592,00.html*.

Sarin, F., Wallin, L., & Widerlöv, B. (2011). Cognitive behavior therapy for schizophrenia: A meta-analytical review of randomized controlled trials. *Nordic Journal of Psychiatry, 65*, 162–174.

Savla, G. N., Vella, L., Armstrong, C. C., Penn, D. L., & Twamley, E. W. (2013). Deficits in domains of social cognition in schizophrenia: A meta-analysis of the empirical evidence. *Schizophrenia Bulletin, 39*, 979–992.

Schmidt, S. J., Mueller, D. R., & Roder, V. (2011). Social cognition as a mediator variable between neurocognition and functional outcome in schizophrenia: Empirical review and new results by structural equation modeling. *Schizophrenia Bulletin, 37*(Suppl. 2), S41–S54.

Schneider, L. C., & Struening, E. L. (1983). SLOF: A behavioral rating scale for assessing the mentally ill. *Social Work Research and Abstracts, 19*, 9–21.

Sensky, T., Turkington, D., Kingdon, D., Scott, J. L., Scott, J., Siddle, R., et al. (2000). A randomized controlled trial of cognitive-behavioral therapy for persistent symptoms in schizophrenia resistant to medication. *Archives of General Psychiatry, 57*, 165–172.

Silverstein, S. M., Schenkel, L. S., Valone, C., & Nuernberger, S. W. (1998). Cognitive deficits and psychiatric rehabilitation outcomes in schizophrenia. *Psychiatric Quarterly, 69*, 169–191.

Smith, T. E., Hull, J. W., Goodman, M., Hedayat-Harris, A., Willson, D. F., Israel, L. M., et al. (1999). The relative influences of symptoms, insight, and neurocognition on social adjustment in schizophrenia and schizoaffective disorder. *Journal of Nervous and Mental Disease, 187*, 102–108.

Tabak, N., Holden, J., & Granholm, E. (2015). Goal attainment scaling: Tracking goal achievement in consumers with serious mental illness. *American Journal of Psychiatric Rehabilitation, 18*(2), 173–186.

Tarrier, N. (2010). Cognitive behavior therapy for schizophrenia and psychosis: Current status and future directions. *Clinical Schizophrenia and Related Psychoses, 4*, 176–184.

Tarrier, N., Beckett, R., Harwood, S., Baker, A., Yusupoff, L., & Ugarteburu, I. (1993). A trial of two cognitive-behavioural methods of treating drug-resistant residual psychotic symptoms in schizophrenic patients: I. Outcome. *British Journal of Psychiatry, 162*, 524–532.

Tarrier, N., Yusupoff, L., Kinney, C., McCarthy, E., Gledhill, A., Haddock, G., et al. (1998). Randomised controlled trial of intensive cognitive behaviour therapy for patients with chronic schizophrenia. *British Medical Journal, 317*, 303–307.

Thase, M. E., Kingdon, D., & Turkington, D. (2014). The promise of cognitive behavior therapy for treatment of severe mental disorders: A review of recent developments. *World Psychiatry, 13*, 244–250.

Tsuang, M. T., Woolson, R. F., & Fleming, J. A. (1979). Long-term outcome of major psychoses: I. Schizophrenia and affective disorders compared with psychiatrically symptom-free surgical conditions. *Archives of General Psychiatry, 36*, 1295–1301.

Turkington, D., Kingdon, D., & Turner, T. (2002). Effectiveness of a brief cognitive-behavioural therapy intervention in the treatment of schizophrenia. *British Journal of Psychiatry, 180*, 523–527.

Turkington, D., Kingdon, D., & Weiden, P. J. (2006). Cognitive behavior therapy for schizophrenia. *American Journal of Psychiatry, 163*, 365–373.

Turkington, D., Munetz, M., Pelton, J., Montesano, V., Sivec, H., Nausheen, B., et al. (2014). High-yield cognitive behavioral techniques for psychosis delivered by case managers to their clients with persistent psychotic symptoms: An exploratory trial. *Journal of Nervous and Mental Disease, 202,* 30–34.

Turkington, D., Sensky, T., Scott, J., Barnes, T. R., Nur, U., Siddle, R., et al. (2008). A randomized controlled trial of cognitive-behavior therapy for persistent symptoms in schizophrenia: A five-year follow-up. *Schizophrenia Research, 98,* 1–7.

Turner, D. T., van der Gaag, M., Karyotaki, E., & Cuijpers, P. (2014). Psychological interventions for psychosis: A meta-analysis of comparative outcome studies. *American Journal of Psychiatry, 171,* 523–538.

Twamley, E. W., Doshi, R. R., Nayak, G. V., Palmer, B. W., Golshan, S., Heaton, R. K., et al. (2002). Generalized cognitive impairments, ability to perform everyday tasks, and level of independence in community living situations of older patients with psychosis. *American Journal of Psychiatry, 159,* 2013–2020.

Twamley, E. W., Jeste, D. V., & Bellack, A. S. (2003). A review of cognitive training in schizophrenia. *Schizophrenia Bulletin, 29,* 359–382.

Ucok, A., Cakir, S., Duman, Z. C., Discigil, A., Kandemir, P., & Atli, H. (2006). Cognitive predictors of skill acquisition on social problem solving in patients with schizophrenia. *European Archives of Psychiatry and Clinical Neuroscience, 256,* 388–394.

VanMeerten, N. J., Harris, J. I., Nienow, T. M., Hegeman, B. M., Sherburne, A., Winskowski, A. M., et al. (2013). Inpatient utilization before and after implementation of psychosocial rehabilitation programs: Analysis of cost reductions. *Psychological Services, 10,* 420–427.

Veltro, F., Mazza, M., Vendittelli, N., Alberti, M., Casacchia, M., & Roncone, R. (2011). A comparison of the effectiveness of problem solving training and of cognitive–emotional rehabilitation on neurocognition, social cognition and social functioning in people with schizophrenia. *Clinical Practice and Epidemiology in Mental Health, 7,* 123–132.

Ventura, J., Hellemann, G. S., Thames, A. D., Koellner, V., & Nuechterlein, K. H. (2009). Symptoms as mediators of the relationship between neurocognition and functional outcome in schizophrenia: A meta-analysis. *Schizophrenia Research, 113,* 189–199.

Wallace, C. J., Lecomte, T., Wilde, J., & Liberman, R. P. (2001). CASIG: A consumer-centered assessment for planning individualized treatment and evaluating program outcomes. *Schizophrenia Research, 50,* 105–119.

Wallace, C. J., Liberman, R. P., Tauber, R., & Wallace, J. (2000). The independent living skills survey: A comprehensive measure of the community functioning of severely and persistently mentally ill individuals. *Schizophrenia Bulletin, 26,* 631–658.

Warner, R. (2004). *Recovery from schizophrenia: Psychiatry and political economy* (3rd ed.). New York: Brunner-Routledge.

Weingardt, K. R., Cucciare, M. A., Bellotti, C., & Lai, W. P. (2009). A randomized trial comparing two models of web-based training in cognitive-behavioral therapy for substance abuse counselors. *Journal of Substance Abuse Treatment, 37,* 219–227.

Weissman, A. R. (1978). The Dysfunctional Attitude Scale: A validation study (doctoral dissertation, University of Pennsylvannia). *Dissertation Abstracts International, 40,* 1389B–1390B.

Weissman, A. R., & Beck, A. T. (1978). *Development and validation of the Dysfunctional Attitude Scale: A preliminary investigation.* Paper presented at the annual meeting of the American Educational Research Association, Toronto, Canada.

Whitehorn, D., Lazier, L., & Kopala, L. (1998). Psychosocial rehabilitation early after the onset of psychosis. *Psychiatric Services, 49,* 1135–1137.

Wiersma, D., Wanderling, J., Dragomirecka, E., Ganev, K., Harrison, G., an der Heiden, W., et al. (2000). Social disability in schizophrenia: Its development and prediction over 15 years in incidence cohorts in six European centres. *Psychological Medicine, 30,* 1155–1167.

Wigfield, A., & Eccles, J. S. (2000). Expectancy-value theory of achievement motivation. *Contemporary Educational Psychology, 25,* 68–81.

Williams, C. H. (2008). Cognitive behaviour therapy within assertive outreach teams: Barriers to implementation: A qualitative peer audit. *Journal of Psychiatric and Mental Health Nursing, 15,* 850–856.

Wykes, T. (2008). Review: Cognitive remediation improves cognitive functioning in schizophrenia. *Evidence-Based Mental Health, 11,* 117.

Wykes, T., Steel, C., Everitt, B., & Tarrier, N. (2008). Cognitive behavior therapy for schizophrenia: Effect Sizes, clincial models, and methodological rigor. *Schizophrenia Bulletin, 34,* 523–537.

Xia, J., & Li, C. (2007). Problem solving skills for schizophrenia. *Cochrane Database of Systematic Reviews, 2,* CD006365.

Zimmermann, G., Favrod, J., Trieu, V. H., & Pomini, V. (2005). The effect of cognitive behavioral treatment on the positive symptoms of schizophrenia spectrum disorders: A meta-analysis. *Schizophrenia Research, 77,* 1–9.

Index

Note. f or *t* following a page number indicates a figure or a table.